Human Osteology

A Clinical Orientation

THIRD EDITION

Human Osteology

A Clinical Orientation

THIRD EDITION

Nafis Ahmad Faruqi
MBBS, MS, MNYAS (USA), Man of YK2 (USA)

Professor
Department of Anatomy
Jawaharlal Nehru Medical College
Aligarh Muslim University
Aligarh 202002, India

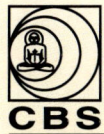

CBS Publishers & Distributors Pvt Ltd

New Delhi • Bengaluru • Chennai • Kochi • Kolkata • Mumbai
Bhopal • Bhubaneswar • Hyderabad • Jharkhand • Nagpur • Patna • Pune • Uttarakhand • Dhaka (Bangladesh)

Disclaimer

Science and technology are constantly changing fields. New research and experience broaden the scope of information and knowledge. The author has tried his best in giving information available to him while preparing the material for this book. Although, all efforts have been made to ensure optimum accuracy of the material, yet it is quite possible some errors might have been left uncorrected. The publisher, the printer and the author will not be held responsible for any inadvertent errors, or inaccuracies.

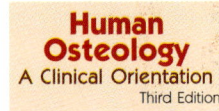

ISBN: 978-93-86310-72-9

Copyright © Author and Publisher

Third Edition: 2017
   Reprint: 2018, 2019
First Edition: 1999
Second Edition: 2000

All rights reserved. No part of this book may be reproduced or transmitted in any form or by any means, electronic or mechanical, including photocopying, recording, or any information storage and retrieval system without permission, in writing, from the author and the publisher.

Published by Satish Kumar Jain and produced by Varun Jain for

CBS Publishers & Distributors Pvt Ltd
4819/XI Prahlad Street, 24 Ansari Road, Daryaganj, New Delhi 110 002, India.
Ph: 23289259, 23266861, 23266867   Website: www.cbspd.com
Fax: 011-23243014   e-mail: delhi@cbspd.com; cbspubs@airtelmail.in.

Corporate Office: 204 FIE, Industrial Area, Patparganj, Delhi 110 092
Ph: 4934 4934   Fax: 4934 4935   e-mail: publishing@cbspd.com; publicity@cbspd.com

Branches

- **Bengaluru:** Seema House 2975, 17th Cross, K.R. Road,
  Banasankari 2nd Stage, Bengaluru 560 070, Karnataka
  Ph: +91-80-26771678/79   Fax: +91-80-26771680   e-mail: bangalore@cbspd.com
- **Chennai:** 7, Subbaraya Street, Shenoy Nagar, Chennai 600 030, Tamil Nadu
  Ph: +91-44-26680620, 26681266   Fax: +91-44-42032115   e-mail: chennai@cbspd.com
- **Kochi:** 42/1325, 1326, Power House Road, Opp KSEB Power House, Ernakulam 682 018, Kochi, Kerala
  Ph: +91-484-4059061-65   Fax: +91-484-4059065   e-mail: kochi@cbspd.com
- **Kolkata:** 6/B, Ground Floor, Rameswar Shaw Road, Kolkata-700 014, West Bengal
  Ph: +91-33-22891126, 22891127, 22891128   e-mail: kolkata@cbspd.com
- **Mumbai:** 83-C, Dr E Moses Road, Worli, Mumbai-400018, Maharashtra
  Ph: +91-22-24902340/41   Fax: +91-22-24902342   e-mail: mumbai@cbspd.com

Representatives

• **Bhopal**	0-8319310552	• **Bhubaneswar**	0-9911037372	• **Hyderabad**	0-9885175004
• **Jharkhand**	0-9811541605	• **Nagpur**	0-9021734563	• **Patna**	0-9334159340
• **Pune**	0-9623451994	• **Uttarakhand**	0-9716462459	• **Dhaka (Bangladesh)**	01912-003485

Printed at: Shree Maitrey Printech, Noida, UP, India

to

*My beloved classmates of 1972 batch admitted in
Jawaharlal Nehru Medical College
Aligarh Muslim University, Aligarh, UP, India*

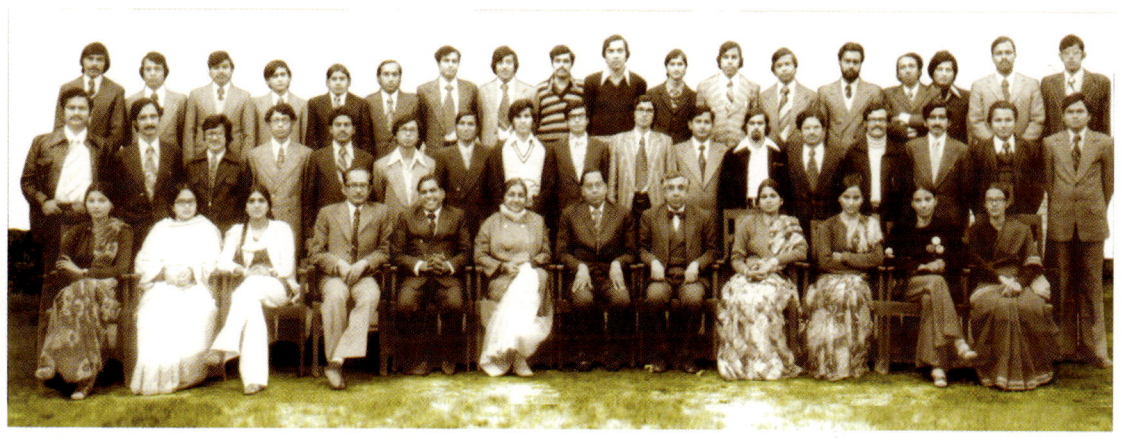

List as Entered In the Record of
Department of Anatomy
Aligarh Muslim University, Aligarh

1. Mr. Abraham George
2. Mr. Aftab Husain
3. Mr. Anil Kumar Gupta
4. Mr. Anil Kumar Malhotra
5. Miss Arfa Begum
6. Miss Asha Rani Agarwal
7. Miss Asha Saxena
8. Mr. Ashok Kumar Agarwal
9. Mr. Chandresh Bhatia
10. Mr. Chhotay Lal Shakia
11. Mr. Deepak Shah
12. Mr. Girish Gupta
13. Mr. Harvinder Paul Singh
14. Mr. Hemant Kumar
15. Mr. Jawed Sabir Hanfi
16. Miss Kalpana Banga
17. Mr. Kamal Ahmad
18. Mr. Khalid Mirza
19. Mr. Md. Afroz Ahmad Farooqi
20. Mr. Md. Ghyasuddin Ansari
21. Mr. Mohd Ismail
22. Mr. Nafis Ahmad Faruqi
23. Mr. Nanak
24. Miss Noor Afshan Siddiqi
25. Mr. Om Prakash Kalra
26. Miss Prabha
27. Mr. Pradeep Kumar Agarwal
28. Mr. Quloobul Hasnain Abidi
29. Mr. Rakesh Maheshwari
30. Mr. Rajendra Kumar Varshney
31. Mr. Rajendra Prasad Singhal
32. Mr. Rakesh Kumar Arya
33. Mr. Ram Kumar
34. Miss Ranjana Kaur
35. Mr. Ratan Prakash Bajaj
36. Mr. Raziuddin Siddiqi
37. Mr. Sanjay Sinha
38. Miss Shahinda Faiyaz
39. Mr. Shekhar Tandon
40. Mr. Shiv Shankar Sanyal
41. Mr. Subhash Chandra Sharma
42. Mr. S. Md. Najeeb Trimizi
43. Mr. Syed Shaida Raza
44. Mr. Raj Kumar Rawal
45. Mr. Talat Halim
46. Miss Tayyaba Abidin
47. Mr. V. Ram Kumar Iyer
48. Mr. Venu Pant
49. Mr. Vinrendra Singh Lohchab
50. Miss Zainab A.S. Essajee
51. Mr. Jalaluddin
52. Mr. Mansoor Ahmad
53. Mr. Zaheer Anwar Khan
54. Mr. Mohd Akhtar
55. Mr. Moazziz Ali Khan

Preface to the Third Edition

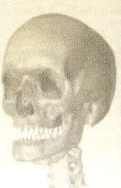

The reception of first and second editions of Human Osteology: A Clinical Orientation prompted the author to enlarge its scope and make it more useful for the students. The clinical information on the subject has been thoroughly revised in the light of recent advances available in literature. A unique feature of the third edition is addition of preliminary information about the joints in the first chapter.

The book has been made more complete and authentic by consulting multiple standard books to specially avoid controversies. All the diagrams have been drawn in colour and nearly 45 more diagrams added to make the book more helpful and attractive.

I hope to get a feedback from my colleagues and students so that the book may be further improved in future.

Nafis Ahmad Faruqi

Preface to the First Edition

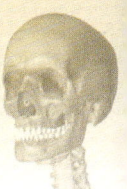

Human Osteology: A Clinical Orientation is a sort of gift to the medical undergraduates and dental surgery students. Adequate coverage on the applied aspect of the subject has considerably increased the value of the book and removed the gaps usually observed in conventional textbooks on the subject. A unique feature of the book is its approximately 450 illustrations which have been drawn by the author himself, minimizing the chances of factual mistakes often discovered in the diagrams made by professional artists. Some of the subjects attracted special attention of the author, e.g. upper and lower jaw bones and teeth which are very relevant to dental students and temporal bones which are of great value for ENT surgeons. Extremely precise treatment of the subject and clarity of linguistic expression have been focussed on in the book.

Towards the end all careful readers of the book may kindly communicate to the author any shortcomings and suggestions regarding the book which may help improve it if the book goes into subsequent editions.

Nafis Ahmad Faruqi

Reader's Comments

Dear Reader,

I will feel honoured if you spare a few minutes from your precious time and comment on this book. Your suggestions will go long way in improving this book in subsequent editions.

Dr Nafis Ahmad Faruqi
Gulfishan
Allahwali Kothi
Dodhpur, Civil Lines,
Aligarh-202001
Mob. 09358256504
WhatsApp no. 07060888167
Email: drnafisahmad@rediffmail.com

Acknowledgements

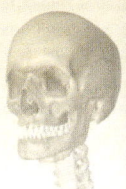

It is rather difficult to have a book of this size prepared and published without collaboration and help from others.

I am first and foremost sincerely thankful to Lt. Gen. (Retd.) Zameer Uddin Shah (Vice-Chancellor, AMU, Aligarh) who granted me 'Leave for Academic Persuit' which made it possible to get the third edition of this book published in the present form.

Dr Krishna Garg, ex-Professor and Head, Department of Anatomy, Lady Hardinge Medical College, New Delhi, and chief editor of *BD Chaurasia's Human Anatomy* volumes and author of many other books on anatomy, is the one who inspired me maximally during the period of my writing recent books. Her enthusiasm and vision have no match, not only in this country but all over the world. I really feel proud of being associated with her.

I do not have words to thank Prof Khursheed Alam, Professor and Head, Department of Anatomy, Patna Medical College, Patna, who liked my books and always encouraged me. His valuable advice was of great help in improving all my books in general and this book in particular. I feel obliged for promotion of my books by him among undergraduate as well as postgraduate students.

My special thanks to Dr SN Kazi (ex-Professor of Anatomy), Director, Kazi Medical Classes Academy and author of multiple books of anatomy, for his valuable suggestions which helped me in improving this book.

I am also thankful to the following teachers who not only personally took interest in my books but also recommended them for undergraduate and postgraduate students.

1. My colleagues Prof Aijaz A. Khan, Prof SM Yunus, Dr Tariq Zaidi, Dr SM Dawar Husain, Dr Farhan Kirmani, Dr Fazal-ur-Rehman, Dr Farah Ghaus, Dr Nema Usman, Dr Nusra Rehman, Dr Mohd. Ajmal and Dr Yasir Salam Siddiqui (orthopaedician).

   Dr Rati Tandon and Dr Mohd. Arshad, senior residents, need special mention for their help during difficult times. I am thankful to them for promoting my book among medical and dental students.

2. Prof SH Zaidi, Department of Anatomy, Rohilkhand Medical College, Bareilly.
3. Prof Namita Malhotra, Department of Anatomy, SHKM Medical College, Mewat, Haryana.
4. Dr Saim Hasan, Department of Anatomy, SHKM Medical College, Mewat, Haryana.
5. Dr Tarun Maheshwari, Department of Anatomy, Govt Doon Medical College, Dehradun.
6. Dr Hamid Ansari, Department of Anatomy, GSVM Medical College, Kanpur.
7. Prof RK Srivastava, Principal, Rama Medical College, Kanpur.
8. Prof Vinod Kumar (retired from Deptartment of Anatomy, GSVM Medical College, Kanpur).
9. Dr Shikky Garg, Department of Anatomy, Govt. Medical College, Agra.

10. Prof Renu Prasad, Department of Anatomy, RIMS, Ranchi.
11. Prof Narendra Thakur, Department of Anatomy, RIMS, Ranchi.
12. Dr K Sandhya, Department of Anatomy, RIMS, Ranchi.
13. Prof Riazul Qamar, Department of Anatomy, MAMC, New Delhi.
14. Prof Daxa Dixit, Department of Anatomy, JNMC, Belgaum.
15. Dr Alka Udainia, Department of Anatomy, Govt. Medical College, Surat.
16. Dr Nidhi Sharma, Department of Anatomy, TMMC, NH-24, Muradabad.
17. Prof Azmi Mohsin, Head, Department of Anatomy, Rajshree Medical College, Bareilly.
18. Dr Makandar UK. Department of Anatomy, Adichunchangiri Institute of Medical Sciences, Mandya, Karnataka.
19. Prof Ram Kumar Ashoka, Department of Anatomy, GFI of Medical Sciences and Research, Faridabad.
20. Prof AK Srivastava, Department of Anatomy, KG Medical University, Lucknow.
21. Prof PK Sharma, Head, Department of Anatomy, Era's Lucknow Medical College and Hospital, Lucknow.
22. Dr Devendra Nath Sinha, B9/84B, Udai Giri Apartment 2, Sector 34, Noida.
23. Dr Manisha Upadhyay, Department of Anatomy, Govt Medical College, Azamgarh.
24. Dr RK Varshney, Managing Director, Mithraj Multispeciality Hospital, Aligarh.
25. Prof Asima Bhattacharya, Department of Anatomy, NEIGRIHMS, Shillong.
26. Prof DK Sharma, Department of Anatomy, AIIMS, Raipur.
27. Dr VK Konuri, Department of Anatomy, AIIMS, Raipur.
28. Dr Rajendra, Department of Anatomy, AIIMS, Mandya, Karnataka.
29. Prof NN Srivastava, Department of Anatomy, UPRIMS and R, Safai, Etawah.
30. Prof TC Singel, Department of Anatomy, MES Medical College, Jamnagar, Gujrat.
31. Dr Divya, Department of Anatomy, AIIMS, Bellur, Karnataka.
32. Dr Zeba Alam, Department of Anatomy, AIIMS, Patna.
33. Prof S.K. Pandey, Department of Anatomy, IMS, BHU, Varanasi.
34. Prof Satyanarayan Shamal, Department of Anatomy, IMS, BHU, Varanasi.
35. Prof Brijendra Singh, Department of Anatomy, AIIMS, Jodhpur.
36. Dr Royana Singh, Dept. of Anatomy, IMS, BHU, Varanasi.
37. Prof Awadhesh Kumar Singh, Dept. of Anatomy, MLN Medical College, Allahabad.
38. Dr Nishtha Singh, Dept. of Anatomy, MLN Medical College, Allahabad.

To my wife Roshan Ara, my children Arsalan Moinuddin and Anam Faruqi, and daughter-in-law Siddiqua Abdullah, I express my grateful appreciation for their patience, love, understanding and support.

Last but not the least my heartfelt thanks are due for the entire CBS team, namely Mr SK Jain, Mr YN Arjuna, Ms Ritu Chawla, Ms Ritu Tiwari, Mr Sanjay Chauhan (Sanju) and Mr Ananda Mohanty. It was their help at different levels that infused strength in me to get my book completed in the present form.

Nafis Ahmad Faruqi

Contents

Preface to the Third Edition   vii
Preface to the First Edition   ix

1. General Considerations of Bone   1
- Properties 1
- Functions 1
- Chemical composition 1
- Structure of bone 1
- Classification of bones 3
- Parts of a young long bone 5
- Features of bones 5
- Blood supply of bones 6
- Joints 7
- Applied anatomy of bones 11

2. The Clavicle   13
- Side determination 13
- Functions 13
- Peculiarities of clavicle 13
- Features and attachments 14
- Ossification 15
- Applied anatomy 16

3. The Scapula   18
- Side determination 18
- Features and attachments 18
- Ossification 24
- Applied anatomy 25

4. The Humerus   26
- Side determination 26
- Features and attachments 26
- Caspular attachments 30
- Angles 31
- Ossification 32
- Applied anatomy 33

5. The Radius   36
- Side determination 36
- Features and attachments 36
- Ossification 40
- Applied anatomy 40

6. The Ulna   44
- Side determination 44
- Features and attachments 44
- Ossification 49
- Applied anatomy 49

7. The Carpal Bones   51
- Carpus 51
- Articulated carpal bones 51
- Individual carpal bones 52
- Ossification 55
- Applied anatomy 56

8. The Metacarpal Bones   58
- Metacarpus 58
- Identifications of metacarpal bones 58
- Features and attachments 59
- Ossification 60
- Applied anatomy 60

9. The Phalanges of the Hand   61
- Characteristics 61
- Ossification 62
- Applied anatomy 62

10. The Hip Bone — 64
Side determination 64
Normal anatomical position 64
Features and attachments 65
Ossification 73
Sexual dimorphism 73

11. The Bony Pelvis — 74
Pelvic girdle 74
Divisions of pelvis 74
Anatomical position 75
Boundaries of pelvic inlet 75
Boundaries of pelvic outlet 76
Boundaries of pelvic cavity 76
Pubic arch and subpubic angle 76
Functions of pelvis 76
Axes of pelvis 77
Pelvic segments 77
Posterior sagittal diameter of Klein 77
Pelvic inclination 78
Planes of pelvic dimensions 78
Conjugate diameters 78
Least diameter 78
Types of pelvis 78
Diameters of pelvis 79
Sex differences in adult pelvis 80
Applied anatomy 81

12. The Femur — 87
Side determintion 87
Anatomical position 87
Angle of femoral torsion 88
Features and attachments 88
Sex differences 95
Ossification 95
Applied anatomy 96

13. The Patella — 102
Peculiarities 102
Side determination 102
Features and attachments 103
Ossification 104
Applied anatomy 104

14. The Tibia — 106
Peculiarities 106
Side determination 106
Features and attachments 106
Capsular attachments 113
Ossification 113
Applied anatomy 113

15. The Fibula — 117
Peculiarities 117
Side determination 117
Features and attachments 118
Ossification 122
Applied anatomy 122

16. The Tarsal Bones — 124
Tarsus 124
Identification of tarsal bones in foot skeleton 124
Individual tarsal bones 124
The talus 124
The calcaneus 128
The navicular bone 131
The cuboid bone 133
The cuneiform bones 135

17. The Metatarsal Bones — 137
Metatarsus 137
Identification of metalarsal bones 137
Features and attachments 138
Ossification 139
Applies anatomy 139

18. The Phalanges of the Foot — 140
Characteristics 140
Ossification 140
Applied anatomy 141

19. The Vertebrae — 142

General considerations 142
Curvatures of vertebral column 143
Movements of vertebral column 143
Features of a typical vertebra 143
Distinguishing features 144
Typical cervical vertebra 145
First cervical vertebra 147
Second cervical vertebra 149
Typical thoracic vertebra 151
Atypical thoracic vertebrae 153
Typical lumbar vertebra 154
Atypical (5th) lumbar vertebra 157
Sacrum 157
Coccyx 162
Ossification of vertebrae 163
Applied anatomy 164

20. The Sternum — 176

Terminology 176
Features and attachments 176
Manubrium (presternum or episternum) 176
Body (mesosternum or gladiolus) 178
Xiphoid process (xiphisternum or metasternum or ensiform cartilage) 180
Sex differences 180
Ossification 180
Applied anatomy 180

21. The Ribs — 182

General considerations 182
Classification of ribs 183
Typical rib 183
First rib 188
Second rib 190
Tenth rib 191
Eleventh rib 192
Twelfth rib 192
Ossification of ribs 193
Applied anatomy 194

22. The Hyoid — 198

Location 198
Features and attachments 198
Ossification 200
Applied anatomy 200

23. The Mandible — 201

Peculiarities 201
Features and attachments 201
Ossification 206
Age changes in mandible 206
Applied anatomy 207

24. The Maxillae — 211

Location 211
Features and attachments 211
Ossification 214
Age changes in maxilla 214
Applied anatomy 214

25. The Parietal Bones — 217

Side determination 217
Features and attachments 217
Ossification 219
Age changes 219
Applied anatomy 219

26. The Frontal Bone — 221

Location 221
Features and attachments 221
Frontal sinus 224
Ossification 224
Applied anatomy 224

27. The Temporal Bones — 226

Side determination 226
Features and attachments 226
Spaces and canals 233
External acoustic meatus 233
Middle ear space (tympanic cavity) 234
Mastoid antrum 236
Bony labyrinth (osseous labyrinth) 237
Ossification 239
Applied anatomy 239

28. The Auditory Ossicles — 241
- Terminology 241
- Features and attachments 241
- Malleus 241
- Incus 242
- Stapes 242
- Ossification 242
- Functions 242
- Applied anatomy 243

29. The Occipital Bone — 244
- Locations 244
- Features and attachments 244
- Ossification 248
- Applied anatomy 249

30. The Zygomatic Bones — 250
- Terminology 250
- Features and attachments 250
- Ossification 252
- Applied anatomy 252

31. The Nasal Bones — 254
- Location 254
- Features and attachments 254
- Ossification 255
- Applied anatomy 255

32. The Lacrimal Bones — 257
- Terminology 257
- Peculiarities 257
- Location 257
- Features and attachments 257
- Ossification 258
- Applied anatomy 258

33. The Ethmoid Bone — 260
- Terminology 260
- Location 260
- Features and attachments 260
- Ossification 262
- Applied anatomy 262

34. The Inferior Nasal Conchae — 264
- Terminology 264
- Location 264
- Features and attachements 264
- Ossification 265
- Applied anatomy 265

35. The Vomer — 266
- Terminology 266
- Location 266
- Features and attachments 266
- Ossification 267
- Applied anatomy 267

36. The Sphenoid Bone — 269
- Terminology 269
- Anatomical position 269
- Articulations 269
- Features and attachments 269
- Ossification 275
- Applied anatomy 276

37. The Palatine Bones — 277
- Terminology 277
- Location 277
- Features and attachments 277
- Ossification 280
- Applied anatomy 280

38. The Skull (General Features) — 282
- Introduction 282
- Neurocranium 283
- Facial skeleton (viscerocranium or splanchnocranium) 283
- Anatomical position of skull 283
- Applied anatomy 284

39. The Exterior of the Skull — 286
- Norma verticalis 286
- Norma occipitalis 288
- Norma frontalis 290
- Norma lateralis 294
- Norma basalis 298

40. The Orbital Cavity 308
- Definition 308
- Shape and parts 308
- Bony contributions 308
- Communications 309
- Measurements 310
- Features 311
- Applied anatomy 321

41. The Nasal Cavity 315
- Features 315
- Applied anatomy 317

42. Interior of the Cranial Vault 320
- Definition 320
- Shape 320
- Bones 320
- Sutures 320
- Features 320
- Applied anatomy 321

43. Interior of the Base of the Skull 322
- Definition 322
- Subdivisions 322
- Anterior cranial fossa 322
- Middle aranial fossa 324
- Posterior cranial fossa 327
- Applied anatomy 330

44. Ossification at a Glance 332
- Definition 332
- Centre of ossification 332
- Primary and secondary centres 332
- Fusion of ossification centres 332
- Fusion between adjacent bones 332
- Epiphysis and diaphysis 332
- Clinical significance 333
- Cartilaginous nasal capsule 333
- Appearance of primary centres in appendicular skeleton (weeks of intrauterine life) 334
- Times of the fusion of epiphyses with diaphysis (in years) 335
- Ossification of clavicle 335
- Ossification of bones of upper limb (except clavicle) 336
- Ossification of bones of lower limb 337
- Ossification of sternum, ribs and vertebrae 338
- Ossification of mandible, hyoid, parietal bone and frontal bone 339
- Ossification of occipital bone and sphenoid 340
- Ossification of temporal bone, palatine bone, lacrimal bone, zygomatic bone and maxilla 341
- Fate of cartilaginous nasal capsule 342

Index *343*

CHAPTER 1

General Considerations of Bone

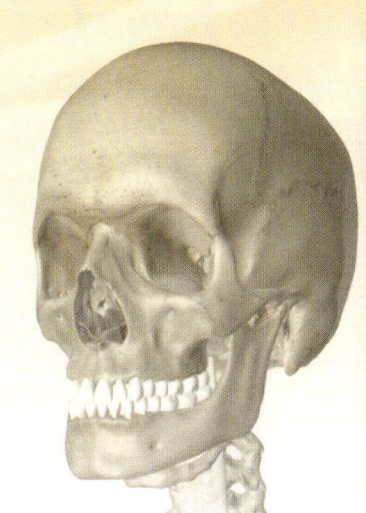

DEFINITION

Bone is the hard part of the body providing dynamic framework to it.

PROPERTIES

1. Bone is a living tissue.
2. Bone is supplied by arteries and nerves.
3. Bone is drained by veins.
4. Bone grows with age.
5. Bone is subject to disease.
6. Bone regenerates when damaged. It has greater regenerative power than any other tissue of the body, except blood.
7. Fractured bone heals leading to union.
8. Bone can undergo remodelling.
9. Bone can withstand strains and stresses.
10. Bone can atrophy or hypertrophy.

FUNCTIONS

1. Bones provide framework to the body.
2. Bones accord shape to the body.
3. Bones act as levers for muscles and therefore help in the movements of the body.
4. Bones provide protection to number of viscera, e.g. brain, lungs and heart.
5. Bone is site of blood formation.
6. Bone plays important role in the immune responses of body by producing cells of reticuloendothelial system.
7. Bones are store houses of calcium and phosphorus.

CHEMICAL COMPOSITION

Bone is one-third organic and two-thirds inorganic. Inorganic calcium salts [calcium phosphate, calcium carbonate and crystals of hydroxyapatite, i.e. $Ca_{10}\{PO_4\}_4(OH)_2$] make it hard and rigid. The organic connective tissue (collagen fibres) makes it tough and resilient. The collagen protein of collagen fibres is characterised by hydroxyproline aminoacid.

STRUCTURE OF BONE

I. Macroscopically

There are two types of bones, spongy or cancellous bone and compact or dense bone. Outer covering of all bones is made up of compact bone (Fig. 1.1). Cancellous bone fills up the interior of the bone except the following.

   i. In the shaft of long bone it is replaced by medullary cavity. This is filled with red marrow in new born but replaced by yellow or fatty marrow in adults.

Human Osteology

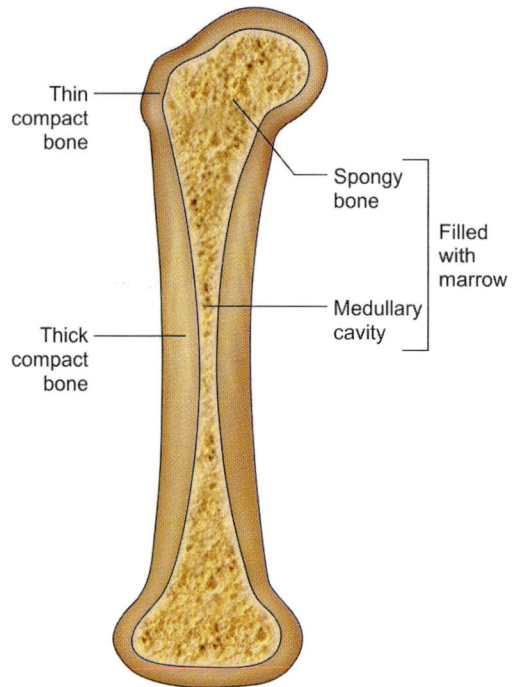

Fig. 1.1: Longitudinal section through a long bone

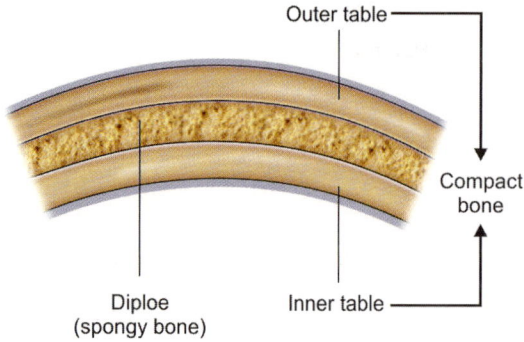

Fig. 1.2: Structure of the flat bone of calva

ii. In maxilla, sphenoid, ethmoid and frontal bones, it is replaced by large air spaces called *sinuses*.

iii. At many places the cancellous bone is replaced by marrow. The red marrow is active in hematopoiesis. Yellow marrow is mainly inert and fatty.

The flat bones of skull cap (calva) have spongy bone (*diploe*) sandwiched between two compact bones called *outer and inner tables* (Fig. 1.2). Red marrow persists in spongy bone throughout life.

The compact bone is more radio-opaque, while spongy bone is relatively more radiolucent. In radiograph, therefore, the compact bone looks more white than spongy bone which appears relatively darker.

II. Microscopically

Microscopically the bones can be classified into four types,

i. *Lamellar bone:* Most of the mature human bones, both compact and spongy, are of this type.
ii. *Fibrous bone:* It is found in early foetuses.
iii. *Dentine:* It is found in teeth.
iv. *Enamel:* It is found in teeth.

The compact bone shows typical Haversian systems each of which is comprised of a central canal along the long axis of bone surrounded by concentric lamellae. Volkmann's canals connect the adjacent Haversian canals. Osteocytes are located in the small spaces (lacunae) between adjacent lamellae (Fig. 1.3). The cytoplasmic processes of osteocytes extend into canaliculi diverging from lacunae. Circumferential lamellae adjoin the surface or medullary cavity of long bones. Interstitial lamellae fill the spaces between Haversian systems.

Spongy bone differs from compact bone in 'lacking Haversian systems' and 'having irregularly arranged bony lamellae'

Periosteum, the outer covering of bone, consists of an external collagen fibrous layer and inner osteogenic cellular layer. Collagen fibres from periosteum piercing the bone are called Sharpey's fibres. Periosteum has a rich nerve supply which makes it most sensitive part of bone.

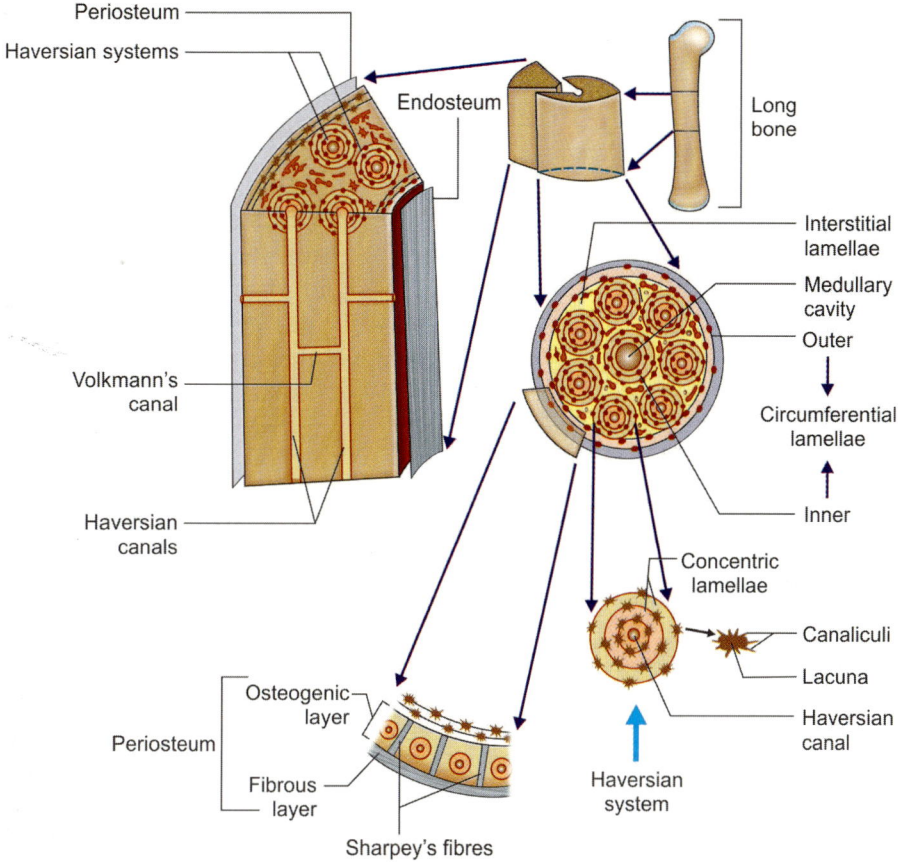

Fig. 1.3: Microscopic structure of compact bone

CLASSIFICATION OF BONES

Bones may be classified according to their development, shape or location.

I. Phylogenetic classification

From comparative anatomy point of view skeleton may be classified as:

a. Exoskeleton

Nails, hairs and enamel of teeth are the only remnants of exoskeleton observed in human being.

b. Endoskeleton

It includes most of the bones.

II. Developmental classification

Developmentally bones may be classified as:
  a. Cartilaginous bones
  b. Membranous bones

III. Morphological classification

According to shape, the bones may be classified as:

a. Long bones – Femur, humerus
b. Short bones – Carpal and tarsal bones
c. Miniature long bones – Metacarpals and metatarsals
d. Flat bones – Parietal bone
e. Irregular bones – Hip bone
f. Pneumatic bones – Maxilla, ethmoid, sphenoid and frontal bone.

IV. Regional classification

Bones may be classified regionally as:

a. Axial bones

It includes 80 bones as shown below:
- i. Skull bones — 22
- ii. Vertebrae — 26
- iii. Ribs — 24
- iv. Sternum — 1
- v. Auditory ossicles — 6
- vi. Hyoid — 1

b. Appendicular bones

It includes 126 bones which are further subgrouped as:
- i. Upper limb bones – 64
- ii. Lower limb bones – 62

Total number of bones is 206

V. Miscellaneous classification

a. Accessory bones

An accessory bone is a small piece of bone which develops from a separate centre of ossification but fails to unite with the main mass of bone, e.g. sutural (Wormian) bones and interparietal bones (Fig. 1.4).

b. Sesamoid bones (Table 1.1)

A sesamoid bone is a bone usually small, developing in the tendon of a muscle, ligament or joint capsule. They ossify after birth and are devoid of periosteum. Sesamoid bones possibly resist pressure, they alter the direction of pull of muscle and minimize the friction.

Table 1.1: Some examples of sesamoid bones

Sesamoid bone	Tendon of muscle
i. Patella	Quadriceps
ii. Pisiform	Flexor carpi ulnaris
iii. Fabella	Lateral head of gastrocnemius
iv. Rider's bone	Adductor longus

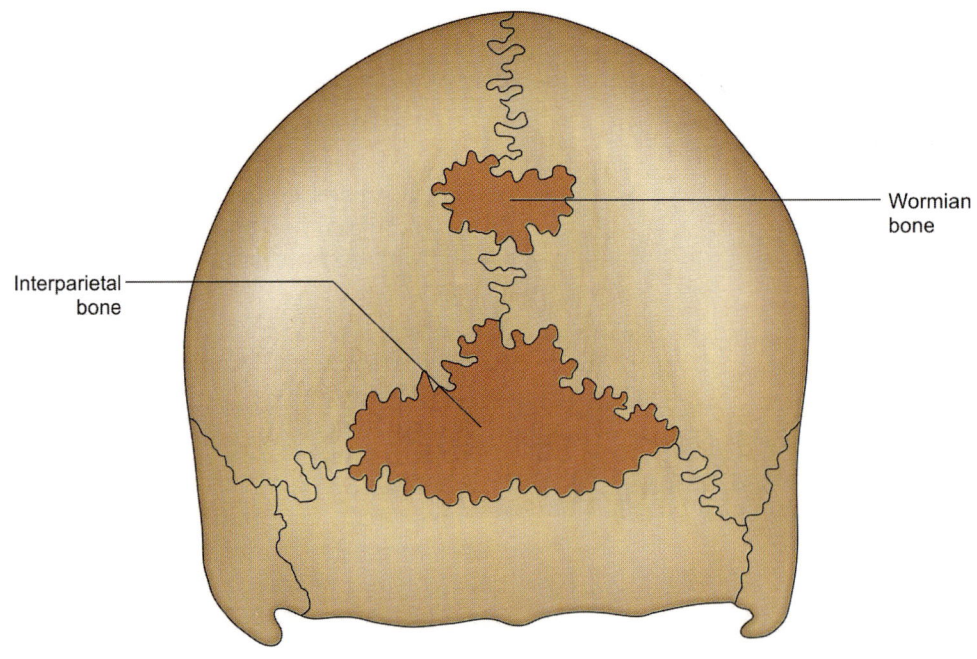

Fig. 1.4: Accessory bones

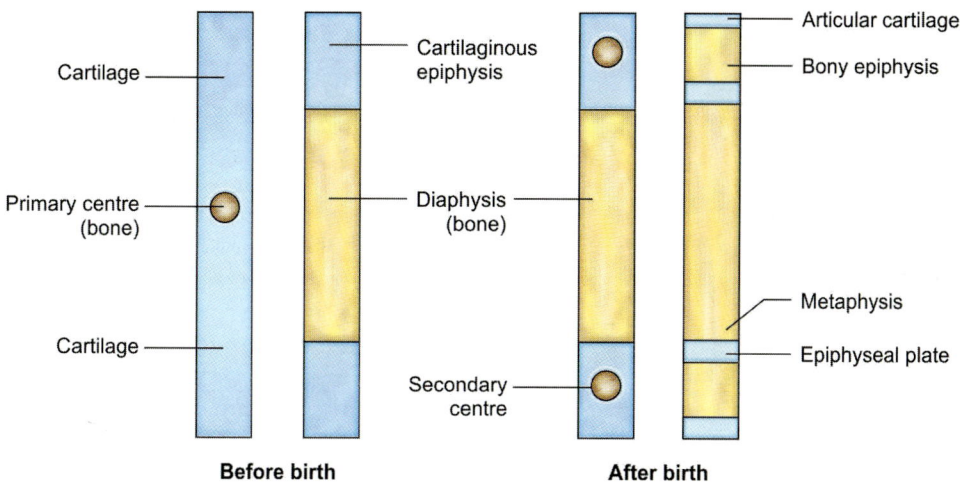

Fig. 1.5: Developing long bone

PARTS OF A YOUNG LONG BONE

1. **Epiphysis (G. epi : upon + physis : growth)**

   At birth both the ends of a long bone are cartilaginous, known as *cartilaginous epiphyses*. After birth these ends undergo ossification resulting into formation of *bony epiphyses*. Epiphysis can be classified as:

   i. *Pressure epiphysis:* Located adjacent to articulation and helps in transmission of weight, e.g. head of femur, lower end of radius, talus.

   ii. *Traction epiphysis (apophysis):* Located at the site of attachment of tendon, e.g. lesser trochanter, tibial tuberosity, tubercles of humerus.

   iii. *Atavistic epiphysis:* Located in that part of a developing bone which was phylogenetically an independent bone, e.g. coracoid process of scapula and os trigonum (lateral tubercle) of talus.

   iv. *Aberrant epiphysis:* It is not always present, e.g. epiphysis at the head of 1st metacarpal and bases of other metacarpals.

2. **Diaphysis (G. dia: in between + physis: growth)**

   It is the region between the two epiphyses of a developing long bone. It corresponds to the shaft of a long bone (Fig. 1.5).

3. **Epiphyseal plate (Growth cartilage, Growth plate, Physis)**

   The cartilaginous plate between epiphysis and diaphysis is called the epiphyseal plate. This is responsible for longitudinal growth of long bones. Epiphyseal plate is nourished by both epiphyseal and metaphyseal arteries.

4. **Metaphysis**

   The epiphyseal end of diaphysis is called metaphysis.

FEATURES OF BONES (Fig. 1.6)

1. **Articular surface** – This is smooth surface participating in the formation of a joint.
2. **Condyle** – This is a large portion at the end of a long bone which is partly articular.
3. **Epicondyle** – It is a small projection from the condyle.
4. **Facet** – It is a small articular surface.
5. **Fossa** – This is a localized depression on the surface.

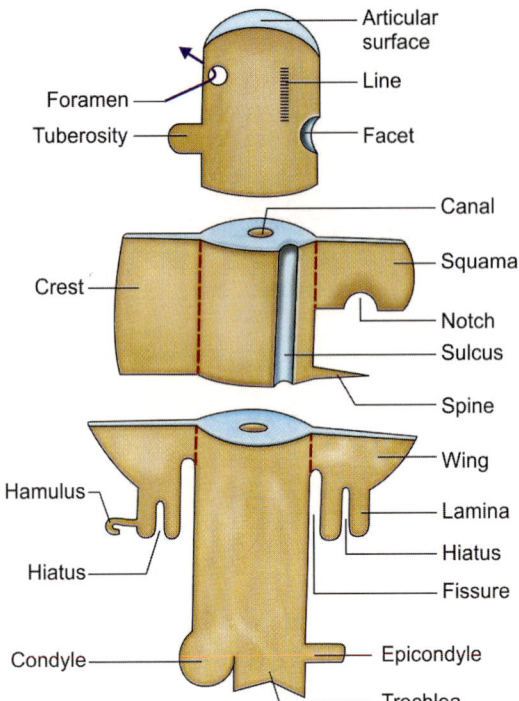

Fig. 1.6: Features of bones

6. **Sulcus/Groove** – This is a linear depression.
7. **Tuberosity/Tubercle/Trochanter/Process**– This is a localized projection.
8. **Trochlea** – A structure which is pulley like.
9. **Foramen** – This is an entry point in the bone.
10. **Canal** – It is a tunnel in the bone.
11. **Notch/Incisure** – This is a marked depression along margin.
12. **Hiatus** – This is a gap in the bone.
13. **Fissure** – A cleft between two adjacent bones is called fissure.
14. **Spine** – It is a pointed process.
15. **Hamulus/Cornu** – This is a hook like projection.
16. **Line** – It is a linear roughness on the surface of bone.
17. **Crest** – This is an elongated flat projection.
18. **Lamina/Plate** – It is a flat piece of bone.
19. **Squama** – This is a large lamina.
20. **Wing** – It is a lateral projection from a midline bone.

BLOOD SUPPLY OF BONES

I. **Long bones:** Following arteries supply a long bone (Fig. 1.7):
   a. *Nutrient artery:* It enters the *nutrient foramen* and runs in the nutrient canal to reach the medullary cavity where it divides into ascending and descending branches (nutritiae). It supplies medullary cavity, inner 2/3rd of the compact bone and metaphysis. It is tortuous to allow the movement of bone.
   b. *Periosteal arteries:* Several periosteal arteries supply the periosteum and outer 1/3rd of compact bone of diaphysis. Periosteal arteries are especially numerours beneath the ligamentous and muscular attachments.
   c. *Epiphyseal arteries:* These are derived from periarticular vascular arcades (circulus vasculosus articuli). These supply the epiphysis.

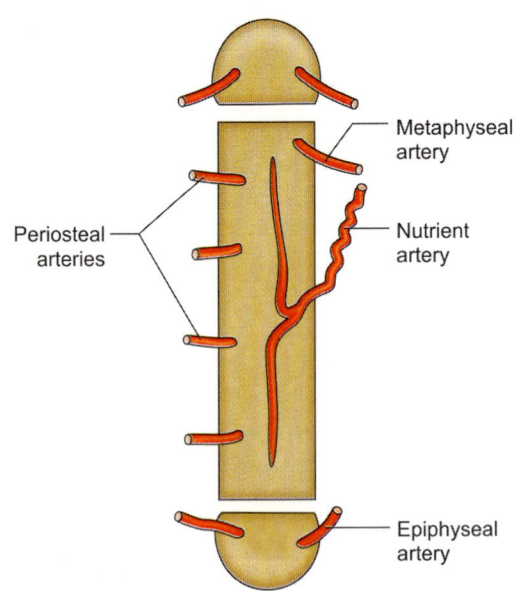

Fig. 1.7: Arteries supplying a long bone

d. *Metaphyseal arteries:* These are derived from neighbouring systemic vessels to supply the metaphysis.

II. **Short bones**

These are supplied by numerous periosteal vessels.

III. **Vertebrae**

The body of vertebra is supplied by the anterior and posterior vessels (Fig. 1.8). The vertebral arch is supplied by large vessels entering through the bases of transverse processes.

IV. **Ribs:** These are supplied by nutrient and periosteal vessels.

V. **Flat bones:** These are supplied by nutrient and periosteal vessels.

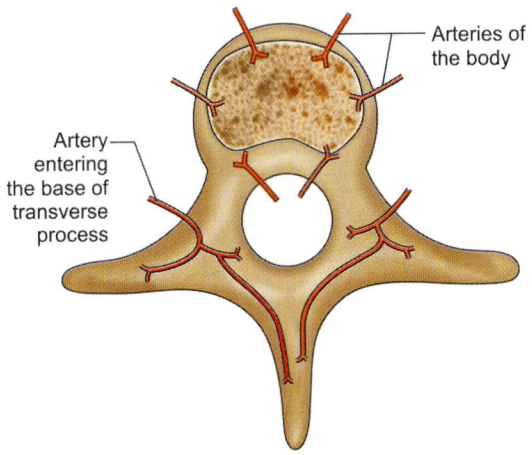

Fig. 1.8: Arterial supply of vertebra

NERVE SUPPLY OF BONES

Nerves accompany the blood vessels of bone. Periosteal nerves are sensory (carry pain) while others are vasomotor in nature.

LYMPHATIC DRAINAGE OF BONES

Lymphatics have not been demonstrated within bone but these are very much present in periosteum which drain into regional lymph nodes.

OSSIFICATION OF BONES

1. Bones ossify from centres of ossification from where laying down of long lamellae starts by osteoblasts.
2. Centres of ossification may be primary or secondary. *Primary centre* appears before birth, usually during 8th week of intrauterine life and gives rise to diaphysis. *Secondary centre* appears at or after birth and gives rise to epiphysis.
3. Most of the long bones have epiphysis at each end but the growth in length occurs mainly at one end. This end is called *growing end*. Here, the epiphysis usually appears earlier and fuses with the body later than that at the non-growing end.

GROWTH OF A LONG BONE

Bone grows in length by multiplication of cells in the epiphyseal plate. Bone grows in thickness by multiplication of cells in the periosteum. Excess bone is removed by osteoclasts, a process called *remodelling*.

SOME INTERESTING DEFINITIONS

Fracture: It is a break in surface of bone.

Dislocation: It is a complete and persistent separation of articulating surfaces of bones forming joints.

Subluxation: It is a partial separation of articulating surfaces of bones participating in formation of a joint.

Sprain: It is temporary subluxation associated with ligament tear.

Strain: It is a tear in muscles.

JOINTS

Joints are the sites where two or more bones meet. A joint formed by two bones is called *simple joint*. A joint formed by more than two bones is called *compound joint*. Bones are held together by intervening connective tissue (*fibrous joint*) or cartilage (*cartilaginous joint*) or capsule (*synovial joint*) (Fig. 1.9). Fibrous joint is least mobile, cartilaginous joint is moderately mobile while synovial joint is maximally mobile. A capsule of a synovial joint is a fibrous tubular sheath whose margins are attached to articulating bones at or beyond articular margins.

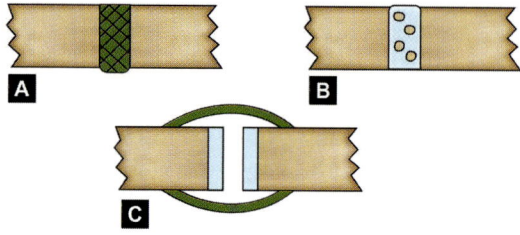

Fig. 1.9: Different types of joints (A) Fibrous joint; (B) Cartilaginous joint; (C) Synovial joint

Table 1.2: The structural classification (Fig. 1.10) of synovial joints in tabulated form

S. No.	Type	Movements	Examples
1.	Plane	Gliding	Intercarpal Carpometacarpal Cuneonavicular
2.	Hinge	Flexion and Extension along transverse axis	Elbow Interphalangeal
3.	Pivot	Rotation along vertical axis	Radioulnar Atlantoaxial between dens of axis and anterior arch of atlas.
4.	Condylar	Flexion Extension Rotation	Knee
5.	Ellipsoid	Flexion Extension Abduction Adduction	Wrist Metacarpophalangeal Metatarsophalangeal
6.	Saddle	Flexion Extension Abduction Adduction Rotation	1st Carpometacarpal
7.	Ball and socket	Greater range of–Flexion Extension Abduction Adduction Rotation	Shoulder Hip

Contd.

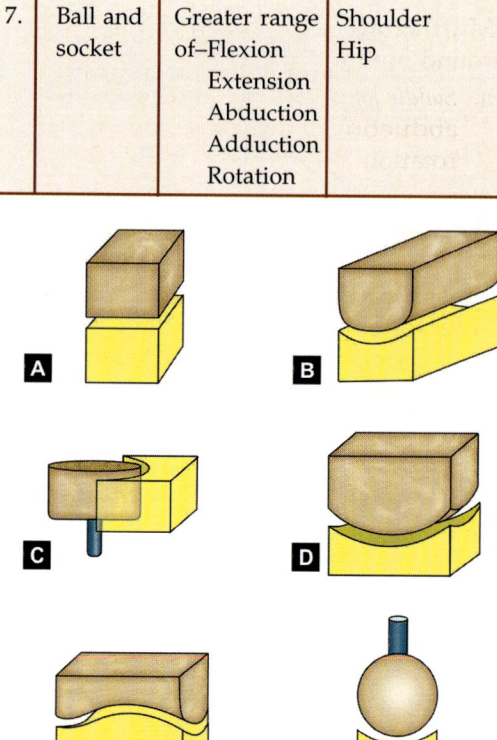

Fig. 1.10: Different types of synovial joints. (A) Plane; (B) Hinge; (C) Pivot; (D) Ellipsoid; (E) Saddle; (F) Ball and socket

Synovial joints can also be classified on the basis of axes involved during movements as mentioned below (Table 1.2),

1. **Plane joint** – Allows only gliding movement and thus no definite axis involved.
2. **Uniaxial joint** – Allows movements around single axis.
   a. *Hinge joint.* Allows flexion and extension around transverse axis.
   b. *Pivot joint* – Allows rotation around vertical axis.
3. **Biaxial joint** – Allows movements around two axes.
   a. *Condylar joint* - Allows flexion, extension and limited rotation.
   b. *Ellipsoid joint* – Allows flexion, extension, abduction and adduction.

4. **Multiaxial joint** – Allows movements around multiple axes.
   a. *Saddle joint* – Allows flexion, extension, abduction, adduction and conjunct rotation.
   b. *Ball and socket joint* – Allows flexion, extension, abduction, adduction, circumduction and rotation.

Table 1.3: Range of movements at different synovial joints of limbs (Apley's System of Orthopaedics and Fractures, 9th Edition)* (American Academy of Orthopaedic Surgeons)**

S. No.	Joints	Movements	Range
1.*	Shoulder (Movements considered in the plane of scapula)	Abduction	0–180°
		Adduction	0–45°
		Flexion	0–180°
		Extension	0–40°
		Lateral rotation	0–80°
		Medial rotation	0–70°
2.*	Elbow	Flexion	0–140°
3.*	Radio-ulnar (From midprone position)	Pronation	0–90°
		Supination	0–90°
4.*	Wrist	Flexion (Palmar flexion)	0–60°
		Extension (Dorsiflexion)	0–50°
		Abduction (Radial deviation)	0–15°
		Adduction (Ulnar deviation)	0–50°
5.**	Thumb joints		
	Interphalangeal	Flexion	0–80°
	Metacarpophalangeal	Flexion	0–50°
	Carpometacarpal	Abduction	0–70°
		Flexion	0–15°
		Extension	0–20°
6.**	Metacarpophalangeal joints of hand (Medial four)	Flexion	0–90°
7.**	Hip	Flexion	
		Knee flexed	0–140°
		Knee extended	0–90°
		Extension	0–10°
		Abduction	0–45°
		Adduction	0–30°
		Rotation (Hip 90° flexed)	
		Medial	0–40°
		Lateral	0–50°
		Rotation (Hip extended)	
		Medial	0–40°
		Lateral	0–40°

Contd.

Table 1.3: Range of movements at different synovial joints of limbs (Apley's System of Orthopaedics and Fractures, 9th Edition)* (American Academy of Orthopaedic Surgeons)** (Contd.)

S. No.	Joints	Movements	Range
8.*	Knee	Flexion	0–150°
		Extension (Hyperextension)	0–20°
9.*	Ankle	Plantar flexion	0–45°
		Dorsiflexion	0–30°

CLOSE PACKED POSITION

This is the most congruent position in which contact areas of articular surfaces reach maximum resulting in the greatest mechanical stability for that joint.

Table 1.4: Close packed positions of some of the synovial joints (Neumann DA 2002)

S.No.	Name of the joint	Close packed position
1.	Glenohumeral	Abduction of 90° and full external rotation
2.	Humero-ulnar	Full elbow extension and full supination
3.	Wrist	Full wrist extension
4.	Knee	Full knee extension
5.	Talocrural (Ankle)	Full ankle dorsiflexion
6.	Subtalar	Full foot supination
7.	Hip	90° flexion, slight abduction and slight external rotation

CLASSIFICATION OF FRACTURES

I. *On the basis of etiology*
  1. *Traumatic fracture*
     Fracture of normal bone due to excessive external force.
  2. *Pathological fracture*
     Fracture of diseased bone due to even trivial force.

II. *On the basis of relationship with external environment (Fig. 1.11)*

1. *Closed or simple fracture*
   Surface skin is intact so no communication with external environment.
2. *Open or compound fracture*
   There is break in overlying skin therefore fracture communicates with external environment.

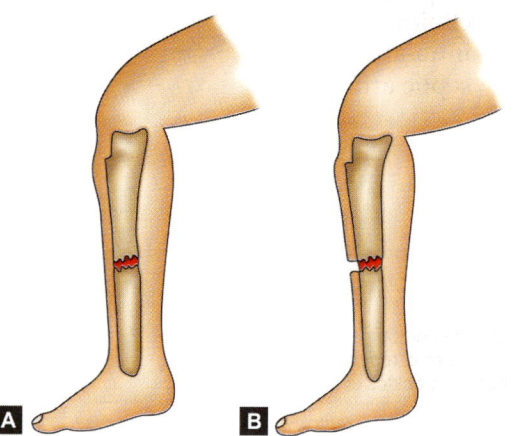

Fig. 1.11: Fractures; (A) Closed or simple; (B) Open or compound

III. *On the basis of displacement*
  A. *Undisplaced fracture*
     On the basis of pattern it can be,
     1. Transverse fracture
     2. Oblique fracture
     3. Spiral fracture

4. Comminuted fracture
5. Segmental fracture
B. *Displaced fracture*
   On the basis of form it can be,
   1. Shift
   2. Angulation
   3. Rotation

APPLIED ANATOMY OF BONES

1. Organic matter in the bone is greatest in childhood making it more flexible.
2. In *rickets* and *osteomalacia* there is inadequate calcium in bone leading to knock-knees and bow-legs (Fig. 1.12).
3. Metaphysis is the commonest site of infection due to rich vascular anastomosis which has relatively less lymphocytes and has hairpin loop arrangement of blood vessels.
4. Capsular relations of metaphysis are clinically important. The inflammation of intra-articular metaphysis may result into septic arthritis, e.g. upper end of femur.
5. Injury of the growing ends of long bones is more dangerous in young children because it will directly affect the growth.
6. In certain conditions (e.g. *pernicious anaemia*) the yellow marrow is replaced by red marrow to enhance the formation of red blood cells.
7. Some interesting facts regarding fractures in young children are as follows:
   i. It is more common due to care-free activities.
   ii. *Green-stick fracture* (incomplete fracture with bending) is common in children due to excessive elasticity in bone.
8. In old age there is generalized skeletal atrophy called *osteoporosis* which makes the bone very weak. *Osteoporosis* is relatively more common in females therefore fracture of femoral neck is more common in elderly lady.
9. In *sternal puncture* the needle pierces the compact bone to reach central spongy bone from where red marrow is aspirated

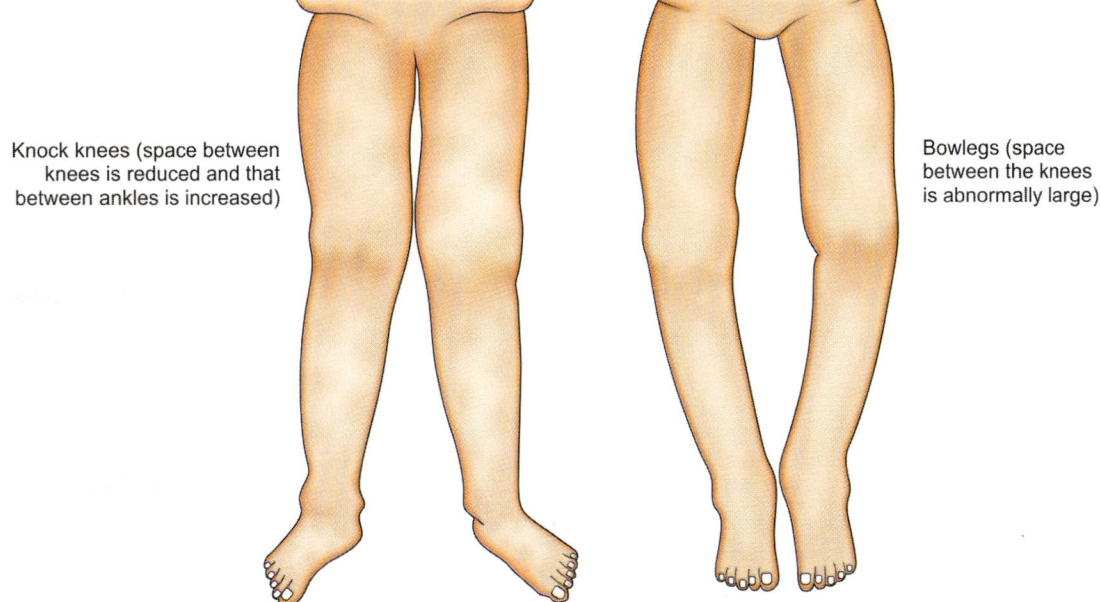

Knock knees (space between knees is reduced and that between ankles is increased)

Bowlegs (space between the knees is abnormally large)

Fig. 1.12: Deformities of the lower limb in *rickets* and *osteomalacia*

for hematological examination. The same procedure is used for bone marrow transplantation.
10. For perfect healing, the fractured ends of a bone should be properly aligned. This is called *reduction*. Healing is difficult and defective if the bony ends are mobile. To make them immobile, a hard cast is made around the fractured site and adjacent joints. This is called *plaster immobilization*.
11. Age of a person can be determined by observing the ossification centres of the bones and their fusion in the radiographs. This is of *medicolegal importance*.
12. Part of a bone may be deprived of blood supply after fracture. This leads to *avascular necrosis*. The best example of avascular necrosis is head of femur after fracture of neck.
13. Fibrous capsule is the most sensitive structure in a joint.
14. Bone cyst is the most common cause of pathological fracture in child.
15. Increased density in metaphysis is seen in *hypervitaminosis*.
16. *Senile osteoporosis* is radiologically manifested only when 30% of skeleton has been lost.
17. Multiple bone fracture in a new born is seen in *osteogenesis imperfecta*.
18. Two interesting facts regarding *Ewing's tumour* are:
    a. It arises from diaphysis.
    b. It is very sensitive to radiotherapy.

CHAPTER
2

The Clavicle

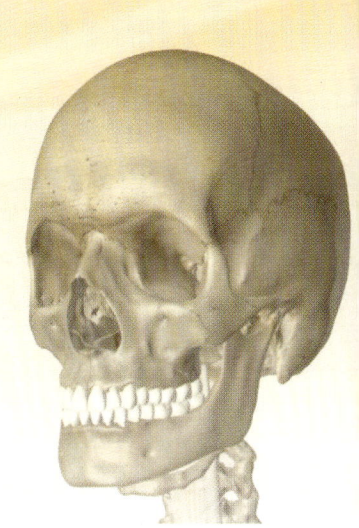

TERMINOLOGY

Clavicle is a Latin word means 'little key'.

SIDE DETERMINATION

1. Curvatures lie in horizontal plane.
2. Flattened end is lateral.
3. Roughened areas near the ends and longitudinal groove in the middle 3rd, face inferiorly.
4. Medial 2/3rd of the clavicle shows convexity forwards.

ANATOMICAL POSITION

The clavicle extends laterally almost horizontally at the root of neck (Fig. 2.1).

FUNCTIONS

1. It acts as a strut for holding the upper limb free from the trunk.
2. It transmits weight of upper limb to axial skeleton (sternum).
3. It provides area for the attachment of muscles.

PECULIARITIES OF CLAVICLE

1. It is the only long bone lying horizontally in the body.

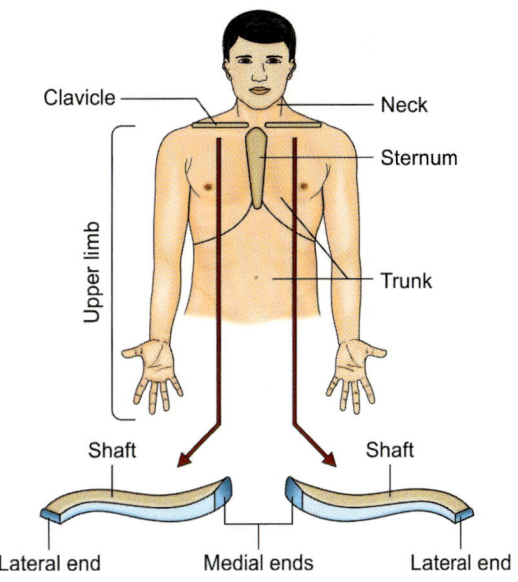

Fig. 2.1: Clavicle: Anatomical position.

2. It has no medullary cavity.
3. The whole clavicle is almost visible through skin and can be easily palpated.
4. It is first bone to start ossification in the body (the second bone to ossify is mandible).
5. It is the only long bone which ossifies by two primary centres.
6. It is the only long bone which ossifies in membrane (long bones ossify in cartilage).

7. It may be pierced by a cutaneous nerve (intermediate supraclavicular nerve).

FEATURES AND ATTACHMENTS

Clavicle has two ends and a shaft (Fig. 2.2).

I. ENDS
A. Lateral end
1. This is also called *acromial end*.
2. It is flattened from above downwards.
3. It meets with acromion process to form *acromio-clavicular joint*.

B. Medial end
1. This is also called *sternal end*.
2. It meets with sternum to form *sterno-clavicular joint*.
3. It receives following attachments (Fig. 2.3):
    i. *Fibrous capsule*
    ii. *Articular disc*
    iii. *Interclavicular ligament*

II. SHAFT
A. Lateral 1/3rd of clavicle
It is flattened from above downwards. It has two surfaces (superior and inferior) and two borders (anterior and posterior).

a. Superior surface (Figs 2.4 and 2.5)
It is subcutaneous.

b. Inferior surface
It has a *conoid tubercle* and a *trapezoid ridge* which provide attachments to conoid and trapezoid parts of *coraco-clavicular ligament* respectively (Fig. 2.6).

c. Anterior border
It is concave forwards and provides origin to *deltoid* muscle.

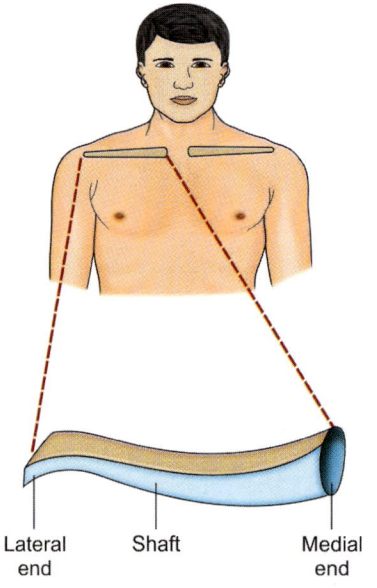

Fig. 2.2: Parts of right clavicle

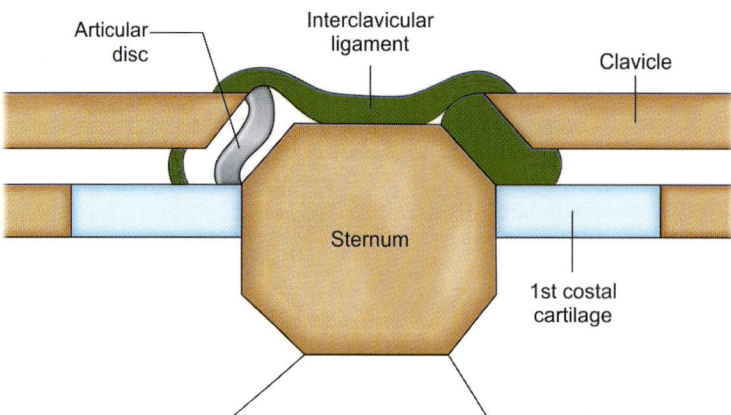

Fig. 2.3: Attachments to the medial end of clavicle

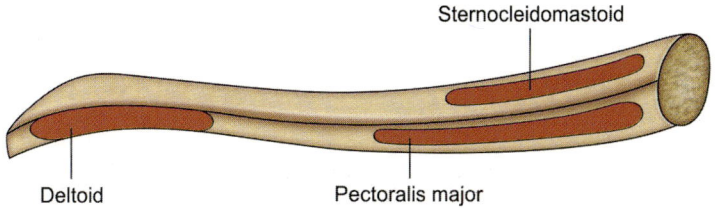

Fig. 2.4: Right clavicle : Anterosuperior aspect

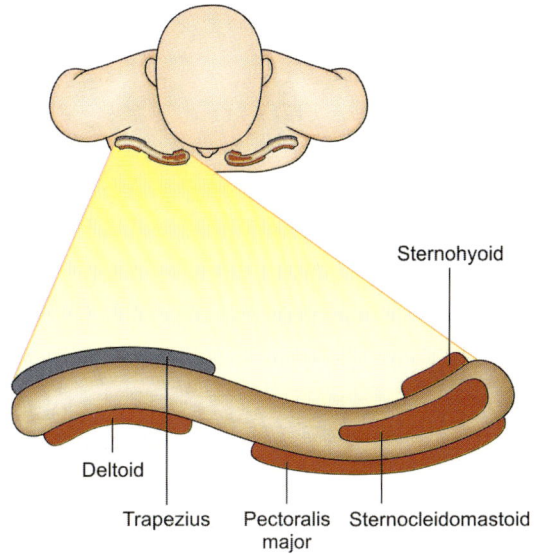

Fig. 2.5: Right clavicle : Superior aspect

d. Posterior border
It shows convexity backwards and provides insertion to *trapezius* muscle.

B. Medial 2/3rd of clavicle
It is quadrilateral in shape and thus has four surfaces, i.e., anterior, posterior, superior and inferior.

a. Anterior surface
It shows convexity forwards. It gives origin to clavicular head of *pectoralis major*.

b. Posterior surface
It exhibits concavity backwards. The origin of *sternohyoid* muscle extends on this surface

medially. It is related to the following structures:
   i. *Divisions of trunks of brachial plexus*
   ii. *3rd Part of subclavian artery*
   iii. *Internal jugular vein*
   iv. *Subclavian vein*
   v. *Brachiocephalic vein*

c. Superior surface (Figs 2.4 and 2.5)
The clavicular head of *sternocleido-mastoid* muscle originates from this surface medially.

d. Inferior surface (Fig. 2.6)
1. *Costoclavicular ligament* is attached to a rough oval impression at its medial end.
2. *Subclavian groove* on its lateral half is for insertion of *subclavius*.
3. *Clavipectoral fascia* is attached to the margins of subclavian groove.
4. *Nutrient foramen* is on the lateral end of subclavian groove. *Nutrient artery* of clavicle arises from suprascapular artery.

OSSIFICATION
It has two primary and one secondary centres for ossification.

A. Primary centres
Two centres appear in shaft during 5th-6th week of intrauterine life. They fuse on 45th day of intrauterine life.

B. Secondary centre
Appearance : One centre at the medial end appears at puberty.
Fusion : 20 years.

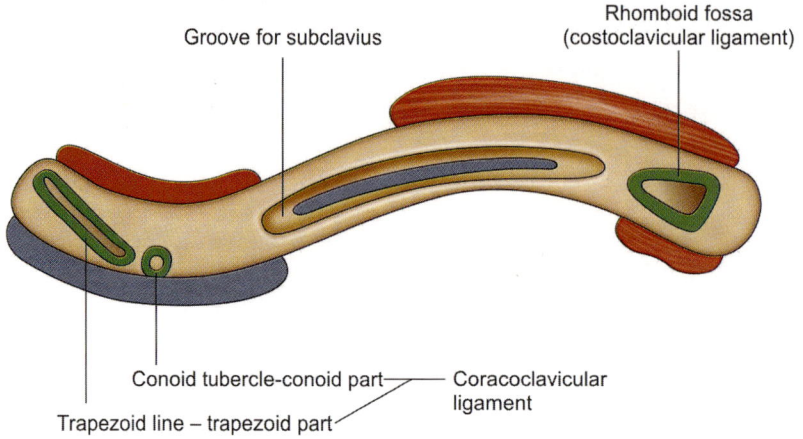

Fig. 2.6: Right clavicle: Inferior aspect

APPLIED ANATOMY

1. Clavicle is the most common bone to fracture in body.
2. Clavicle is the most common bone to fracture during birth.
3. Most common fracture site is at the junction of medial 2/3rd and lateral 1/3rd, because:
   i. This is the site of weight transmission through coracoclavicular ligament.
   ii. Here the two curvatures of clavicle meet (Fig. 2.7).

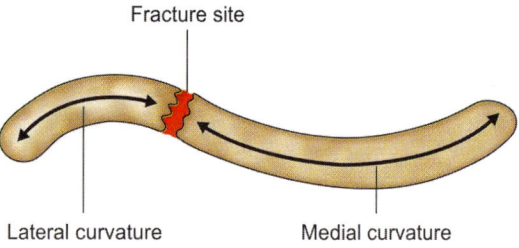

Fig. 2.7: Fracture of clavicle

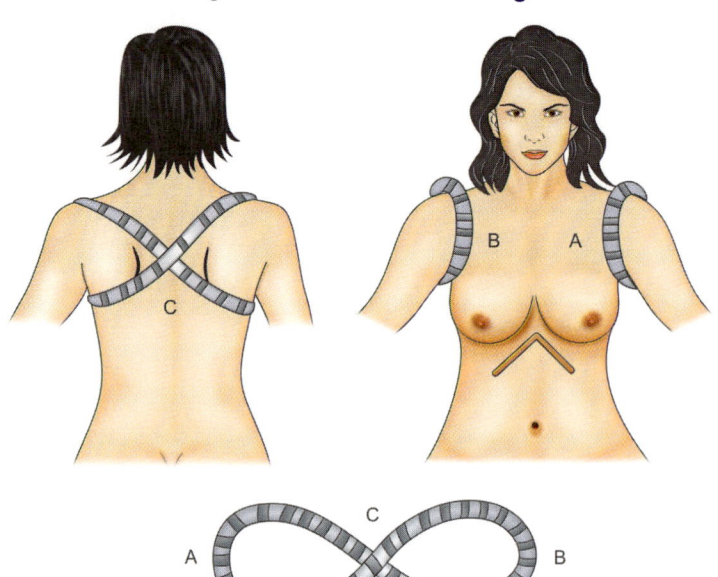

Fig. 2.8: Figure of 8 bandage

4. Fracture commonly occurs due to fall on the outstretched hand.
5. Fracture is treated by immobilization with figure of 8 bandage (Fig. 2.8).
6. After fracture, deformity is downward displacement of lateral fragment due to weight of limb, a condition called *drooping of shoulder* (Fig. 2.9).
7. Fracture of clavicle is often incomplete in children *(green-stick fracture)*.
8. Delayed union and nonunion are rare in clavicular fractures.
9. After clavicular fracture, the medial segment is raised by sternocleidomastoid muscle (Fig. 2.9).
10. A vein connecting cephalic vein with external jugular vein is sometimes present (Fig. 2.10). If so, it crosses the front of clavicle and may be torn during fracture of clavicle leading to severe bleeding.

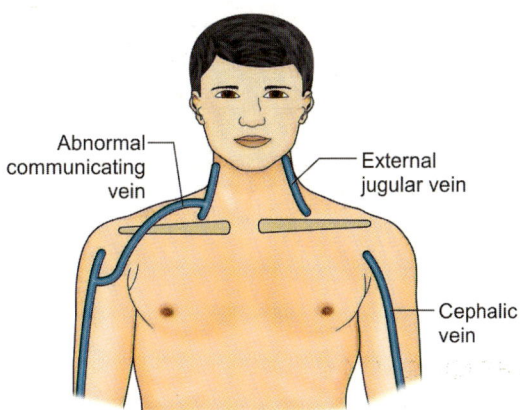

Fig. 2.10: Abnormal communicating vein

11. *Malunion* is very common in clavicular fractures and therefore it often heals with a *'bump'* which is very common (Fig. 2.11).

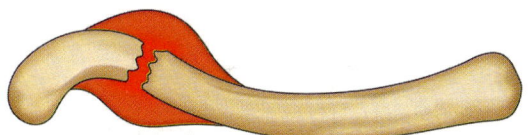

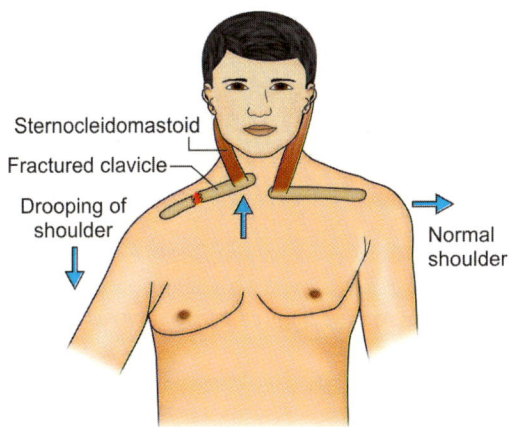

Fig. 2.9: Deformities in clavicular fracture

Fig. 2.11: A 'bump' at the site of clavicular fracture

CHAPTER 3
The Scapula

TERMINOLOGY

Scapula is also called as *shoulder blade*.

SITUATION

Scapula is located on the posterolateral aspect of thorax against the 2nd to 7th ribs (Fig. 3.1).

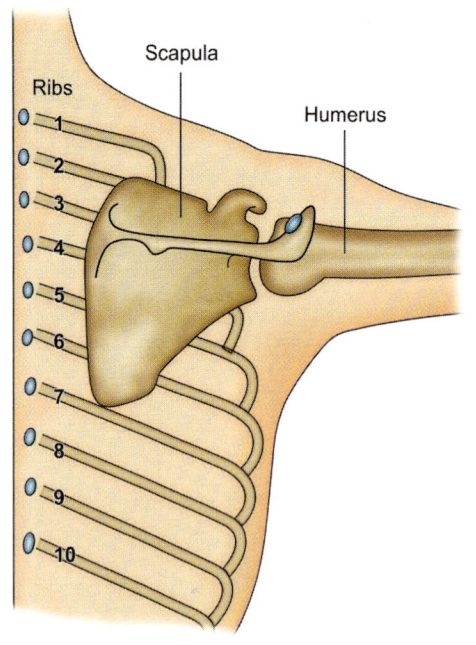

Fig. 3.1: Situation of scapula

SIDE DETERMINATION (Fig. 3.2)

1. The truncated angle (*glenoid cavity*) of triangular scapula faces laterally.
2. A bracket like projection (*spine*) from surface of scapula, is directed posteriorly.
3. Scapula's upper border is marked by a hook like projection (*coracoid process*) adjacent to glenoid cavity and a notch (*suprascapular notch*) near the root of coracoid process.

ANATOMICAL POSITION

Keep the scapula on the back of thorax in such a way that,
1. Glenoid cavity looks laterally, forwards and slightly upwards.
2. Coracoid process is directed forwards.

FEATURES AND ATTACHMENTS

Scapula has two surfaces (costal and dorsal), three borders (superior, medial and lateral), three angles (superior, inferior and lateral) and three processes (spine, acromion and coracoid).

I. Surfaces

A. Costal surface (subscapular fossa)

1. It is concave.
2. It is directed medially and forwards.

The Scapula

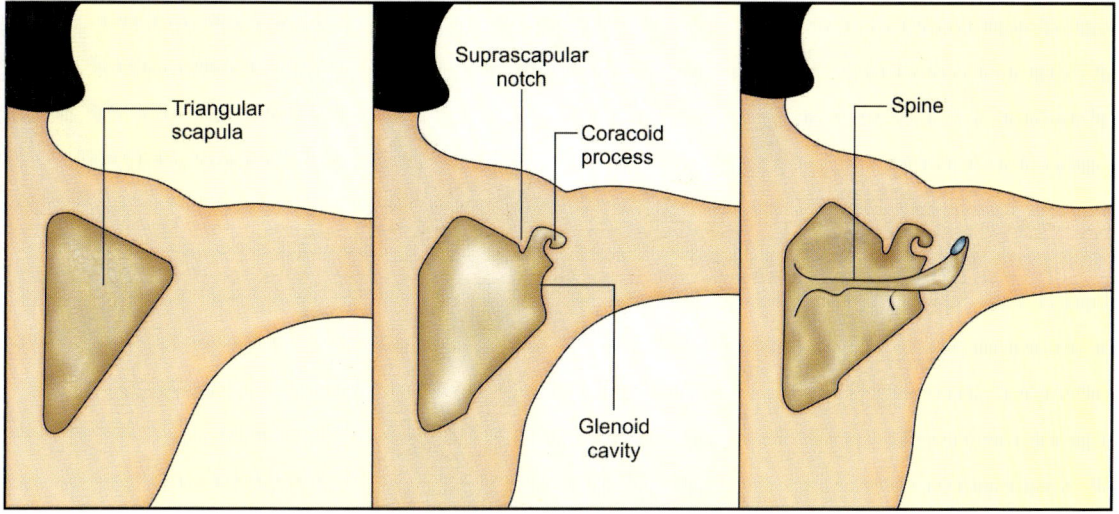

Fig. 3.2: Determination of side of scapula

3. It is subdivided by 3 longitudinal ridges into smooth areas. These ridges provide attachments to *intramuscular tendons of subscapularis* (Fig. 3.3).
4. *Subscapularis*, a multipennate muscle, is attached to the medial 2/3rd of subscapular fossa including the vertical grooved area near the lateral border (Fig. 3.4).
5. *Subscapular bursa* is related to scapula near the glenoid cavity.

B. Dorsal surface (Figs 3.5 and 3.6)

1. It is convex.
2. Spine divides it into *supraspinous* and *infraspinous fossae*.
3. *Spinoglenoid notch* is the connection between two fossae on the back of glenoid cavity.

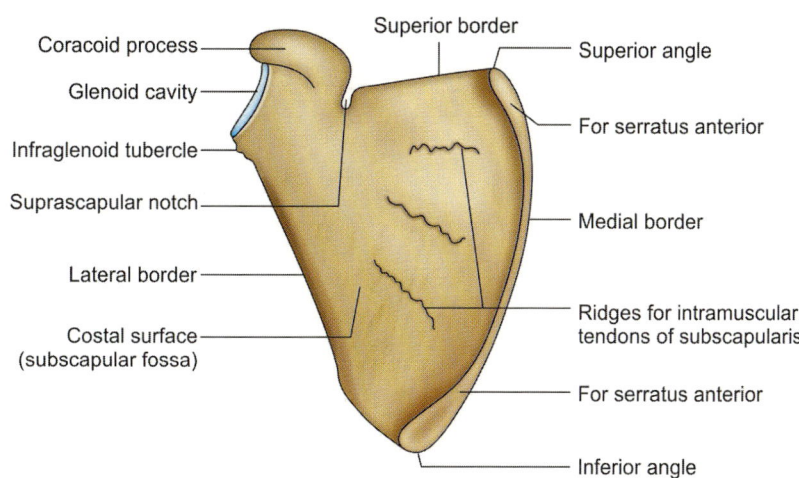

Fig. 3.3: Right scapula : Ventral aspect

Human Osteology

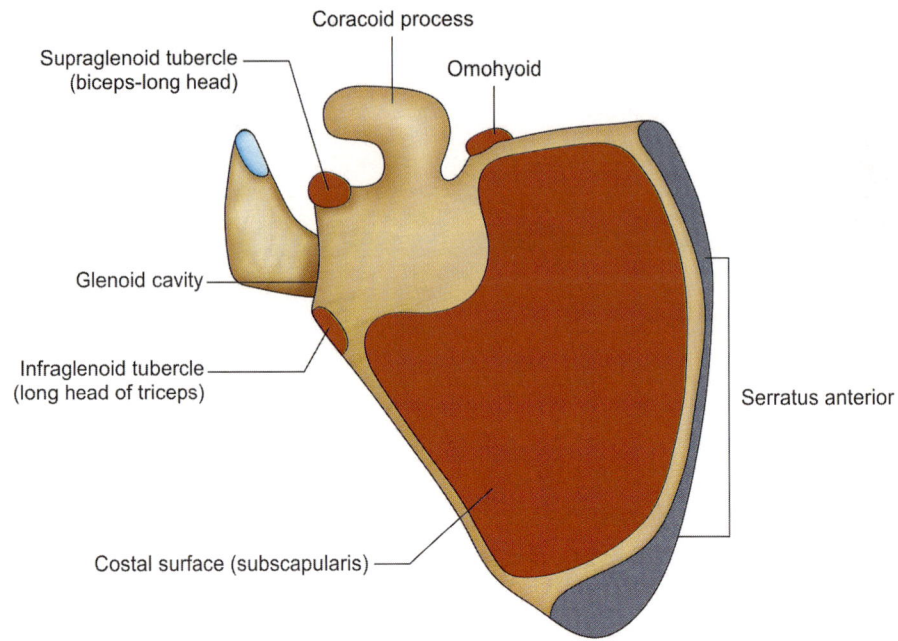

Fig. 3.4: Right scapula : Ventral aspect

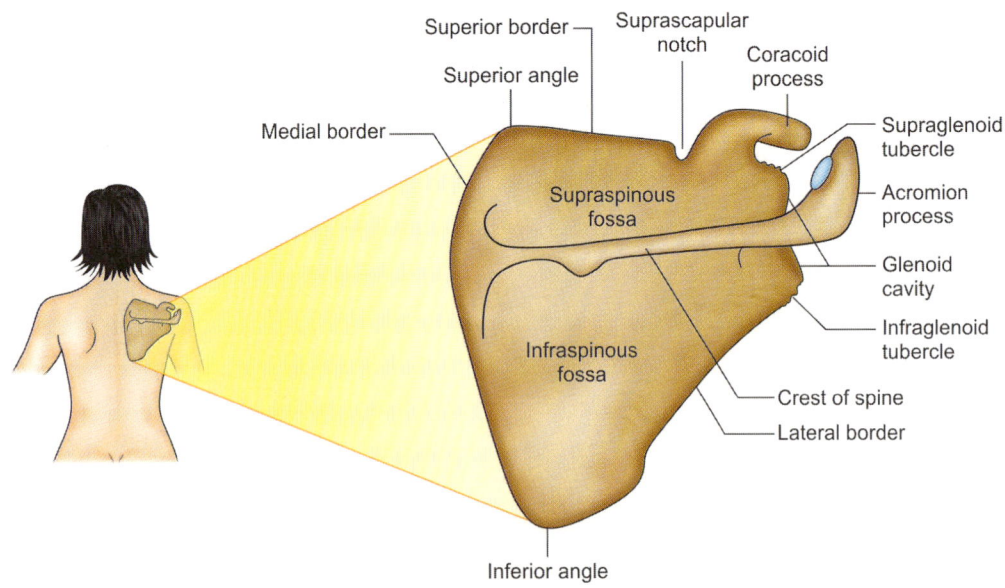

Fig. 3.5: Right scapula: Dorsal aspect

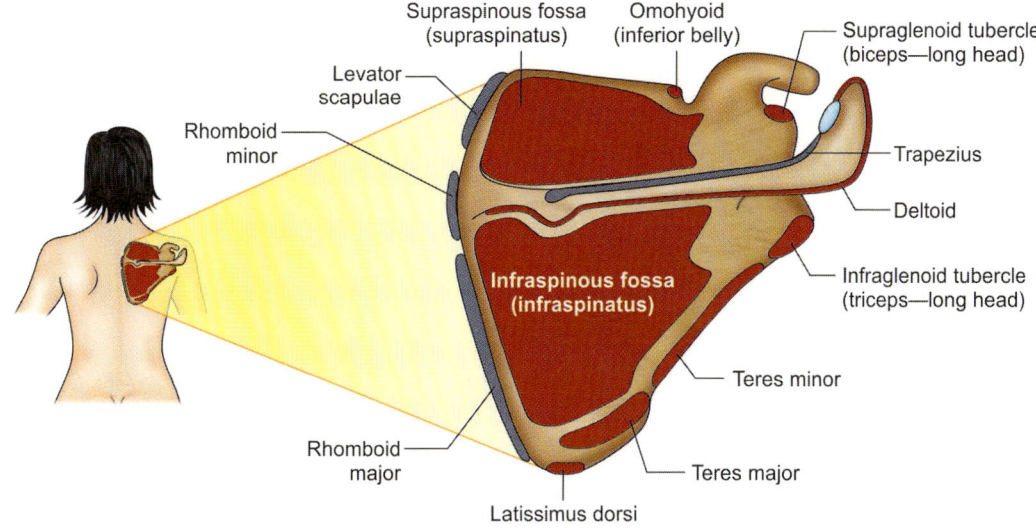

Fig. 3.6: Right scapula : Dorsal aspect

4. *Supraspinatus* is attached to medial 2/3rd of supraspinous fossa.
5. *Infraspinatus* is attached to medial 2/3rd of infraspinous fossa.
6. *Teres minor* is attached to the upper 2/3rd of the dorsal surface of lateral border. This origin is interrupted by the circumflex scapular artery.
7. *Teres major* is attached to the lower 1/3rd of the dorsal surface of lateral border and inferior angle.

Note: *Remember that child is always carried by adults in their arms, therefore minor is above major*

8. *Latissimus dorsi* also originates from dorsal surface of the inferior angle by a small slip.

II. Borders

A. Superior border

1. It is the shortest border.
   Note: Superior begins with 'S' and 'Shortest' also begins with 'S'
2. *Suprascapular notch* is present near the root of coracoid process.
3. *Superior transverse (suprascapular) ligament* converts the suprascapular notch into suprascapular foramen.
4. *Suprascapular artery* passes above the ligament and *suprascapular nerve* passes below the ligament, through foramen.

Note: *To remember this fact think that Air Force flies above the Navy, i.e. A=Artery is above and N = Nerve is below*

5. *Inferior belly of omohyoid* is attached to the superior border near the suprascapular notch.

B. Lateral border

1. It is the thickest border.
2. *Infraglenoid tubercle* is present at its upper end, just below the glenoid cavity.
3. *Long head of triceps* originates from infraglenoid tubercle.

C. Medial border (vertebral border)

1. It extends from superior angle to inferior angle.
2. *Serratus anterior* is inserted to the costal surface of the medial border and the inferior angle.

3. *Levator scapulae* is attached to the medial border above the root of spine.
4. *Rhomboid minor* is attached to the medial border opposite the root of spine.
5. *Rhomboid major* is attached to the medial border below the root of spine.

Note: *Levator scapulae has to elevate the scapula and therefore is always superior most, rhomboid minor has to be superior to rhomboid major as the baby is carried by adults in their arms, i.e. minor is above the major.*

III. Angles

A. Superior angle
It is covered by trapezius.

B. Inferior angle
It is covered by latissimus dorsi.

C. Lateral angle (glenoid angle)
1. It bears the *glenoid cavity*, a pear shaped concave articular surface.
2. It is also known as the *head of scapula*.
3. *Labrum glenoidale* is attached to the margins of glenoid cavity deepening its concavity which receives the convexity of humerus to make shoulder joint.
4. *Capsule of shoulder joint* is attached to labrum and bone beyond it.
5. Long head of biceps originates from the *supraglenoid tubercle* (a small tubercle just above the glenoid cavity) which is intra-capsular (Fig. 3.7).

Note: *Glenoid tubercles are always meant for long heads, since 2 comes before 3, i.e. 2 is above 3 therefore biceps is attached to supraglenoid tubercle and triceps to infraglenoid tubercle.*

IV. Processes

A. Spinous process
1. It is a bracket like projection from upper part of dorsal aspect of scapula, also called *spine of scapula*

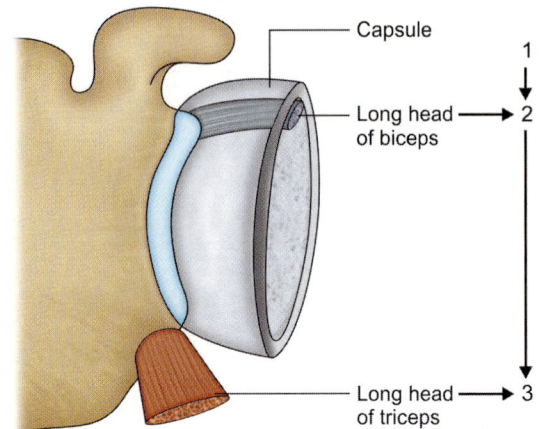

Fig. 3.7: Attachments of long heads of biceps (2) and triceps (3)

2. It divides the dorsal surface of scapula into *supraspinous* and *infraspinous fossae* (Fig. 3.8 and 3.9).
3. Spine has 2 surfaces (superior and inferior) and 3 borders (anterior, posterior and lateral).

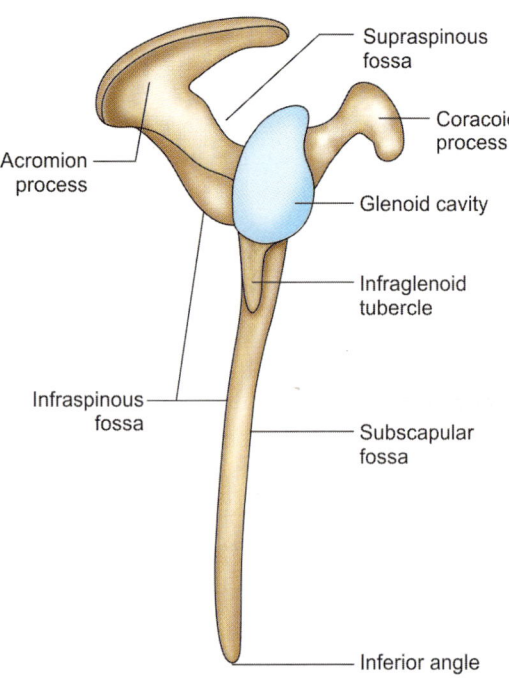

Fig. 3.8: Right scapula : Lateral view

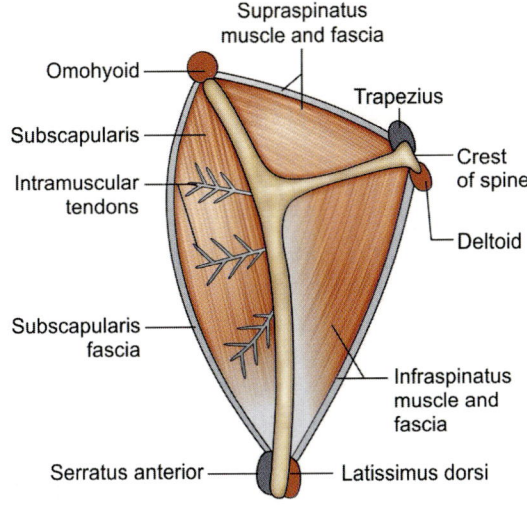

Fig. 3.9: Vertical sectional view of scapula

4. Its superior surface contributes to *supraspinous fossa* whose medial 2/3rd provides attachment to *supraspinatus* while lateral 1/3rd is related to *suprascapular nerve* and *vessels* (Fig. 3.10).

5. Inferior surface of spine contributes to *infraspinous fossa* whose medial 2/3rd gives attachment to *infraspinatus*.

6. Anterior border of spine is attached to dorsal surface of scapula.

7. Lateral border of spine bounds *spinoglenoid notch* meant for the passage of *suprascapular nerve and vessels*.

8. Posterior border of spine is also called *crest of spine*. *Trapezius* is attached to the upper lip of crest of spine while posterior fibres of *deltoid* are attached to its lower lip.

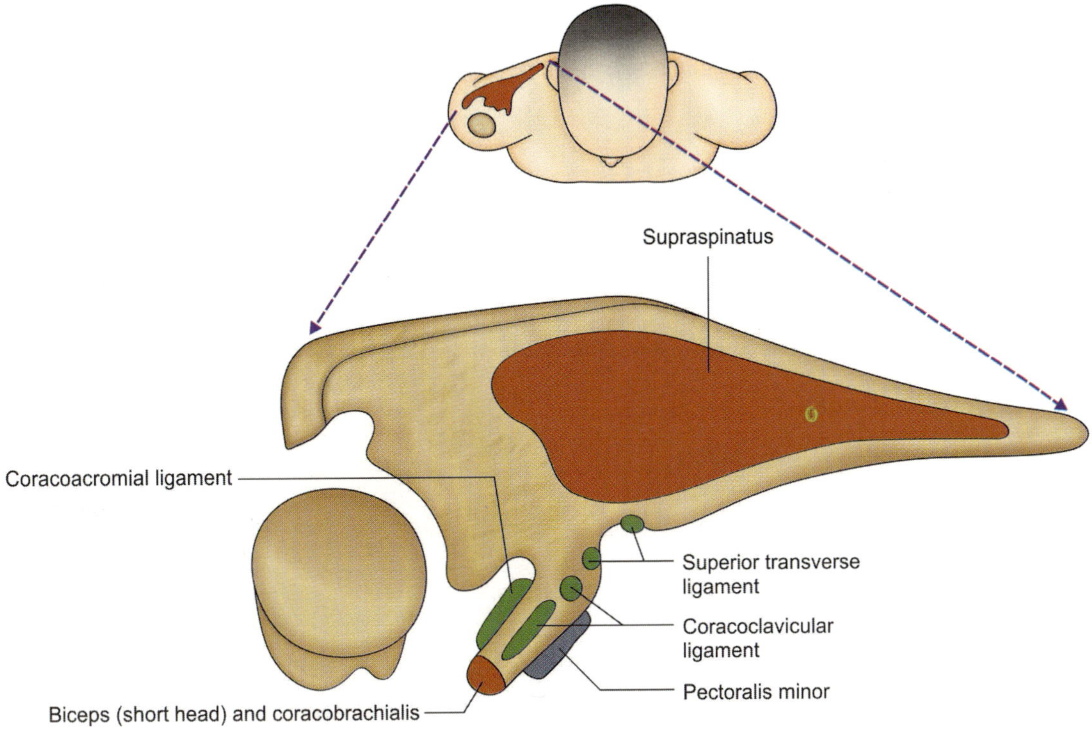

Fig. 3.10: Right scapula : Superior aspect

B. Acromion (acromial process)

1. It projects forwards from lateral end of spine.
2. It overhangs the glenoid cavity.
3. It is subcutaneous.
4. It has 2 borders (medial and lateral), 2 surfaces (superior and inferior) and a tip.
5. Medial and lateral borders continue with the upper and lower lips of the crest of spine respectively.
6. Superior surface is subcutaneous.
7. Inferior surface is related to *subacromial bursa*.
8. *Trapezius* is attached to the medial border in continuation of its attachment to the upper lip of crest of spine.
9. *Deltoid's middle fibres* are attached to the lateral border in continuation of its attachment to the lower lip of crest of spine.
10. *Coracoacromial ligament* is attached to the medial side of tip.
11. A small articular facet on its medial border just behind the tip meets with lateral end of clavicle to form *acromio-clavicular joint*.

C. Coracoid process (Fig. 3.11)

1. It lies below the junction of lateral 1/4th with the rest of clavicle.
2. It is directed forwards and slightly laterally.
3. It arises from upper part of glenoid cavity.
4. *Short head of biceps* and *coracobrachialis* arise from its tip by a common tendon.
5. *Pectoralis minor* is inserted to its medial border.
6. *Coracoacromial ligament* is attached to its lateral border.
7. *Conoid part of coraco-clavicular ligament* is attached to its knuckle.
8. *Trapezoid part of coracoclavicular ligament* is attached to a ridge on its superior aspect between the attachments of pectoralis minor and coracoacromial ligament.
9. *Coracohumeral ligament* is attached to its root adjacent to glenoid cavity.

OSSIFICATION

A. Primary centre

One centre appears in the body during 8th week of intrauterine life.

B. Secondary centres: 7 in all,

Appearance : 1st Secondary centre appears in the middle of coracoid process during 1st year.

Following 6 centres appear at puberty:

1 for root of coracoid process (Subcoracoid centre),

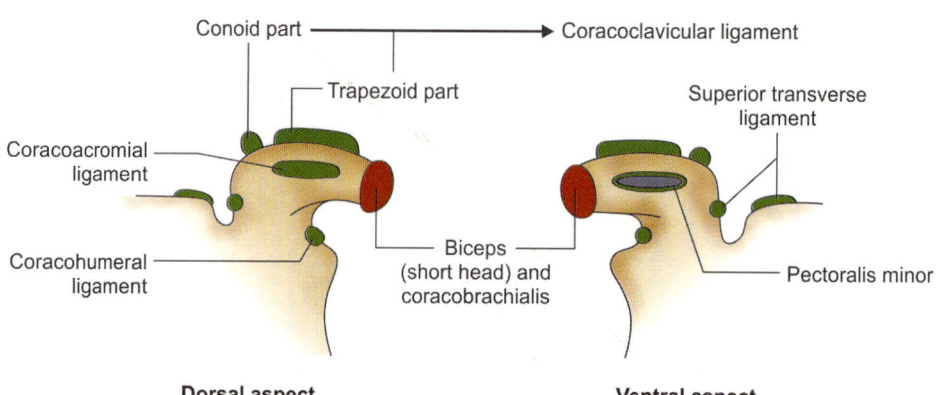

Fig. 3.11: Coracoid process of right scapula

Fusion: 2 for acromion process,
1 for medial border,
1 for inferior angle,
1 for lower 2/3rd of rim of glenoid cavity.
Subcoracoid centre fuses with rest of bone by 15th year. All other centres fuse by 20th year.

APPLIED ANATOMY

1. *Winging of scapula*: It is due to the paralysis of serratus anterior muscle. It usually results from injury of the long thoracic nerve of Bell which supplies the serratus anterior. In winging, the medial border of scapula becomes unduly prominent especially when the patient is asked to push against a wall.
2. In case of *paralysis of serratus anterior* the patient is unable to raise the arm above the head as the paralysed muscle can no more rotate the scapula.
3. *Scaphoid scapula*: It is a developmental defect leading to the formation of scapula with concave medial border.
4. Sometimes acromion remains separated from the spine by a cartilage or a synovial joint.
5. Rarely a joint separates the coracoid process and the body of scapula. In certain mammals this condition is maintained throughout life. In reptiles, coracoid is a separate bone. In human it is represented by *atavistic epiphysis*.
6. *Sprengel's shoulder* is due to failure of the descent of scapula from neck downwards during the development (Fig. 3.12).

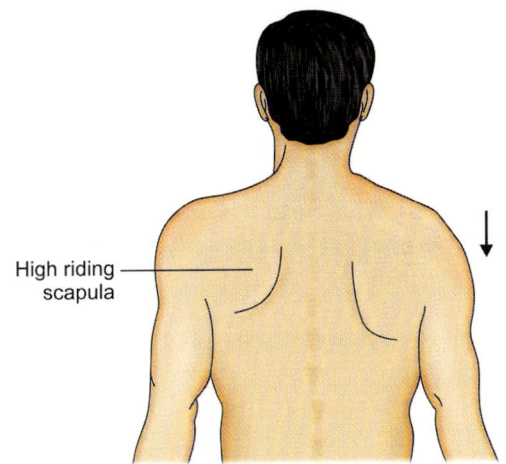

Fig. 3.12: Sprengel's shoulder

7. *Scapular fractures* are seldom displaced due to thick muscles surrounding it.

CHAPTER 4

The Humerus

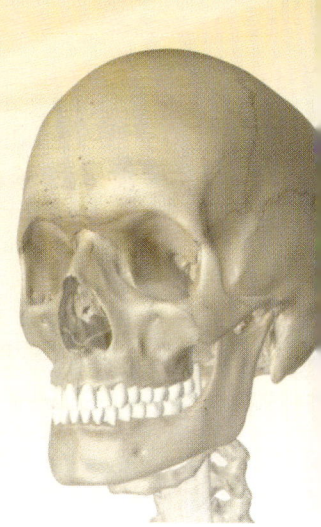

Humerus is the vertical bone located in the arm. It is said to be largest and longest bone of upper limb.

SIDE DETERMINATION (Fig. 4.1)

1. The rounded end (the end with head) is superior.
2. The head is directed medially.
3. Lesser tuberosity at the upper end faces forwards.

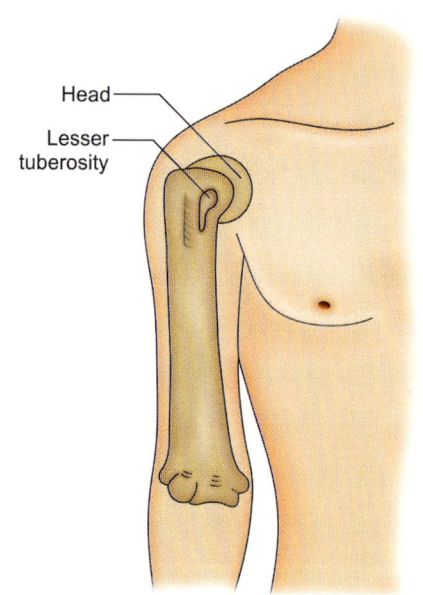

Fig. 4.1: Determination of side of humerus

ANATOMICAL POSITION

Humerus is placed vertically in such a way that the head at its upper end faces medially, backwards and upwards.

FEATURES AND ATTACHMENTS

Humerus has two ends (upper and lower) and a shaft.

I. Upper end

It includes head, neck, greater and lesser tubercles and intertubercular sulcus.

A. Head

1. It is 1/3rd of a sphere.
2. It is covered by articular cartilage.

B. Neck

3 necks are described.

a. Anatomical neck

1. It is adjacent to head.
2. Capsular ligament of shoulder joint is attached to anatomical neck. Capsular attachment is deficient at the upper end of intertubercular sulcus for the passage of tendon of long head of biceps. Medially the capsule extends for about 2 cm on the shaft thus enclosing the medial part of epiphyseal line (Fig. 4.2).

The Humerus 27

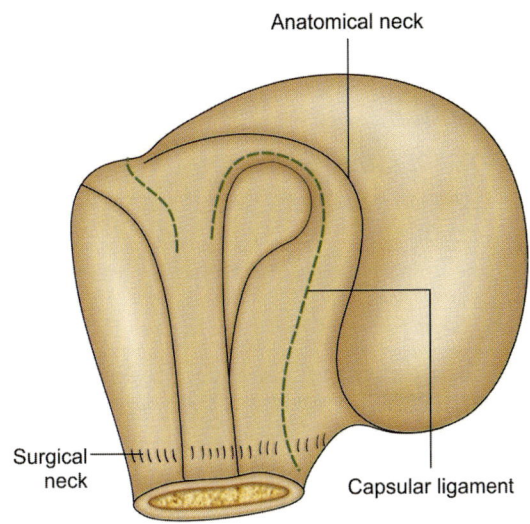

Fig. 4.2: Upper end of right humerus: Anterior aspect

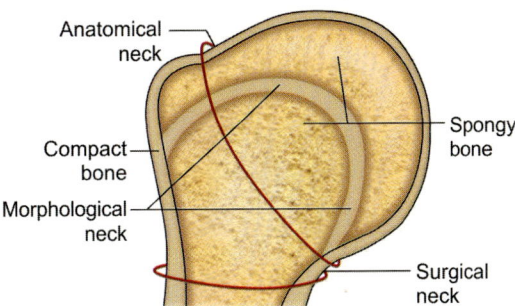

Fig. 4.3: Longitudinal section through upper end of humerus

Note: *Remember the term 'SIT' for greater tuberosity where 'S' stands for Supraspinatus, 'I' for Infraspinatus and 'T' for Teres minor.*

3. It is covered by *subacromial bursa*.

D. Lesser tubercle
1. *Subscapularis* is inserted on it.
2. *Transverse humeral ligament* is attached to it.

E. Intertubercular sulcus (Fig. 4.4)
1. It is also called bicipital groove due to its relation with the long head of biceps.

b. Surgical neck
1. It is the junction of upper end and the shaft.
2. It is related to axillary nerve and posterior circumflex humeral vessels.

Note: *Remember, it is the anatomy which is taught 1st and surgery is taught afterwards in medical curriculum, therefore the 1st constriction from head is the anatomical neck and the next constriction is surgical neck.*

c. Morphological neck
The upper convex end of diaphysis is received by concavity of the epiphysis at the upper end of humerus. This junction is called morphological neck which can be appreciated only in vertical sectional view (Fig. 4.3).

C. Greater tubercle
1. It is the lateral most point in the shoulder region.
2. There are three impressions on the greater tubercle-upper, middle and lower. These impressions provide attachments to *supraspinatus, infraspinatus* and *teres minor* respectively.

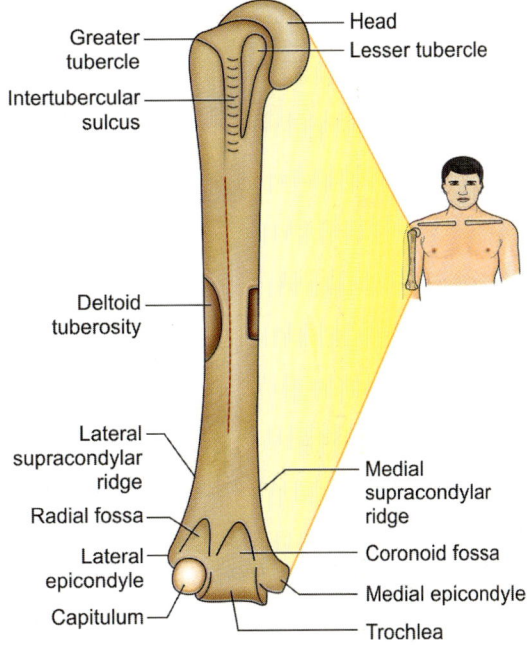

Fig. 4.4: Right humerus : Anterior aspect

2. It is between greater and lesser tubercles.
3. *Pectoralis major* is attached to its lateral lip by a trilaminar tendon.
4. *Latissimus dorsi* is attached to its floor.
5. *Teres major* is inserted on the medial lip.

> **Note:** *For remembering the attachments of muscles in relation to bicipital groove, keep in mind the axiom "LADY between two MAJORS." LADY stands for Latissimus dorsi while Majors are Pectoralis Major and Teres Major.*

6. Contents of bicipital groove:
   i. *Long head of biceps.*
   ii. *Synovial sheath of this tendon.*
   iii. *Ascending branch of anterior circumflex humeral artery.*

II. Shaft

1. It is rounded in upper half.
2. It is triangular in lower half.
3. It has 3 borders, anterior, medial and lateral.
4. It has 3 surfaces, anterolateral, anteromedial and posterior (Fig. 4.5).

A. Borders

a. Anterior border

1. It continues with lateral lip of bicipital groove.
2. *Brachialis muscle* arises from its lower half.

b. Lateral border

1. It is prominent only in the lower part where it forms the *lateral supracondylar ridge*.
2. *Radial groove* crosses its middle.
3. *Lateral intermuscular septum* is attached to the whole extent of lateral supracondylar ridge.
4. *Brachioradialis* originates from the upper 2/3rd of lateral supracondylar ridge.
5. *Extensor carpi radialis longus* arises from lower 1/3rd of lateral supracondylar ridge.

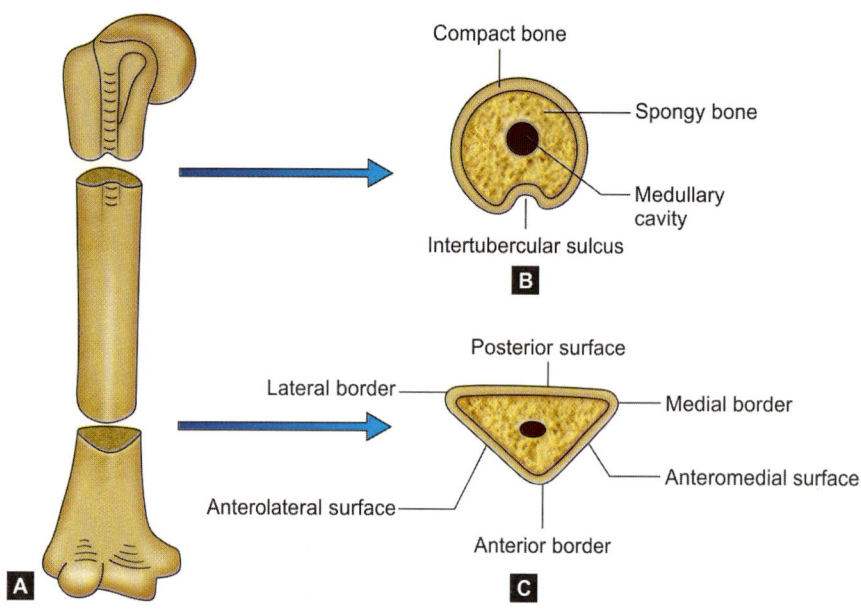

Fig. 4.5: Right humerus: (A) Anterior view; (B) Upper cross section; (C) Lower cross section

c. Medial border
1. It continues with medial lip of bicipital groove.
2. *Coracobrachialis* is inserted in its middle.
3. It is prominent below as *medial supracondylar ridge*.
4. *Medial intermuscular septum* is attached to the whole extent of medial supracondylar ridge.
5. *Pronator teres* (humeral head) arises from its lower part.

B. Surfaces
a. Anterolateral surface
1. It lies between anterior and lateral borders.
2. A 'V' shaped *deltoid tuberosity* is located in its upper half for the attachment of *deltoid*.
3. Radial groove runs downwards and forwards behind the deltoid tuberosity.
4. *Brachialis muscle* arises from the lower part of this surface.

b. Anteromedial surface
1. It is between anterior and medial borders.
2. *Nutrient foramen* is located in its middle. Nutrient canal is directed downwards.

> **Note:** *Nutrient canal is directed opposite to the growing end. To remember the direction of nutrient canal remember the rhyme "Towards the Elbow I go, from Knee I Flee". For remembering the rhyme think that you go to someone who calls you by using upper limb and you flee when someone kicks you.*

3. *Brachialis* arises from its lower half (Fig. 4.6).

c. Posterior surface
1. It is between lateral and medial borders.
2. *Lateral head of triceps* arises from an oblique ridge in its upper part.
3. *Radial groove* runs downwards and laterally in its middle 1/3rd. Contents of radial groove are:
   i. *Radial nerve*
   ii. *Profunda brachii vessels*
4. *Medial head of triceps* arises from the triangular area below the radial groove (Fig. 4.7).

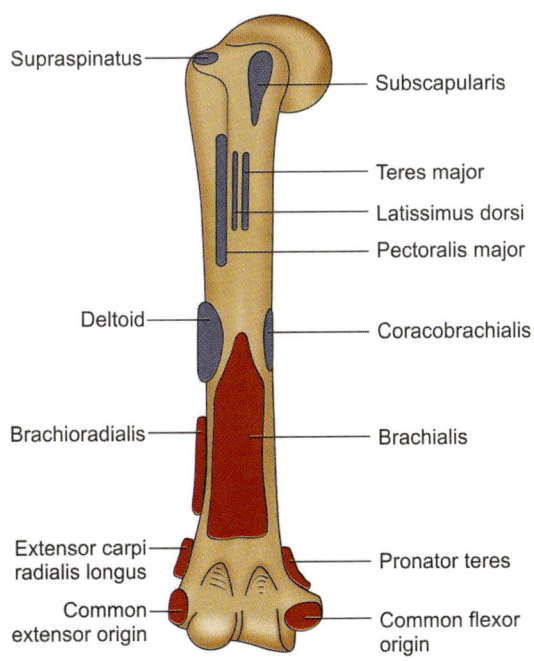

Fig. 4.6: Right humerus : Anterior aspect

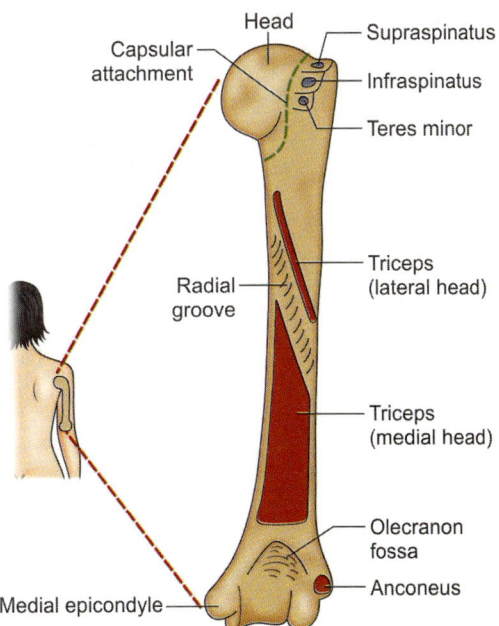

Fig. 4.7: Right humerus: Posterior aspect

III. Lower end
1. It is flattened from before backwards.
2. It is expanded from side to side.
3. It has articular and nonarticular parts.

A. Articular parts
It includes capitulum and trochlea.

a. Capitulum
1. It is rounded projection anteroinferiorly.
2. It is articular anteriorly and inferiorly.
3. It articulates with the head of radius.

b. Trochlea
1. It is shaped like a pulley, that is why it is called trochlea.
2. It is articular anteriorly, inferiorly as well as posteriorly.
3. It articulates with the trochlear notch of ulna.
4. Trochlea projects 6 mm downwards towards its medial end as compared to its lateral end. Carrying angle in the extended and supinated forearm is due to this downward projection of trochlea medially.

B. Non-articular parts
It includes epicondyles (medial and lateral) and fossae (coronoid, radial and olecranon).

a. Medial epicondyle
1. It is subcutaneous
2. It projects on the medial side of elbow.
3. *Ulnar nerve* is related to the posterior surface of medial epicondyle.
4. Its anterior surface provides an area of *common flexor origin* for *flexor carpi radialis, palmaris longus, flexor carpi ulnaris* and *flexor digitorum superficialis*.
5. *Ulnar collateral ligament* of elbow is attached to its apex.

b. Lateral epicondyle
1. It is small and less prominent than the medial epicondyle.
2. Its anterolateral part provides an impression of *common extensor origin* for *extensor carpi radialis brevis, extensor digitorum, extensor digiti minimi* and *extensor carpi ulnaris*.
3. *Anconeus* arises from its posterior surface.
4. *Radial collateral ligament* of elbow is attached to the tip of lateral epicondyle.

c. Coronoid fossa
1. It is situated above the trochlea anteriorly.
2. Coronoid process of ulna fits into it during flexion of elbow.

d. Radial fossa
1. It is situated above capitulum anteriorly.
2. Head of radius fits into it during flexion of elbow.

e. Olecranon fossa
1. It is situated posteriorly, above the trochlea.
2. Olecranon process of ulna fits into it during extension at elbow.
3. Sometimes the bony septum between coronoid and olecranon fossae is perforated. This is called *supratrochlear foramen* or the *septal aperture*.

CAPSULAR ATTACHMENTS (Fig. 4.8)
1. The capsule of shoulder joint is attached to the anatomical neck. It is deficient at the upper end of intertubercular sulcus in order to allow the passage of the tendon of long head of biceps along with its synovial sheath. Inferiorly the capsular ligament extends down the medial side of the shaft for about 2 cm.
2. The capsule of elbow joint encloses the capitulum, trochlea, coronoid fossa, radial fossa and olecranon fossa.

The Humerus

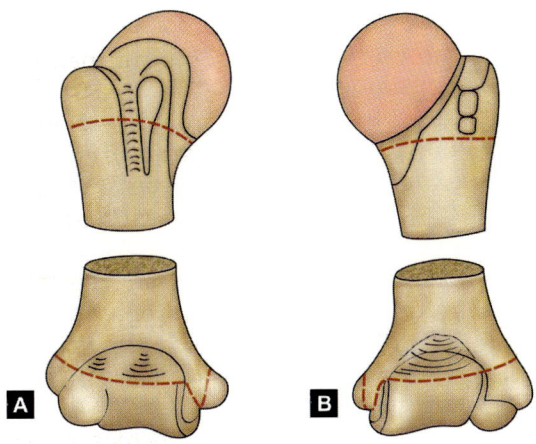

Fig. 4.8: Epiphyseal lines and capsular attachments of right humerus. (A) Anterior view; (B) Posterior view. Continuous lines, capsular attachments; Dotted lines, epiphyseal lines

ANGLES

I. Carrying angle (Fig. 4.9)

1. It is an angle observed between long axis of arm and long axis of forearm.
2. It is seen in fully extended and fully supinated forearm.
3. It is due to the downward projection of the medial part of trochlea.
4. It is about 15°.
5. It is more in female than male.

II. Angle of humeral torsion (Fig. 4.9)

1. It is the angle between the long axes of upper and lower ends of humerus.
2. In quadrupeds it is 90°, while in human being it is about 164°.
3. It is more in males than females.

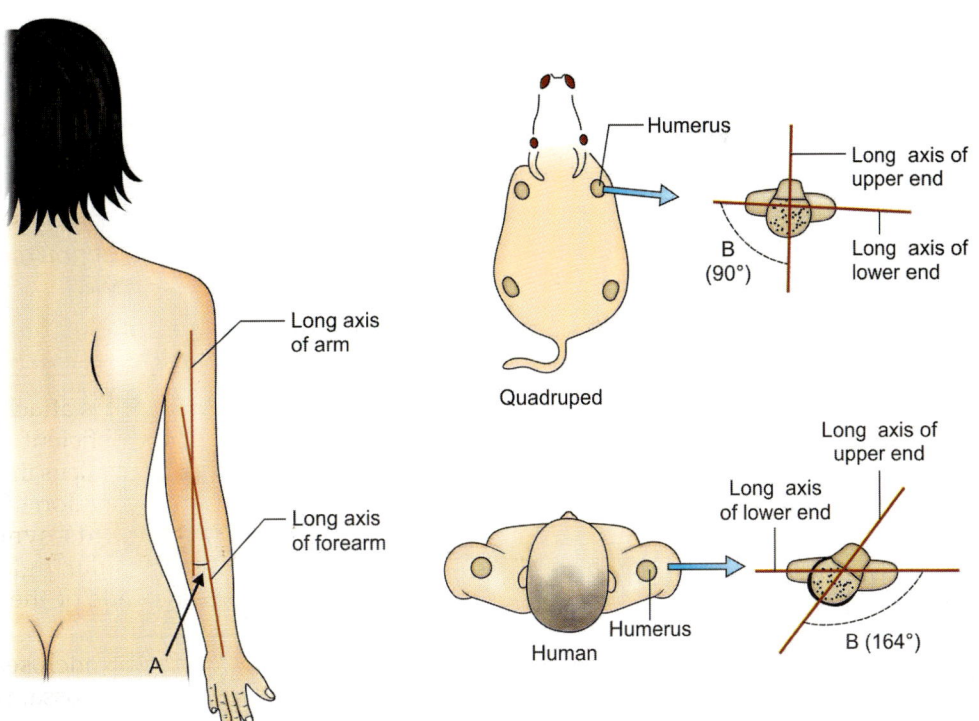

Fig. 4.9: Angles: (A) Carrying angle (posterior view of right upper limb); (B) Angle of humeral torsion (superior view of right humerus)

OSSIFICATION

A. Primary centre
One centre appears for the shaft during 8th week of intrauterine life.

B. Secondary centres
Seven secondary centres appear in all, of which three appear for the upper end and four for the lower end.

> **Note:** *For remembering the ossification, keep in mind that a part which is larger requires more time to ossify in comparison to a part which is smaller, therefore the centre for the larger parts appear early as compared to the centres for smaller parts, in other words remember, bigger the size, earlier the appearance.)*

a. Upper end
3 secondary centres,

Appearance

Head – 1st year
Greater tubercle – 3rd year
Lesser tubercle – 5th year

Fusion

All three centres at the upper end fuse together at 7 years to form conjoint epiphysis which itself fuses with the shaft by 20th year.

> **Note:** *To remember the appearance of secondary centres at the upper end of humerus, start from '1' and go on adding '2', i.e. 1^{+2} 3^{+2} 5^{+2} 7.*

b. Lower end
4 Secondary centres,

Appearance

Medial epicondyle – 5th year
Lateral epicondyle – 12th year
Capitulum and lateral
  flange of trochlea – 2nd year
Medial part of trochlea – 12th year

Fusion

Two epiphyses are formed at the lower end, one for medial epicondyle and other for the rest. The centres for lateral epicondyle, capitulum and trochlea fuse with each other during the 14th year, the epiphysis thus formed fuses with the shaft at 16th year. Medial epicondyle fuses with shaft at 18th year.

> **Note:** *'Medial epicondyle is located below lesser tubercle therefore centre appears at the same time, i.e. 5th year. There is one centre for TWO parts, i.e. capitulum and lateral part of trochlea and therefore the time of appearance is TWO years.*

For the secondary centres at lower end and their fusions, formula of '2' can be applied which is as follows:

Centre for medial part of trochlea
Centre for lateral epicondyle
  12 years
Fusion of lateral 3 centres to form big lateral epiphysis at lower end
  12 + 2 = 14 years
Fusion of lateral epiphysis with shaft
  14 + 2 = 16 years
Fusion of medial epiphysis or epicondyle with shaft
  16 + 2 = 18 years

For remembering the time of fusion of epiphysis of long bones with the shaft in cases of the limbs, following formula (Fig. 4.10) can be remembered:

Table 4.1: Time of fusion of epiphyses with shaft of long bones of limbs

Region	Time of fusion
Shoulder	20 years
Elbow	18 years
Wrist	20 years
Hip	18 years
Knee	20 years
Ankle	18 years

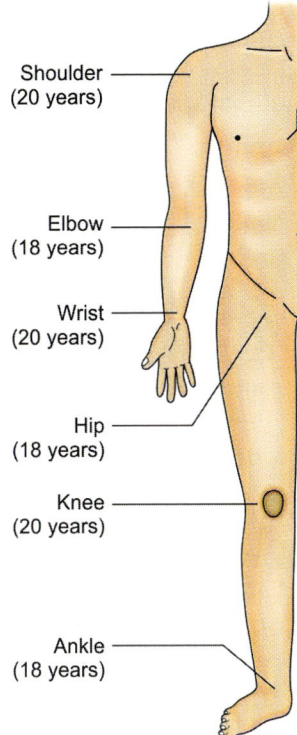

Fig. 4.10: Time of fusion of epiphyses with shaft of long bones of limbs

APPLIED ANATOMY

1. Commonest fracture of humerus is the *supracondylar fracture* and not the fracture at surgical neck. Supracondylar fracture may be of extension type (80%) or flexion type (20%). In former the distal segment is extended or tilted backwards. In latter the distal segment is flexed, i.e. tilted forwards (Fig. 4.11).

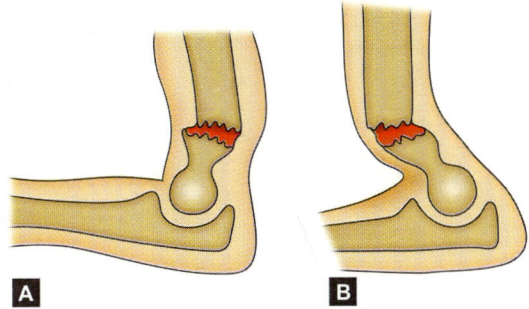

Fig. 4.11: Supracondylar fracture of humerus. (A) Flexion type; (B) Extension type

Note: *Remember the above fact clearly because this is a common mistake committed by students*

2. Shoulder joint is most common joint to undergo dislocation. This is due to loose capsule and disproportional articular surfaces i.e., shallow and smaller glenoid cavity articulating with larger head.
3. Most common type of *shoulder dislocation* is *sub-coracoid*.
4. Positive *Duga's sign* is most interesting sign in shoulder dislocation in which patient is unable to touch the shoulder of normal side with the palm of affected side.
5. Axillary nerve is related to the humerus at surgical neck and therefore may be involved in *fracture of humerus at surgical neck*.
6. Etiology of fracture of surgical neck of humerus differs with age. In children it is due to fall on outstretched hands or bony cyst. In old age it is due to osteoporosis or secondaries.
7. Radial nerve is related to the humerus in the radial groove and might be involved in *fracture of mid shaft*.
8. Medial collateral ligament of elbow is very strong so that the medial epicondyle is torn away in *posterolateral dislocation of elbow*.
9. The trochlea and capitulum lie in a plane anterior to that of shaft of humerus. This increases the range of flexion at elbow.
10. Metaphysis being the sensitive site for inflammation, its relation with capsular attachment is clinically important. The proximal (upper) epiphyseal line is entirely extracapsular except medially. The epiphyseal line for medial epicondyle is extracapsular. Capsule of elbow joint is attached partly to epiphysis and partly to shaft.
11. Ulnar nerve is related to posterior surface of medial epicondyle where it can be palpated easily. Palpation of ulnar nerve is important in cases of *leprosy*. Ulnar

nerve may be involved in humeral fracture.

12. In *supracondylar fracture of humerus*, median nerve is most likely to be damaged.
13. *Nonunion of fracture of humerus* is very common if the fracture is at the junction of upper and middle 3rd due to poor blood supply.
14. *Fracture separation of the epiphysis* at the upper end of humerus may occure in children due to the fact that the shoulder joint capsule is stronger than the epiphyseal cartilage.
15. *Supracondylar fracture of humerus* is prone to vascular (brachial artery) injuries. In *Volkmann's ischaemic contracture* of the forearm, the contracture is the late result of fibrosis of the muscles of the forearm which have undergone ischaemic necrosis. The most important sign in this condition is *Griffith's sign* in which passive stretching of the flexed fingers causes severe pain.
16. Most common site of fracture in humerus during childhood is distal humerus.
17. Most common *recurrent dislocation* is observed in shoulder.
18. If the greater tuberosity of humerus is lost, it will affect abduction and lateral rotation of arm.
19. Fracture of shaft of humerus in children requires operative reduction.
20. Most common site of *bone cyst* is upper end of humerus.
21. Fracture of shaft of humerus is more common in adults than in children.
22. The deformity in case of fracture of shaft of humerus is influenced by the muscles of upper arm as shown below (Fig. 4.12).
23. Triceps muscle acts as an internal splint in *supracondylar humeral fracture* when flexed beyond 90°(Fig. 4.13) .

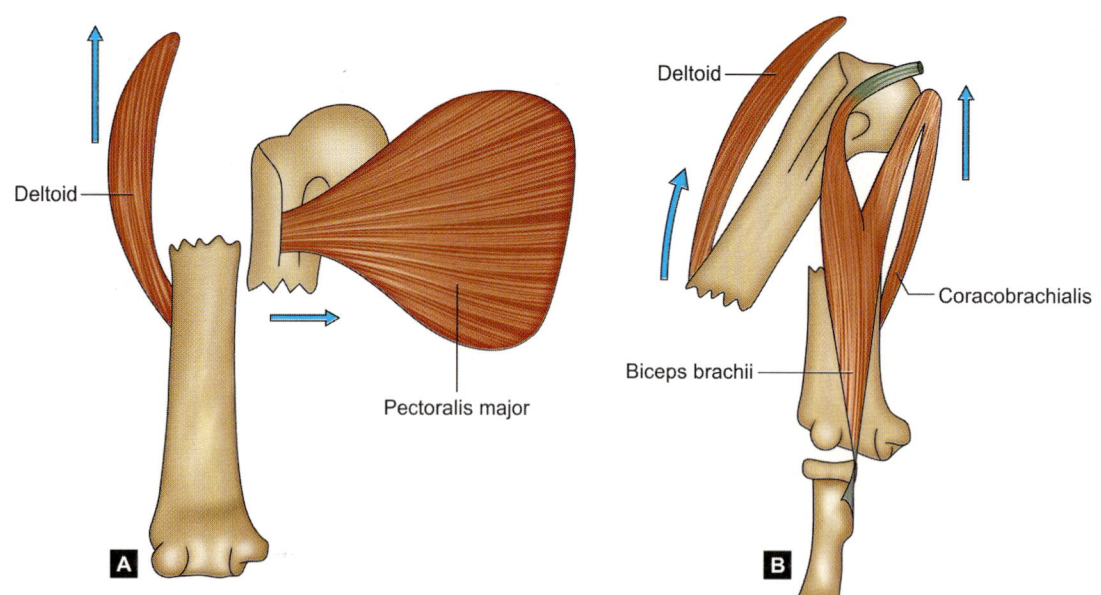

Fig. 4.12: Influence of upper arm muscles on the deformity after fracture of shaft of humerus: (A) Upper fracture; (B) Lower fracture

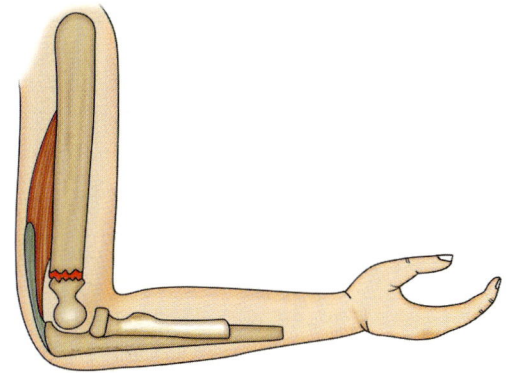

Fig. 4.13: Role of triceps as internal splint in supracondylar fracture of humerus

24. *Fracture of lateral condyle* of humerus accounts for 16.8 per cent of fractures of distal humerus. The fracture is common in children and is due to severe varus force.

25. *Intercondylar fracture in humerus of adult:* The fracture line may take the shape of a 'T' or 'Y' (Fig. 4.14)

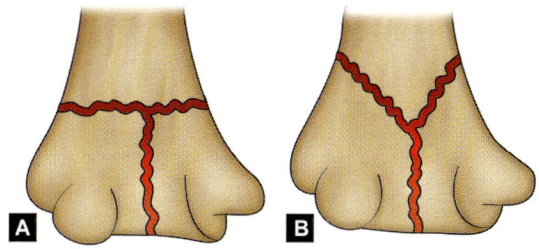

Fig. 4.14: Types of intercondylar fractures of humerus; (A) 'T' type; (B) 'Y' type

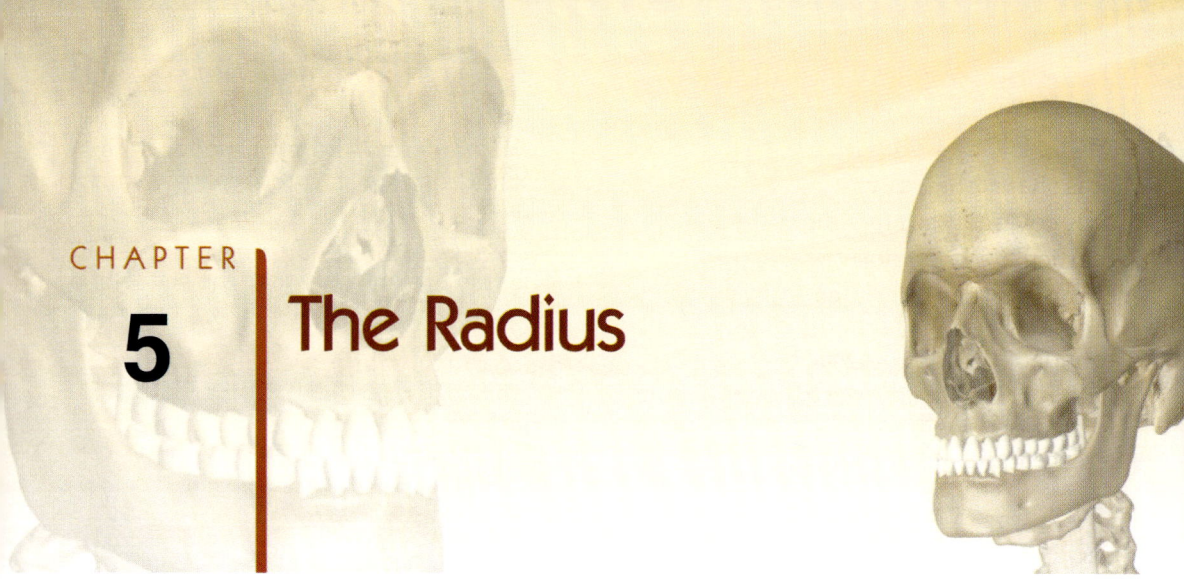

CHAPTER
5
The Radius

It is the lateral bone of forearm and is homologous with tibia of leg.

SIDE DETERMINATION (Fig. 5.1)

1. Keep the bone vertically in such a way that the narrow end is superior while the wider end is inferior.
2. Keep the lower end in such a manner that the styloid process is directed laterally and prominent tubercle (Lister's tubercle) faces dorsally.
3. Keep the sharpest border (interosseous border) of shaft medially.

ANATOMICAL POSITION

Radius is vertically placed with the head superior, radial tuberosity and interosseous border medial, styloid process lateral and Lister's tubercle posterior.

FEATURES AND ATTACHMENTS

It has two ends (upper and lower) and a shaft.

I. Upper end

It has head, neck and tuberosity.

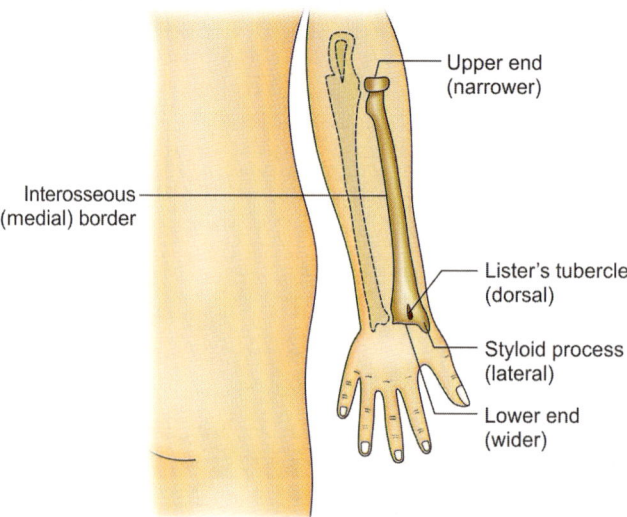

Fig. 5.1: Determination of side of radius

A. Head
1. It is shaped like disc.
2. It is covered with hyaline cartilage.
3. It articulates superiorly with capitulum.
4. Circumference of head articulates medially with ulna, rest of it is surrounded by *annular ligament* (Fig. 5.2).
5. Its superior surface participates in the formation of elbow while the circumference forms *superior radio-ulnar joint*.

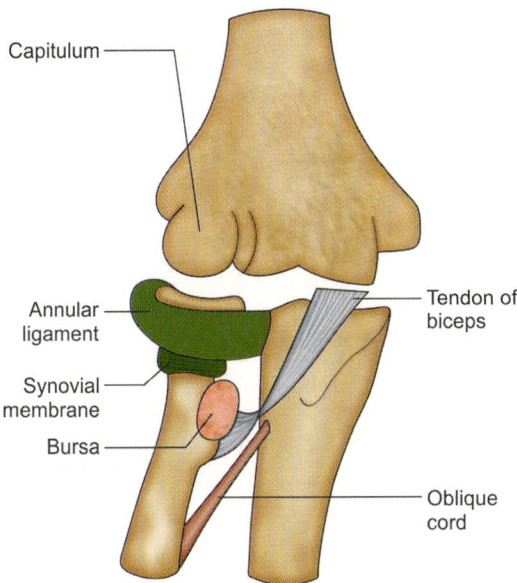

Fig. 5.2: Relations of head of radius

B. Neck
1. It is the constricted part below the head.
2. It is covered by the lower part of *annular ligament*. The *synovial membrane* separates the neck from the annular ligament.
3. *Quadrate ligament* is attached to the medial part of the neck.
4. Head and neck rotate freely within the annular ligament because they are free from capsular ligament.

C. Tuberosity
1. It is situated just below the medial part of neck.
2. *Biceps tendon* is attached to the rough, posterior part of radial tuberosity.
3. A *bursa* covers the smooth anterior part of tuberosity.

Note: *Remember that attachment of muscular tendon to bone produces roughness while the part of bone covered by bursa or cartilage is smooth.*

4. *Oblique cord* is attached just below the radial tuberosity.

II. Shaft
It has 3 borders and 3 surfaces.

A. Borders
a. Anterior border
1. It extends from anterior margin of radial tuberosity to the styloid process of radius.
2. *Anterior oblique line* is the oblique upper half of the anterior border (Fig. 5.3.)
3. *Radial head of flexor digitorum superficialis* originates from the anterior oblique line (Fig. 5.4).
4. *Extensor retinaculum* is attached to the lower crest like part of anterior border.

b. Posterior border (Fig. 5.5)
1. It is well demarcated only in its middle 3rd.
2. *Posterior oblique line* is the upper oblique part of posterior border.

c. Medial (interosseous) border
1. It is sharpest amongst all the borders.
2. It extends from radial tuberosity above to the posterior margin of ulnar notch below.
3. *Interosseous membrane* is attached to its lower 3/4th.
   1. In its lower part, it forms the posterior margin of a triangular area.
   2. *Deep fibres of pronator quadratus* are inserted on this triangular area.

Human Osteology

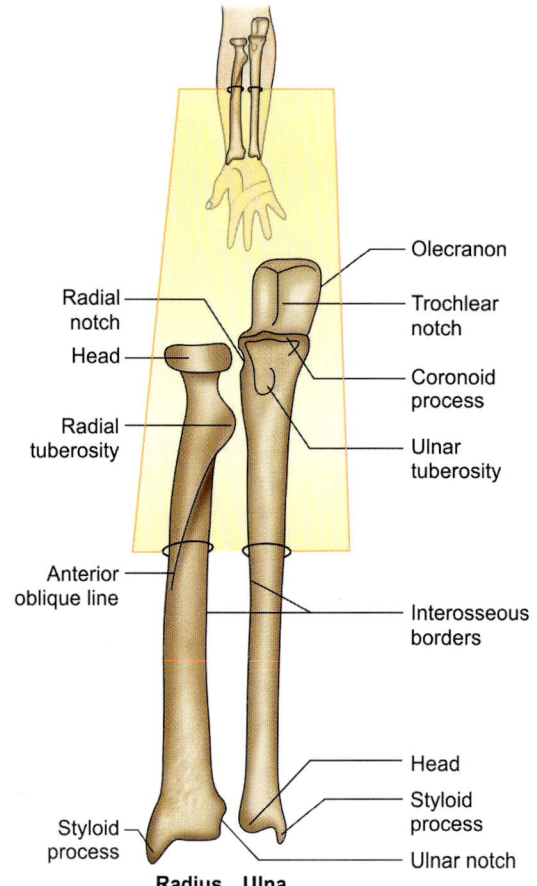

Fig. 5.3: The bones of right forearm: Anterior aspect

B. Surfaces

a. Anterior surface

1. *Flexor pollicis longus* originates from its upper 3/4th.
2. *Pronator quadratus* is inserted on its lower 1/4th.
3. *Nutrient foramen* is situated in its upper part. Nutrient foramen leads into nutrient canal which is directed upwards.

Note: *Remember the axiom "Towards Elbow I go, and from Knee I flee".*

1. *Nutrient artery* for radius is a branch from anterior interosseous artery.

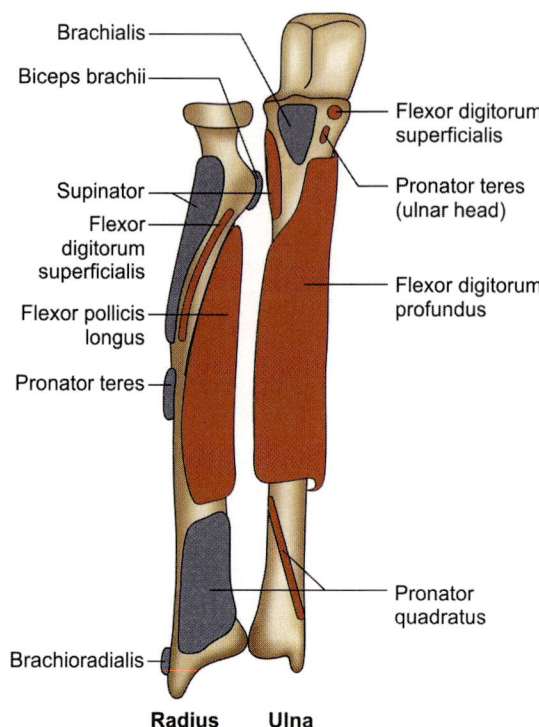

Fig. 5.4: Bones of right forearm: Anterior aspect

b. Posterior surface (Fig. 5.6)

1. *Abductor pollicis longus* arises from the middle 1/3rd of this surface.
2. *Extensor pollicis brevis* originates from posterior surface just distal to the attachment of abductor pollicis longus.
3. Extensor muscles of thumb cover the lower part of posterior surface.

c. Lateral surface

1. *Supinator* is inserted on its upper 1/3rd.
2. *Pronator teres* is inserted on its middle 1/3rd.
3. Extensor tendons cover its lower 1/3rd.

III. Lower end

1. It is the widest part of the bone.
2. It has 5 surfaces (anterior, posterior, medial, lateral and inferior):
   i. *Anterior surface* is in the form of a thick ridge and provides attachment to

The Radius

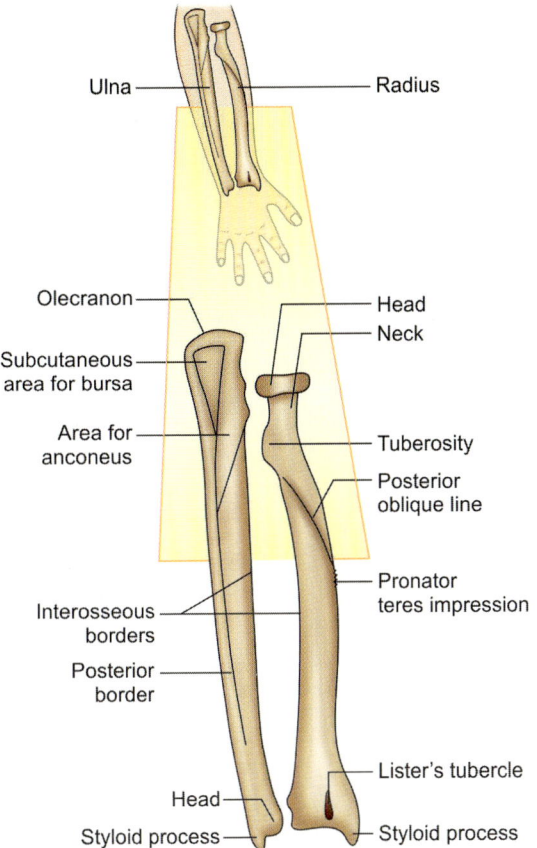

Fig. 5.5: Bones of right forearm: Posterior aspect

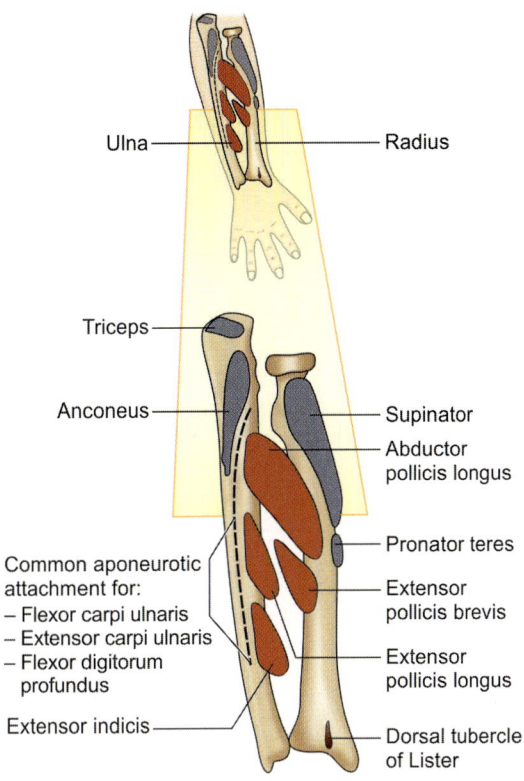

Fig. 5.6: Bones of right forearm: Posterior aspect

palmar radiocarpal ligament of wrist joint.

ii. **Posterior surface** presents four grooves for extensor tendons. *Dorsal tubercle of Lister* is a prominent tubercle on the posterior surface, lateral to the groove for extensor pollicis longus.

Note: *Remember both 'Lister' and 'Longus' start with 'L' showing that 'Extensor pollicis longus grooves Lister's tubercle.*

Groove lateral to Lister's tubercle is traversed by *extensor carpi radialis longus* and *extensor carpi radialis brevis*. The groove medial to groove for extensor pollicis longus, is meant for *extensor digitorum* and *extensor indicis* (Fig. 5.7).

iii. **Medial surface** is occupied by the *ulnar notch* for the head of ulna. Articular disc of inferior radioulnar joint is attached to the lower margin of ulnar notch.

iv. **Lateral surface** is related to tendons of *abductor pollicis longus* and *extensor pollicis brevis*. The lateral surface is prolonged downwards as the *styloid process*. Brachioradialis is inserted on this surface just proximal to the base of styloid process. *Radial collateral ligament* of wrist joint is attached to the tip of styloid process.

v. **Inferior surface** presents a lateral triangular area for scaphoid and a medial quadrangular area for lunate.

Note: *Remember MLA, i.e. Medial is Lunate Area.*

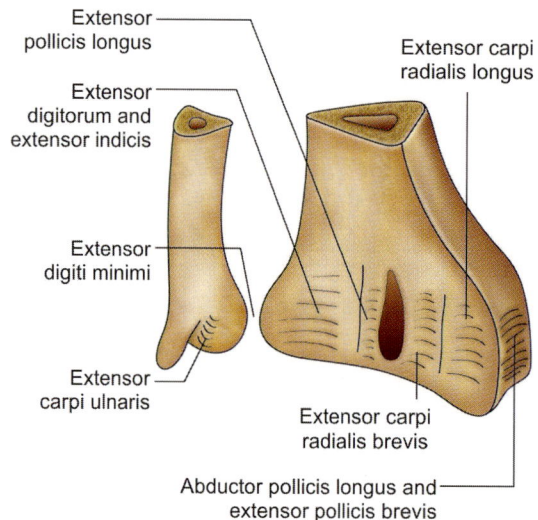

Fig. 5.7: Lower ends of right radius and ulna: Dorsal aspect

OSSIFICATION

A. Primary centre

One centre appears for the shaft during 8th week of intrauterine life.

B. Secondary centres

Two in all, one for upper end and one for lower end.

a. Upper end

Appearance - 4 years
Fusion - 18 years

b. Lower end

Appearance - 2 years
Fusion - 20 years

APPLIED ANATOMY

1. Commonly the head of radius is dislocated anteriorly.
2. The radius can be exposed in its whole length by an incision along the anterior border of the brachioradialis.
3. Fall on out stretched hand leads to *Colles' fracture*. This is the fracture of radius 2 cm above the distal end with upward and posterior displacement of distal segment, leading to characteristic *dinner fork deformity*. This is most common of all fractures after the age of 40 years (Fig. 5.8).
4. *Juvenile Colles'* is an epiphyseal fracture at lower end of radius (Fig. 5.9).
5. *Reflex sympathetic dystrophy (Sudeck's osteodystrophy)* occasionally follows the Colles' fracture. Some believe that it is merely severe disuse atrophy of bone, but others believe that there may be tem-

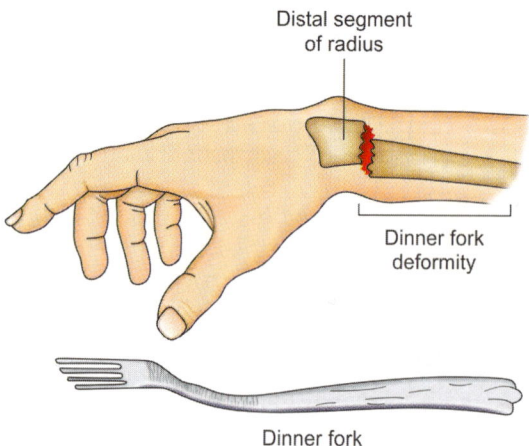

Fig. 5.8: Colles' fracture showing dinner fork deformity

The Radius 41

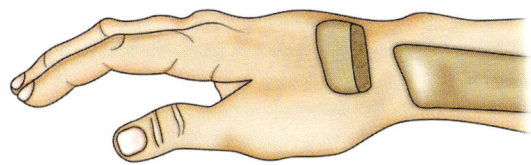

Fig. 5.9: Juvenile Colles'

porary abnormality of the sympathetic nervous supply of the limb causing increased vascularity of the region.

6. *Smith's fracture* results from the fall on dorsum of flexed hand. In this case the distal segment of radius is displaced forwards. In other words the condition is reverse of Colles' fracture.
7. Sudden pull of the hand to raise the body above the ground may displace the head of radius out of annular ligament. The condition is called *pulled elbow* and is only seen in small children <5 yrs of age.
8. Epiphyseal line of the upper end of radius is intracapsular while that at the lower end is extracapsular. This information is important clinically because metaphysis is maximally prone to infection and an intracapsular metaphysis puts the joint at risk (Fig. 5.10).

9. Fall on out stretched hand may fracture the head of radius.
10. Fracture of radial styloid process occurs typically in generator operators and used to be common in drivers in yesteryears. It is also called "Chauffeur's fracture".
11. *Barton's fracture* is a vertical fracture of distal end of radius (Fig. 5.11).

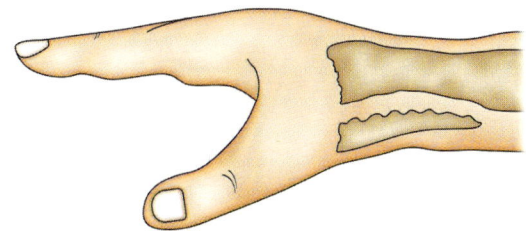

Fig. 5.11: Barton's fracture

12. Fracture of the head of radius can be of three types:
    a. *Chisel slit:* It is an oblique fracture involving head only (Fig. 5.12).
    b. *Marginal fracture*: In this, fracture involves both head and neck (Fig. 5.13).
    c. *Comminuted fracture:* In this, head breaks into multiple pieces (Fig. 5.14).

Fig. 5.10: Epiphyseal lines and capsular attachments of the bones of forearm. (A) Anterior view; (B) Posterior view. Continuous lines, capsular attachments; Dotted lines, epiphyseal lines

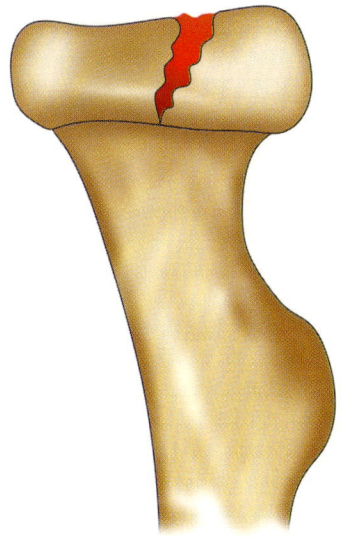

Fig. 5.12: Chisel slit

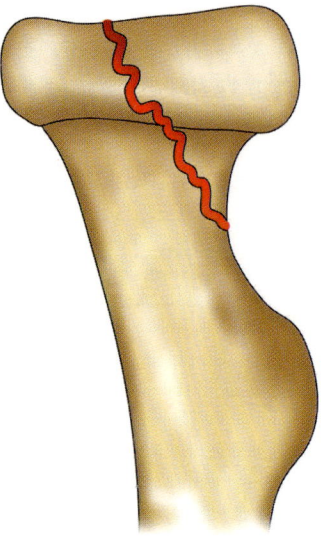

Fig. 5.13: Marginal fracture

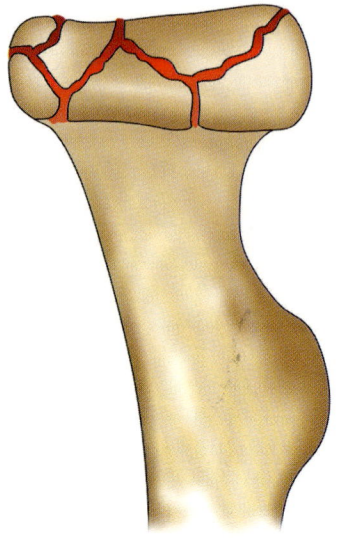

Fig. 5.14: Comminuted fracture

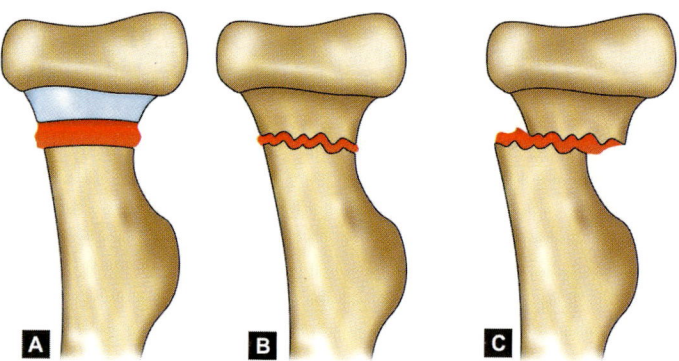

Fig. 5.15: Fracture radial neck. (A) In child; (B) In adult; (C) Displaced fracture

13. *Neck fracture of radius*: In children, line of fracture is epiphyseo-metaphyseal area. In adult line of fracture is somewhere in middle of the neck and it may be with or without displacement (Fig. 5.15).

14. *Essex Lopresti fracture:* It is a comminuted, impacted fracture of radial head and neck with associated distal radio-ulnar joint dislocation (Fig. 5.16).

15. *Hutchinson's fracture (Chauffeur's fracture):* It is a sagitally oriented intra-articular fracture of radial styloid process (Fig. 5.17).

16. *McLaughlin line:* This is long axis of the shaft of radius. It always passes through

17. *Galeazzi fracture:* It is the fracture of radius at the junction of middle and distal third with associated dislocation of distal radioulnar joint.
18. Rarely radius may be completely absent leading to club hand deformity (Fig. 5.19).

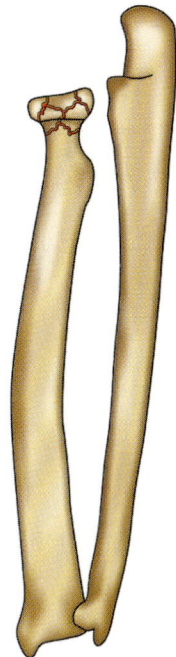

Fig. 5.16: Essex Lopresti fracture

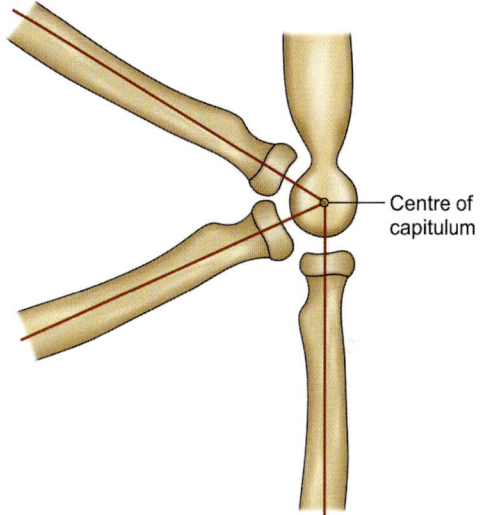

Fig. 5.18: McLaughlin line

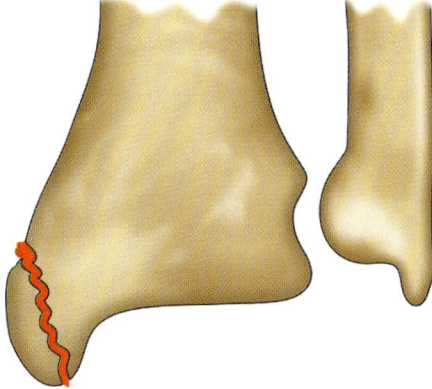

Fig. 5.17: Hutchinson's fracture

the centre of capitulum of humerus irrespective of the position of elbow. This is most useful reference point for diagnosis of dislocation of head of radius (Fig. 5.18).

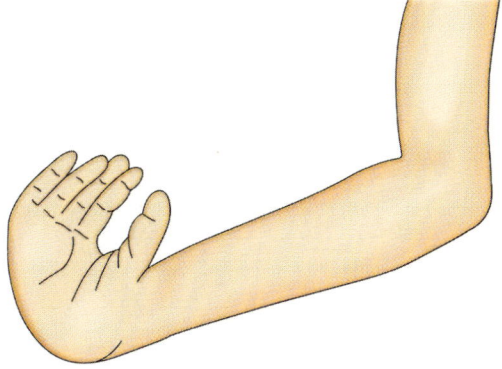

Fig. 5.19: Club hand

CHAPTER 6

The Ulna

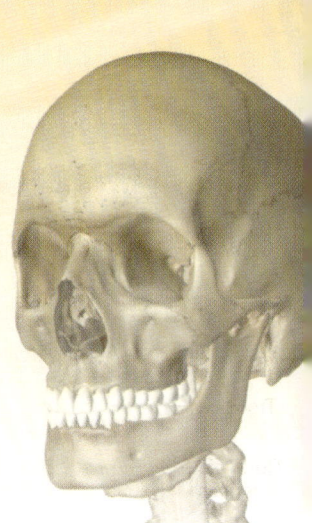

It is the medial bone of forearm and is homologous with fibula of lower limb.

SIDE DETERMINATION (Fig. 6.1)

1. Keep the bone vertically in such a way that the hook-like end is upwards.
2. The concavity of hook and the coronoid process are looking forwards.
3. Sharp crest like border of shaft is directed laterally.

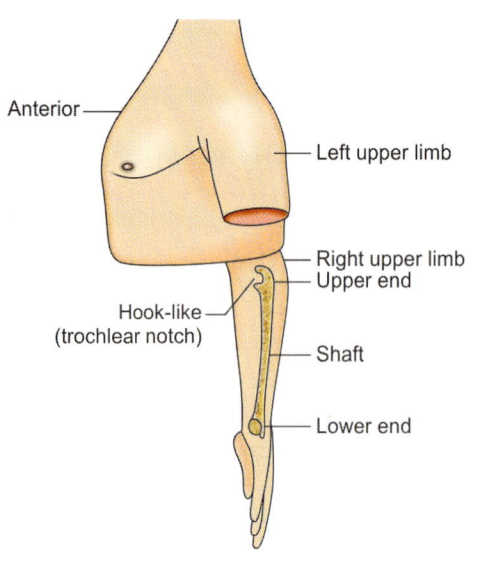

Fig. 6.1: Determination of side of ulna

ANATOMICAL POSITION

Ulna is the medial bone of forearm lying vertically in such a way that the concavity at the upper end faces forwards and interosseous border is directed towards lateral bone of forearm i.e., radius.

FEATURES AND ATTACHMENTS

It has two ends (upper and lower) and a shaft.

I. Upper end

It has two processes (olecranon and coronoid) and two notches (trochlear and radial).

A. Processes

a. Olecranon process (Figs 6.2 and 6.4)

It projects upwards from shaft. It has 5 surfaces:

  i. *Superior surface*
   1. *Triceps* is attached to its rough posterior 2/3rd.
   2. *Capsular ligament* is attached anteriorly to the margins.
   3. A *bursa* is located between tendon of triceps and capsule.
  ii. *Anterior surface*
   It forms the upper part of trochlear notch.

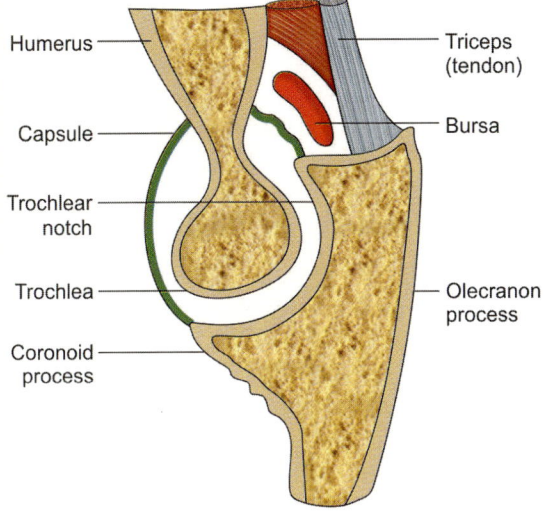

Fig. 6.2: Relations of olecranon process

iii. *Posterior surface*
  1. It forms a triangular subcutaneous area (Fig. 6.3).
  2. A *bursa* separates the posterior surface of the olecranon from the skin.
  3. Its upper part forms the *point of elbow*.

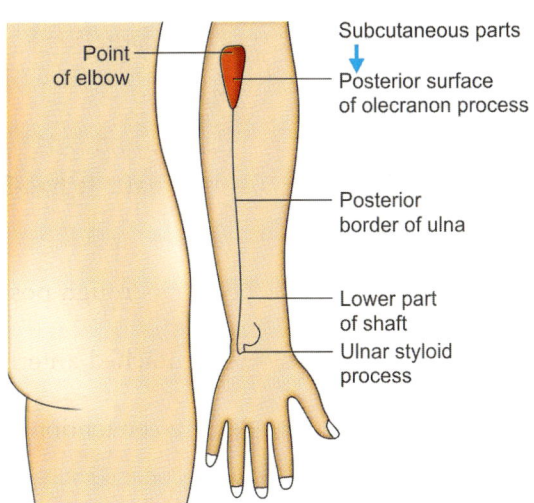

Fig. 6.3: Subcutaneous parts of right ulna

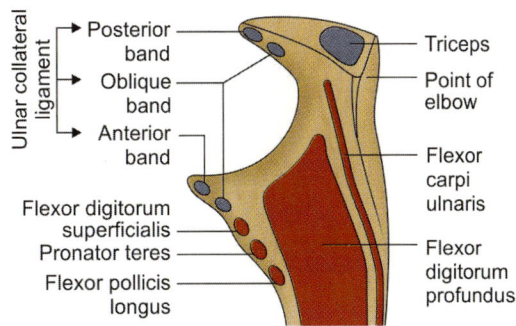

Fig. 6.4: Medial aspect of upper end of right ulna

iv. *Medial surface*
  1. *Flexor carpi ulnaris* originates from its upper part.
  2. *Flexor digitorum profundus* (upper fibres) arises from its lower part.
  3. *Ulnar collateral ligament* (posterior and oblique bands) is attached to its upper part.

v. *Lateral surface*
  Anconeus is inserted on this surface.

b. Coronoid process

It projects forwards from the shaft just below the olecranon process. It has 4 surfaces:

  i. *Superior surface*
    It forms the lower part of *trochlear notch*.

  ii. *Anterior surface*
    1. At the lower corner of this surface there is *ulnar tuberosity* (Fig. 6.5).
    2. *Brachialis* is attached to the whole of the anterior surface including ulnar tuberosity.
    3. The medial margin of the anterior surface is sharp and provides attachments to following from proximal to distal:
      – *Anterior band of ulnar collateral ligament.*
      – *Oblique band of ulnar collateral ligament.*

46 Human Osteology

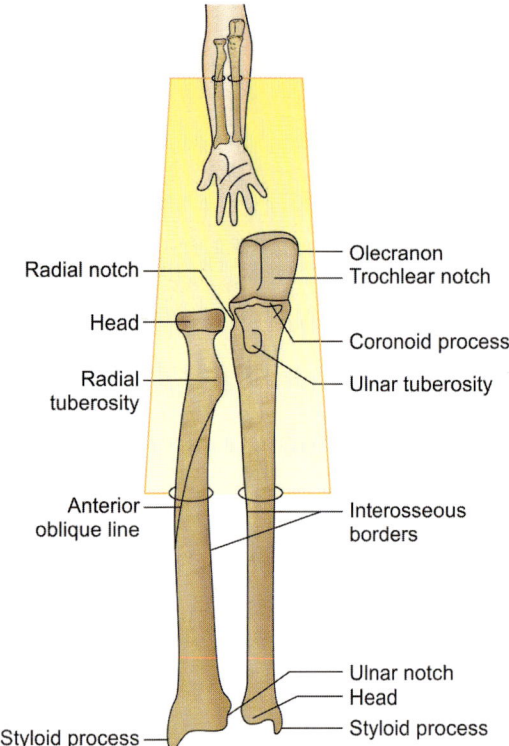

Fig. 6.5: The bones of right forearm: Anterior aspect

- Lower part of humero-ulnar head of flexor digitorum superficialis.
- Ulnar head of pronator teres.
- Very rarely the *ulnar head of flexor pollicis longus*.

iii. Medial surface

It receives attachment of *flexor digitorum profundus*.

iv. Lateral surface

1. The upper part of this surface is articular for the circumference of head of radius and therefore called *radial notch*.
2. *Annular ligament* is attached to the anterior and posterior margins of the radial notch.
3. The lower part of the lateral surface forms a depressed area called *supinator fossa*. The supinator fossa accommodates radial tuberosity.
4. Supinator fossa is limited posteriorly by *supinator crest*. Supinator crest and posterior part of fossa are meant for the origin of deep part of supinator.

B. Notches (articular surfaces)

a. Trochlear notch

1. It articulates with the trochlea of humerus.
2. The capsule of elbow joint is attached to the margins of trochlear notch except laterally where trochlear notch is continuous with the radial notch.

b. Radial notch

1. It articulates with the head of radius to form the superior radio-ulnar joint.
2. *Annular ligament* is attached to the anterior and posterior margins of the notch.

II. Shaft

It has 3 borders (lateral, anterior and posterior) and 3 surfaces (anterior, medial and posterior).

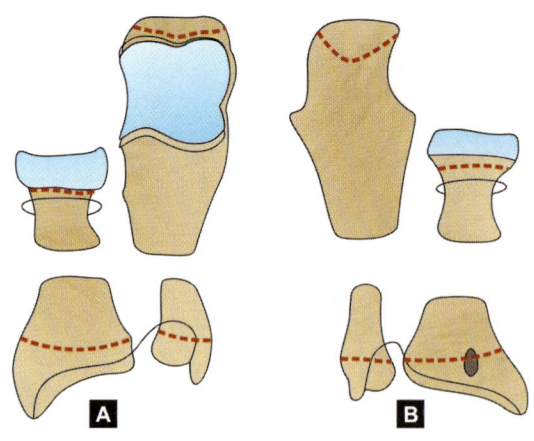

Fig. 6.6: Capsular attachments (continuous lines) and epiphyseal lines (dotted lines) of the radius and ulna. (A) Anterior view; (B) Posterior view.

A. Borders

a. Lateral border
1. This is also called *interosseous border*.
2. It is sharpest in its middle 2/4th.
3. *Interosseous membrane* is attached to it, except at its upper end (Fig. 6.7). The direction of fibres in interosseous membrane is downwards and medial.

b. Anterior border
1. It is thick and round.
2. Its upper 3/4th is covered by the originating fibres of the *flexor digitorum profundus*.

c. Posterior border (Figs 6.3 and 6.8)
1. It is subcutaneous.
2. The deep fascia of forearm is attached to it. The deep fascia acts as common aponeurosis for the attachment of following 3 muscles:
   i. *Flexor digitorum profundus* from its upper 3/4th.
   ii. *Flexor carpi ulnaris* from its upper 3/5th.
   iii. *Extensor carpi ulnaris* from its middle 1/3rd.

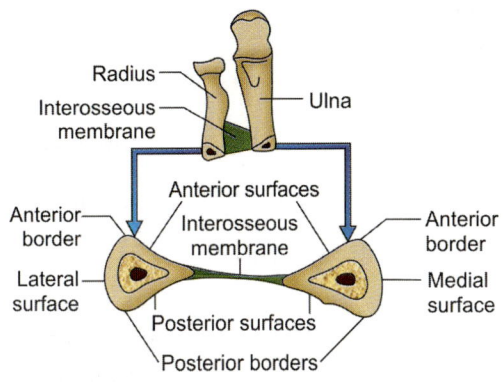

Fig. 6.7: Borders and surfaces of radius and ulna

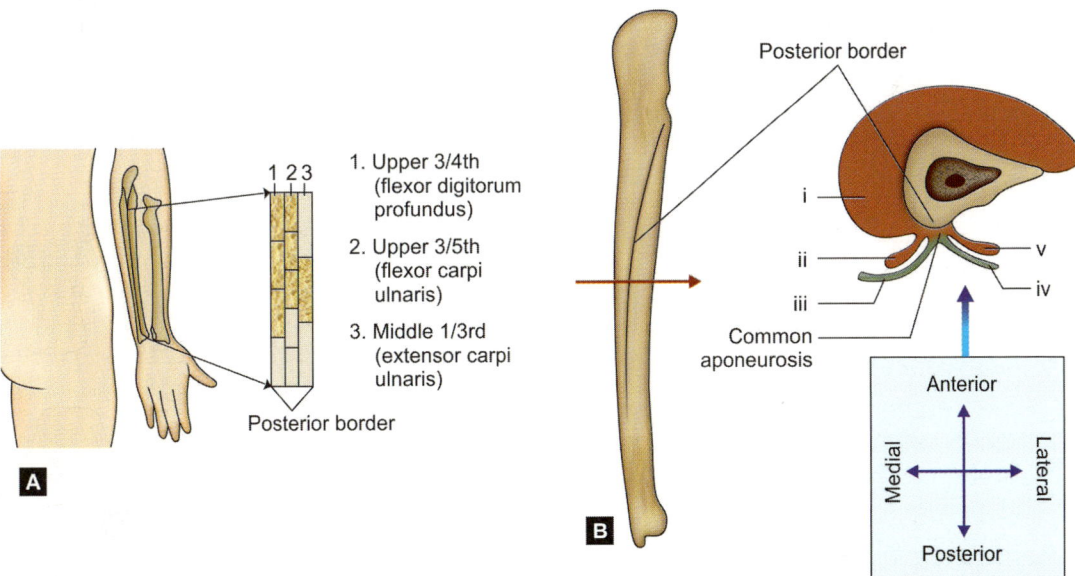

Fig. 6.8: Common aponeurotic attachment to the posterior border of right ulna. (A) Muscles attached; (B) Attachments from medial to lateral; (i) flexor digitorum profundus; (ii) flexor carpi ulnaris; (iii and iv) deep fascia; (v) extensor carpi ulnaris

B. Surfaces

a. Anterior surface (Fig. 6.9)

1. *Flexor digitorum profundus* arises from its upper 3/4th.
2. *Pronator quadratus* originates from an oblique ridge in its lower 1/4th.
3. *Nutrient foramen* is located in its upper part which leads into nutrient canal directed upwards.

Note: *Nutrient canal is directed opposite to the growing end therefore upwards in ulna because lower end is growing end.*

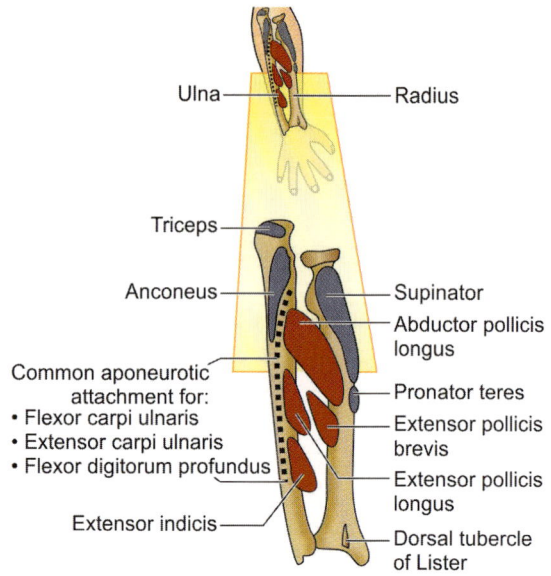

Fig. 6.10: The bones of right forearm: Posterior aspect

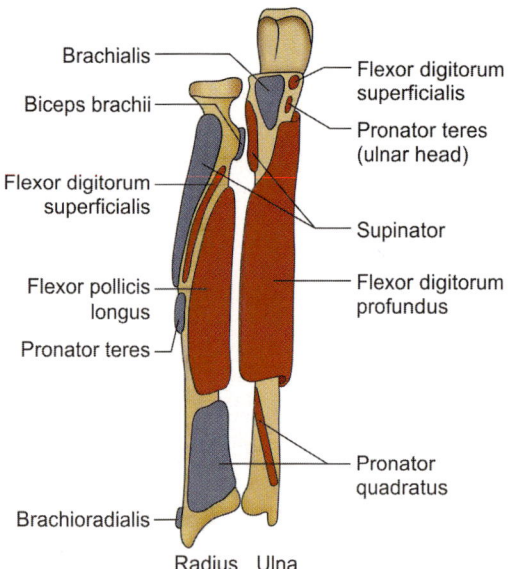

Fig. 6.9: The bones of right forearm: Anterior aspect

b. Medial surface

1. *Flexor digitorum profundus* originates from its upper ¾th.
2. Lower 1/4th of this surface is subcutaneous.

c. Posterior surface (Figs 6.10 and 6.11)

1. It lies between posterior and interosseous borders.
2. It is divided into smaller upper and larger lower part by an oblique line.
3. Area above the oblique line receives insertion of *anconeus*.
4. The posterior surface below the oblique line is divided into medial and lateral areas by a vertical line. The lateral one provides attachments to 3 muscles from proximal to distal:
   – *Abductor pollicis longus*
   – *Extensor pollicis longus*
   – *Extensor indicis*

Note: *Remember the middle 3rd of the posterior surfaces of both radius and ulna are meant for longus tendons of extensor compartment going to thumb. Extensor pollicis longus arises from middle 1/3rd of ulna only. Abductor pollicis longus originates from the upper ulna as well as middle 1/3rd of radius.*

III. Lower end

It includes the head and styloid process.

A. Head

1. It articulates with the ulnar notch of radius and forms the inferior *radio-ulnar joint*.

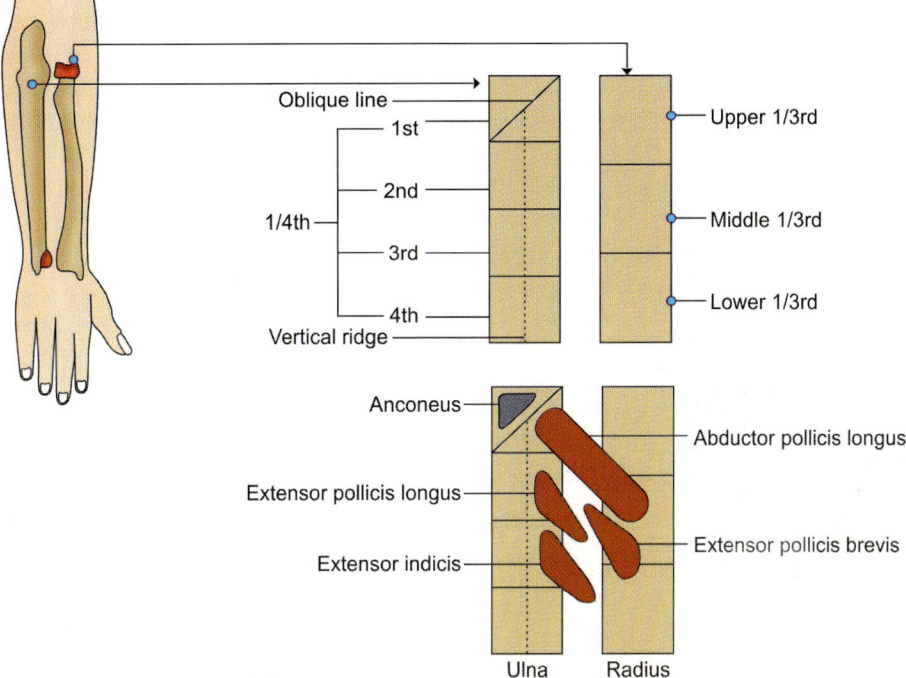

Fig. 6.11: Attachments to the posterior surfaces of radius and ulna

2. Articular disc separates the head from wrist joint.

B. Styloid process

1. It projects downwards from the postero-medial aspect of lower end of ulna.
2. *Medial (ulnar collateral) ligament of wrist joint* is attached to its apex.
3. The *apex of triangular articular disc* is attached to the depression between the head and styloid process.
4. *Tendon of extensor carpi ulnaris* grooves the area between the head and styloid process posteriorly (Fig. 6.12).

OSSIFICATION

A. Primary centre

One centre appears for the shaft during 8th week of intrauterine life.

B. Secondary centres

Two in all, one for upper end and one for lower end.

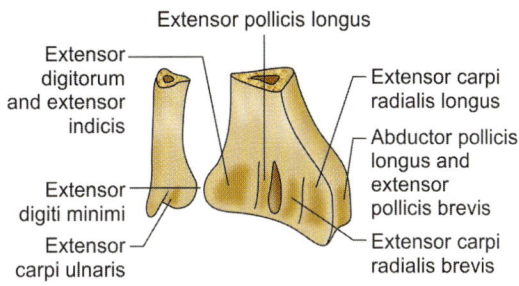

Fig. 6.12: Lower ends of the right radius and ulna: Dorsal aspect

a. Upper end

Appearance : 8 years
Fusion : 18 years

b. Lower end

Appearance : 6 years
Fusion : 20 years.

APPLIED ANATOMY

1. Ulna stabilizes the forearm. Its trochlear notch grips the lower end of humerus.

2. Ulna helps the radius to produce supination and pronation by providing a foundation for the radius to move.
3. If a person falls on the outstretched hand then *dislocation of elbow* may take place. Dislocation is more common if the elbow is slightly flexed.
4. Tip of olecranon process (point of elbow) lies in line with the two epicondyles of humerus in fully extended elbow. In a fully flexed elbow the three bony points form an equilateral triangle. In dislocation of elbow this relationship is altered. While it is maintained in the supracondylar fracture of humerus (Fig. 6.13).

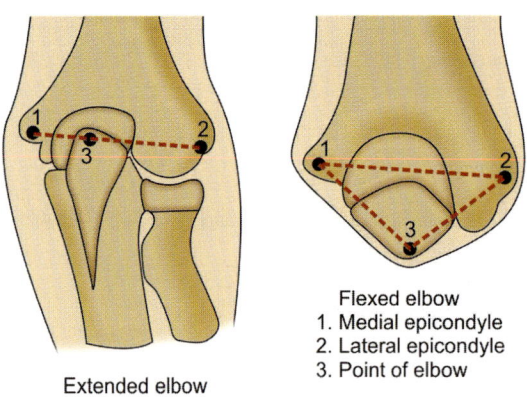

Extended elbow

Flexed elbow
1. Medial epicondyle
2. Lateral epicondyle
3. Point of elbow

Fig. 6.13: Interrelationship of epicondyles of humerus (1 and 2) and point of elbow (3)

5. *Fracture of olecranon* occurs if one falls on the point of elbow.

6. Fracture of olecranon can be classified as (Fig. 6.14);
   a. *Avulsion fracture:* In this case fracture line is close to insertion of triceps and thus displaced by its pull.
   b. *Transverse fracture*: It is located somewhere in the middle.
   c. *Comminuted fracture*: Bone is broken into multiple pieces.
7. Ulna is fractured when the arm is put up to ward off a blow with a stick. This is an example of traumatic fracture due to direct violence. It is seen in night watchman and is called *night stick fracture*.
8. Fracture of shaft of ulna may be alone or in association with the fracture of radius. Usually single bone fractures are very rare.
9. Owing to the shapes of bones, backward dislocation at elbow is often associated with *fracture of coronoid process* of ulna.
10. *In cases of acute synovitis* (inflammation of synovial membrane) of elbow joint, the bulging of the capsule is noticed around olecranon due to collection of fluid inside the joint. Bulging is due to laxity of capsule around olecranon.

The metaphyses at both ends of ulna are extracapsular (Fig. 6.6) and therefore rarely involved in cases of lesions of elbow and inferior radioulnar joints and vice versa.

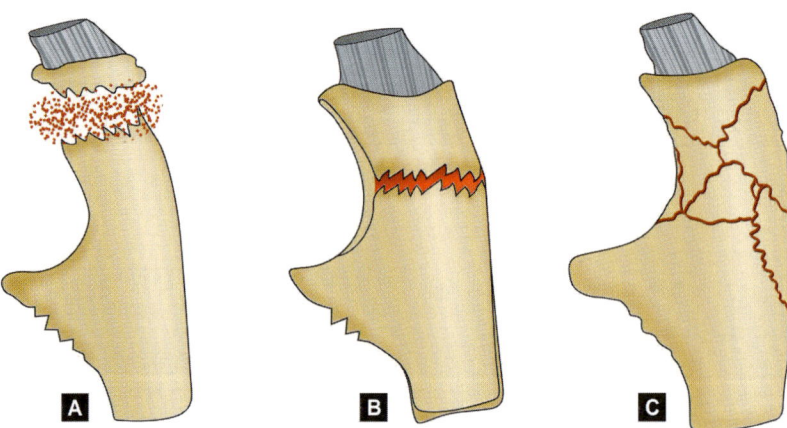

Fig. 6.14: Fractures of olecranon. (A) Avulsion fracture; (B) Transverse fracture; (C) Comminuted fracture

CHAPTER 7
The Carpal Bones

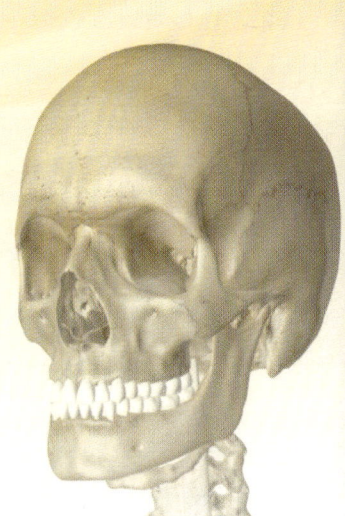

CARPUS

8 carpal bones together constitute the carpus.

NAMES (Fig. 7.1)

The carpal bones are arranged in two rows, proximal and distal. They are named from lateral to medial as follows:

In proximal row – Scaphoid
 Lunate
 Triquetral
 Pisiform
In distal row – Trapezium
 Trapezoid
 Capitate
 Hamate

Note: *To remember the names and the sequences, remember the following; "She Looks Too Pretty, Try To Catch Her".*

ARTICULATED CARPAL BONES (Fig. 7.2)

When all the carpal bones articulate with each other, the carpus in general shows following features:
1. It is semicircular in shape.
2. The circumference of semicircle meets with radius proximally to form wrist joint.

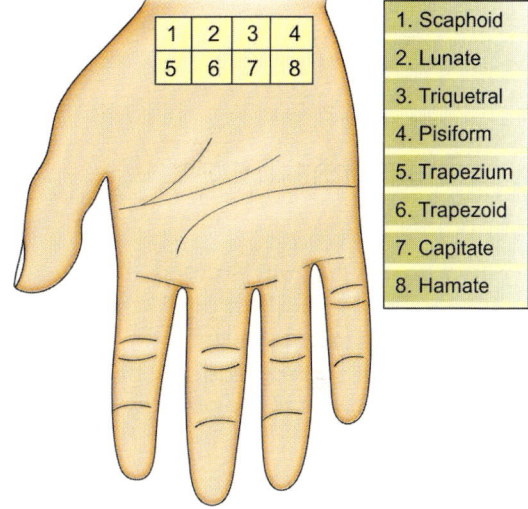

Fig. 7.1: Naming the carpal bones

3. The diameter of semicircle is distal and articulates with bases of 5 metacarpals.
4. The carpus shows overall concavity on the palmar aspect than the dorsal aspect. This concavity forms fibro-osseous tunnel (*carpal tunnel*) with flexor retinaculum.
5. The proximal row is convex proximally and concave distally.
6. The distal row is convex proximally but flat distally.

52 Human Osteology

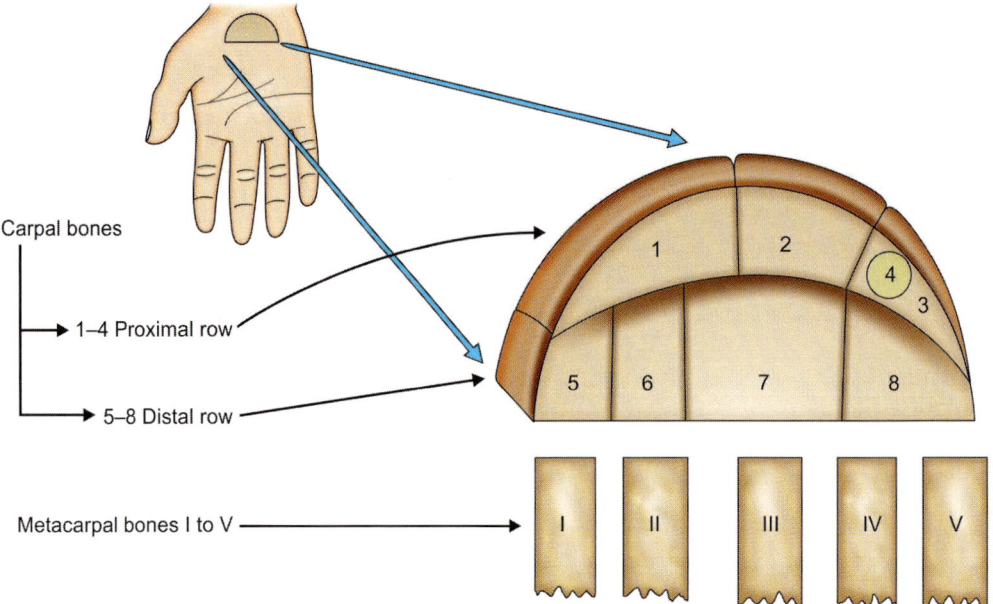

Fig. 7.2: Right carpus: Anterior view

INDIVIDUAL CARPAL BONE

I. Identification

1. *Scaphoid:* It is boat shaped, has a *constriction* (neck) and *tubercle*.
2. *Lunate:* It is half moon shaped.
3. *Triquetral:* It is pyramidal in shape. It has an *oval articular facet* for pisiform.
4. *Pisiform:* It is pea like.
5. *Trapezium:* It is quadrilateral and possesses a *groove* and *crest*.
6. *Trapezoid:* It is shaped like a baby's foot.
7. *Capitate:* It is largest among carpal bones and has a rounded *head*.
8. *Hamate:* It is wedge shaped and has a *hook* like process.

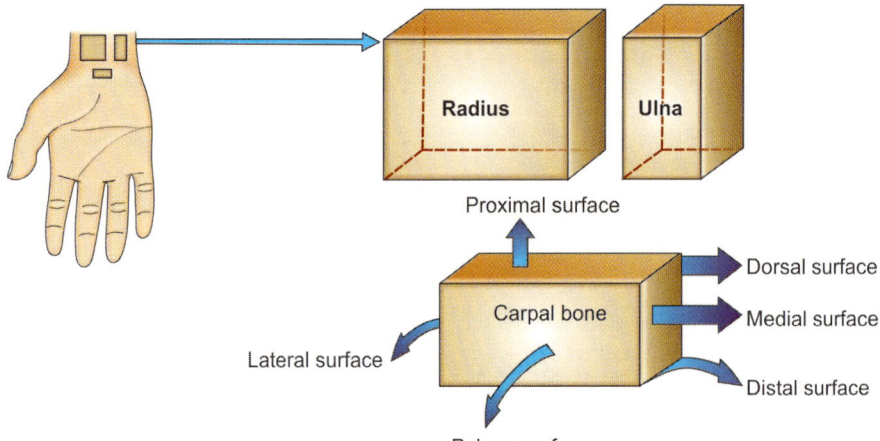

Fig. 7.3: Surfaces of a carpal bone

II. Surfaces (Fig. 7.3)

All the carpal bones in general may be considered to have following 6 surfaces:
1. – Proximal
2. – Distal
3. – Medial
4. – Lateral
5. – Palmar
6. – Dorsal

III. Four bony pillars (Figs 7.4 and 7.5)

Four corners of the carpus on the palmar aspects present four bony pillars. The bony pillars are formed by:
1. Tubercle of scaphoid (Proximal, lateral pillar)
2. Pisiform (Proximal medial pillar)
3. Crest of trapezium (Distal lateral pillar)
4. Hook of hamate (Distal medial pillar)

These pillars increase the concavity of the carpus on palmar aspect and provide attachments to *flexor retinaculum* to form *carpal tunnel*.

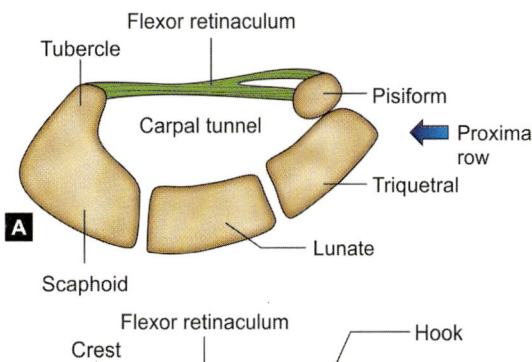

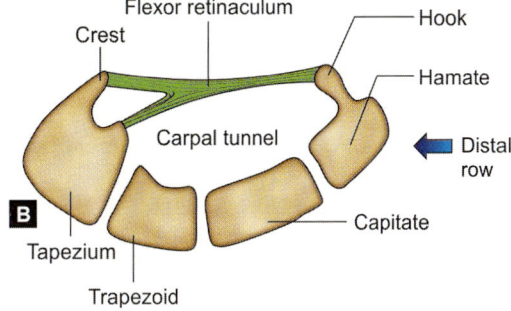

Fig. 7.5: Transverse sections through carpus. (A) Proximal row; (B) Distal row

IV. Articulations

1. *Radiocarpal articulation:* Proximal surfaces of scaphoid, lunate and triquetral form wrist joint with lower end of radius and articular disc. In normal anatomical position, scaphoid is related to radius and

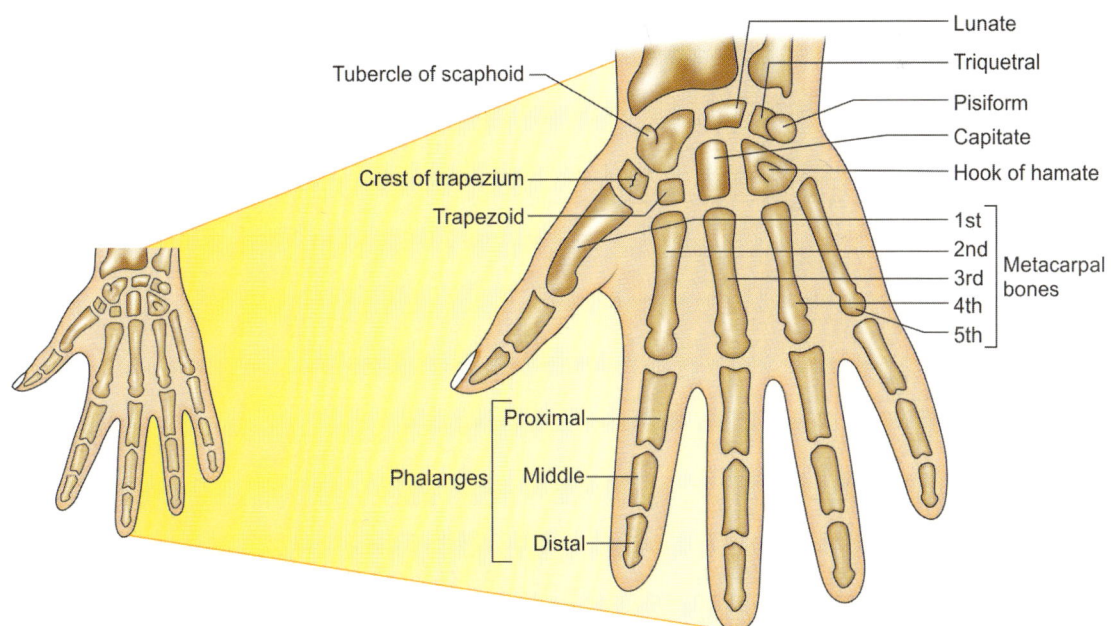

Fig. 7.4: Skeleton of right hand : Palmar aspect

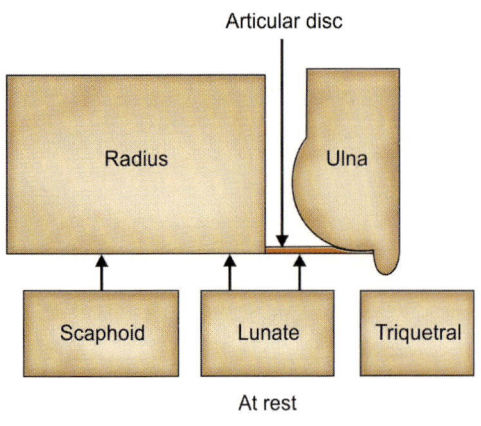 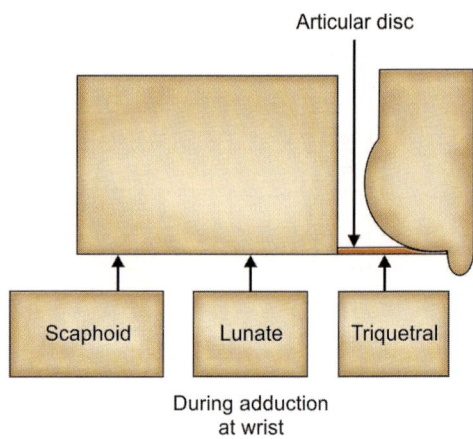

Fig. 7.6: Relations of proximal row of carpal bones to radius and articular disc

lunate to radius and articular disc. During adduction at wrist scaphoid and lunate come to lie under radius while articular disc is related to triquetral (Fig. 7.6).

2. Intercarpal articulations (Table 7.1 and Fig. 7.7)

Table 7.1: Intercarpal articulations

Carpal bones	Surfaces	Adjacent bones
Scaphoid	Medial	Lunate
	Distal	Trapezium, trapezoid, capitate
Lunate	Lateral	Scaphoid
	Medial	Triquetral
	Distal	Capitate
Triquetral	Lateral	Lunate
	Palmar	Pisiform
	Distal	Hamate
Pisiform	Dorsal	Triquetral
Trapezium	Medial	Trapezoid
	Proximal	Scaphoid
Trapezoid	Lateral	Trapezium
	Medial	Capitate
	Proximal	Scaphoid
Capitate	Lateral	Trapezoid
	Proximal	Scaphoid, lunate
	Medial	Hamate
Hamate	Lateral	Capitate
	Proximal	Triquetral

3. *Carpometacarpal articulations*: Distal surfaces of carpal bones of distal row articulate with bases of metacarpals as follows (Table 7.2):

Table 7.2: Carpometacarpal articulations

Carpal bones	Metacarpal number
Trapezium	1st
Trapezoid	2nd
Capitate	3rd
Hamate	4th and 5th

4. *Non-articular surfaces of carpal bones*: These surface provide attachments to palmar, dorsal, interosseous and collateral ligaments (Fig. 7.8).

V. Attachments to bony pillars
A. Tubercle of scaphoid
1. *Flexor retinaculum.*
2. *Abductor pollicis brevis.*

B. Pisiform
1. *Flexor retinaculum.*
2. *Extensor retinaculum.*
3. *Flexor carpi ulnaris.*
4. *Abductor digiti minimi.*
5. *Pisohamate ligament.*
6. *Pisometacarpal ligament.*

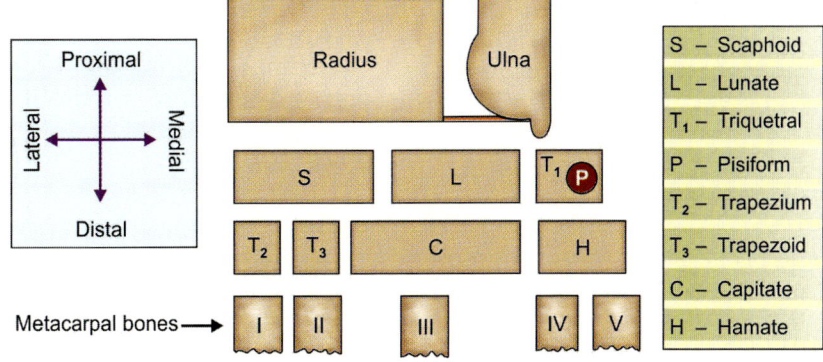

Fig. 7.7: Carpal articulations

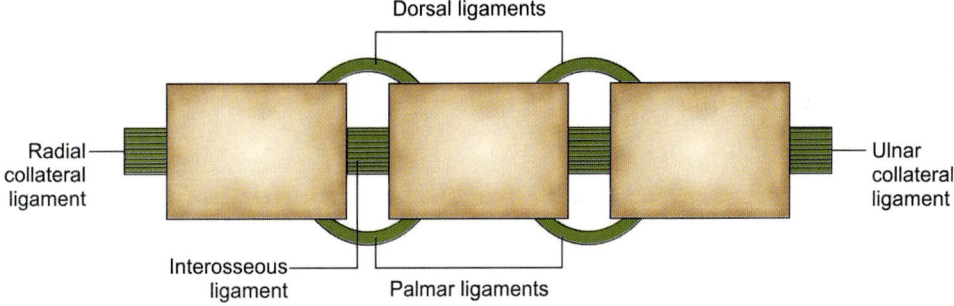

Fig. 7.8: Attachments to nonarticular surfaces of carpal bones

C. Crest of trapezium

1. Flexor retinaculum.
2. Abductor pollicis brevis.
3. Flexor pollicis brevis.
4. Opponens pollicis.

Note: *There is a groove on the palmar aspect of trapezium just medial to its crest. The layers of flexor retinaculum are attached to the margins of groove which itself lodges the tendon of flexor carpi radialis.*

D. Hook of hamate

1. Flexor retinaculum.
2. Flexor digiti minimi.
3. Opponens digiti minimi.

Note: *Deep branch of ulnar nerve grooves it on the medial side)*

OSSIFICATION

Each carpal bone ossifies by single centre. All these centres appear after birth (Table 7.3).

Note: *You can remember like this–Capitate and Hamate are FIRST to ossify therefore in FIRST YEAR. Triquetral is 3rd bone, TRI = 3, therefore during 3rd year. Lunate is 4th bone to ossify therefore in 4th year. Except Pisiform all the rest*

Table 7.3: Ossification of carpal bones

Carpal bones	Time of appearance
Capitate	3rd Month
Hamate	4th Month
Triquetral	3rd Year
Lunate	4th Year
Scaphoid and Trapezoid	5th Year
Trapezium	6th Year
Pisiform	12th Year

(i.e. Scaphoid, Trapezoid and Trapezium) ossify during 5–6 years. Pisiform is the smallest bone, therefore last to ossify. Count the number of alphabets in PISIFORM BONE. It is 12 and therefore centre appears at 12th year.

APPLIED ANATOMY

1. *Fracture of scaphoid* is the most common carpal fracture. It usually occurs due to fall on the outstretched hand.
2. If there is *fracture of scaphoid* then there will be tenderness in the anatomical snuff box (Fig. 7.9) as well as over the volar (palmar) aspect of scaphoid. The latter is more diagnostic.
3. In cases of *fracture of scaphoid, nonunion* is quite common. This is due to the fact that scaphoid has a precarious blood supply.
4. *Avascular necrosis* is most common in scaphoid after fracture due to same reason. Ischaemic necrosis is due to the fact that usually there are two nutrient arteries, one to proximal and other to distal half. Sometimes both the arteries supply distal half and therefore if there is fracture, the proximal segment undergoes necrosis (Fig. 7.10).

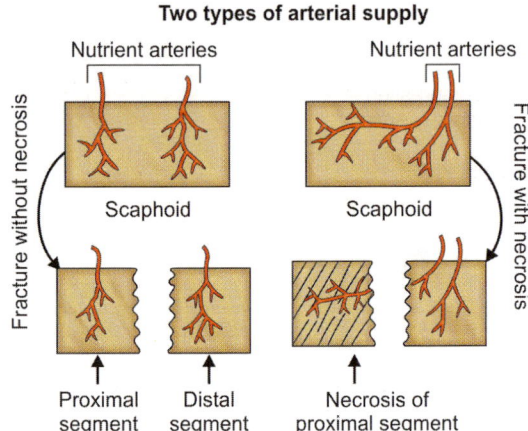

Fig. 7.10: Fracture of scaphoid

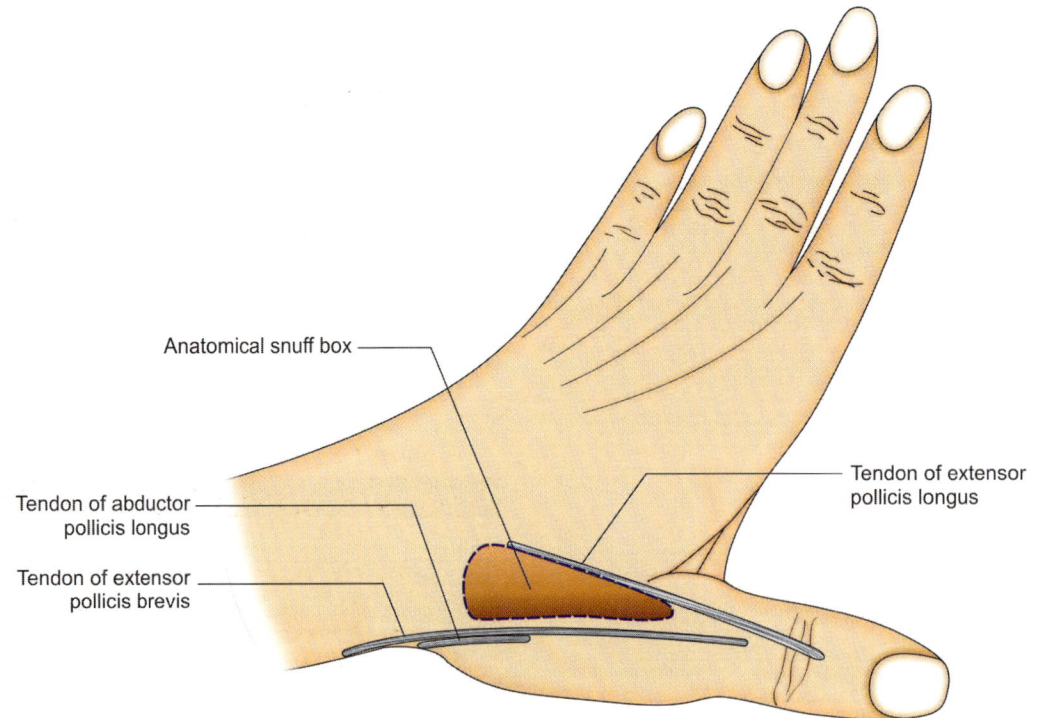

Fig. 7.9: Left anatomical snuff box

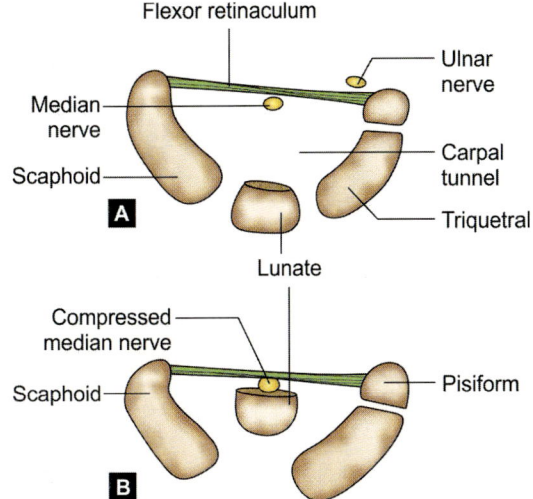

Fig. 7.11: Transverse sectional view of carpal tunnel. (A) Normal; (B) Dislocation of lunate

5. *Fracture of lunate* is uncommon but *forward dislocation* is common leading to *carpal tunnel syndrome*. In carpal tunnel syndrome there is compression over median nerve which passes through the carpal tunnel (Fig. 7.11).

6. *Fracture of triquetral* is associated with pain and tenderness at the back of wrist. A flake of bone is visible dorsally in the lateral radiograph.

7. *Osteochondritis* some times involves lunate bone. This condition is called *Kienbock's disease*. Always think of this condition when there is persisting wrist pain in young adults.

8. Best radiological view for the *fracture of scaphoid* is oblique view.

CHAPTER

8 | The Metacarpal Bones

METACARPUS

Five metacarpal bones together constitute the metacarpus.

NAMING THE METACARPAL BONES

Metacarpal bones are named by numbering them. They are numbered from lateral to medial, i.e. the metacarpal bone along thumb is called 1st metacarpal bone and the metacarpal bone along little finger is known as 5th metacarpal bone.

IDENTIFICATION OF METACARPAL BONES (Fig. 8.1)

I. **First metacarpal bone**
   1. It is smallest.
   2. Facet on the proximal surface of base is concavo-convex.

II. **Second metacarpal bone:** Its base is grooved.

III. **Third metacarpal bone**
   Its base has a styloid process.

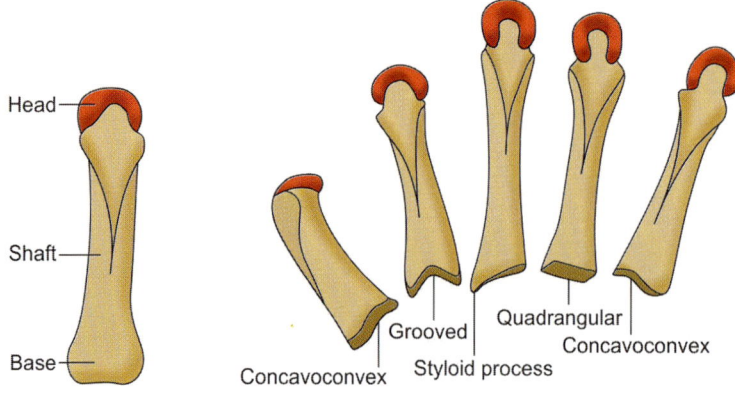

Fig. 8.1: Right metacarpal bones : Dorsal view

IV. **Fourth metacarpal bone:** The proximal surface of its base has large quadrilateral surface.

V. **Fifth metacarpal bone:** The base shows concavoconvex facet on its proximal surface and an elongated facet on one side of it.

FEATURES AND ATTACHMENTS

Metacarpal bones are miniature long bones. Each metacarpal bone has got a distal end (head), a proximal end (base) and a shaft.

I. Head

1. It is covered with *articular area* which is more extensive on palmar aspect.
2. It articulates with the base of proximal phalanx.
3. The heads of medial four metacarpal bones form knuckles of hand.
4. On the dorsal surface on each side there is a small *tubercle for collateral ligament*.

II. Shaft (body)

1. It is concave on the palmar aspect contributing to the hollow of palm.
2. It is also concave on its sides for the attachments of *interossei*.
3. The dorsal surface presents a triangular area distally.
4. *Transverse head of adductor pollicis* arises from the anterior surface of shaft of 3rd metacarpal bone.
5. *Opponens pollicis* is inserted on the shaft of 1st metacarpal bone.
6. *Opponens digiti minimi* is inserted on the shaft of 5th metacarpal bone.

III. Base

1. Its proximal surface articulates with the adjacent carpal bone as follows:
   1st metacarpal bone - with trapezium
   2nd metacarpal bone - with trapezoid
   3rd metacarpal bone - with capitate
   4th metacarpal bone - with hamate
   5th metacarpal bone - with hamate
2. Except the base of 1st metacarpal bone, adjacent sides of bases of rest of the metacarpal bones articulate with each other (Fig. 8.2).
3. *Oblique head of adductor pollicis* arises from bases of 2nd and 3rd metacarpal bones.
4. *Abductor pollicis longus* is attached to the base of 1st metacarpal bone.
5. *Flexor carpi radialis* gets attached to the bases of 2nd and 3rd metacarpal bones on their palmar aspects.

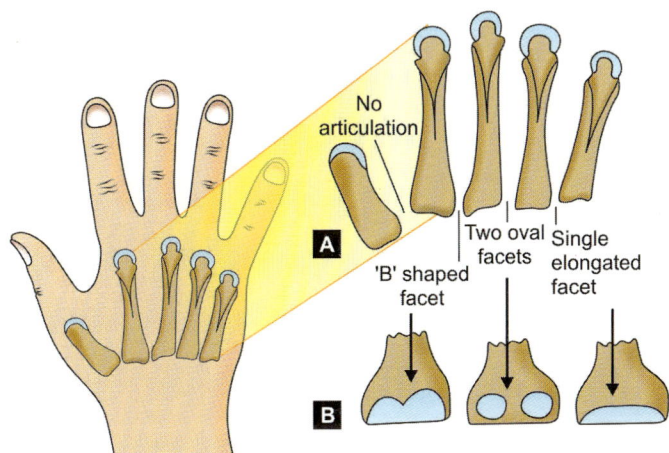

Fig. 8.2: Right metacarpal bones: (A) Dorsal aspect; (B) Adjacent bases

6. *Extensor carpi radialis longus* is attached to base of 2nd metacarpal bone on its dorsal aspect.
7. *Extensor carpi radialis brevis* is attached to the base of 3rd metacarpal bone on its dorsal aspect.
8. Both *flexor carpi ulnaris* (indirectly via pisometacarpal ligament) and *extensor carpi ulnaris* (directly) are attached to the base of 5th metacarpal bone on its palmar and dorsal aspects respectively.

PECULIARITIES OF 1ST METACARPAL BONE

1. It is placed more anteriorly than the rest of the metacarpal bones.
2. It is rotated medially through 90°. This facilitates the opposition of thumb.
3. Its base does not articulate with adjacent metacarpal bone making it free to move.

OSSIFICATION

A. Primary centre

One centre appears for shaft during 9th week of intracterine life.

B. Secondary centres

Only one secondary centre appears for each metacarpal bone. This is located in the base of the 1st metacarpal bone and heads of rest of the metacarpal bones.
Appearance : 2 years

Fusion : 1st Metacarpal bone - 16 years
Rest of the metacarpal bones - 18 years

APPLIED ANATOMY

1. *Bennett's fracture* – It is an oblique fracture involving the ulnar side of the base of 1st metacarpal bone, with intra-articular extension (Fig. 8.3).

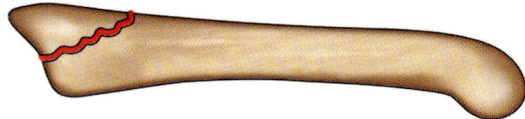

Fig. 8.3: Bennett's fracture

2. *Rolando's fracture* is an extra-articular fracture across the base of the first metacarpal bone (Fig. 8.4).

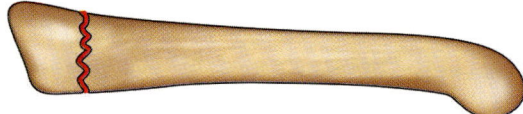

Fig. 8.4: Rolando's fracture

3. Occasionally the 1st metacarpal bone may bifurcate distally.
4. Street fighters commonly fracture the distal end of their 5th metacarpal bone. In this type of fracture the head of metacarpal bone is bent towards the palm.
5. *Boxer's fracture*: It is a tranverse fracture through metacarpal neck resulting in volar angulation of head.

CHAPTER 9

The Phalanges of the Hand

The total number of phalanges in each hand is 14. Thumb has got only two phalanges i.e., proximal and distal. Rest of the fingers have got three phalanges each, i.e. proximal, middle and distal (Fig. 9.1).

CHARACTERISTICS (Figs 9.2 and 9.3)

1. Each phalanx has:
    a. A proximal end – *base*
    b. An intervening part – *shaft*
    c. A distal end – *head*

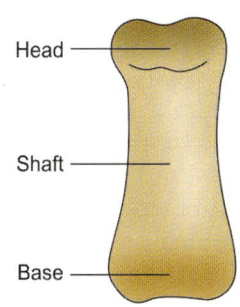

Fig. 9.2: Parts of phalanx

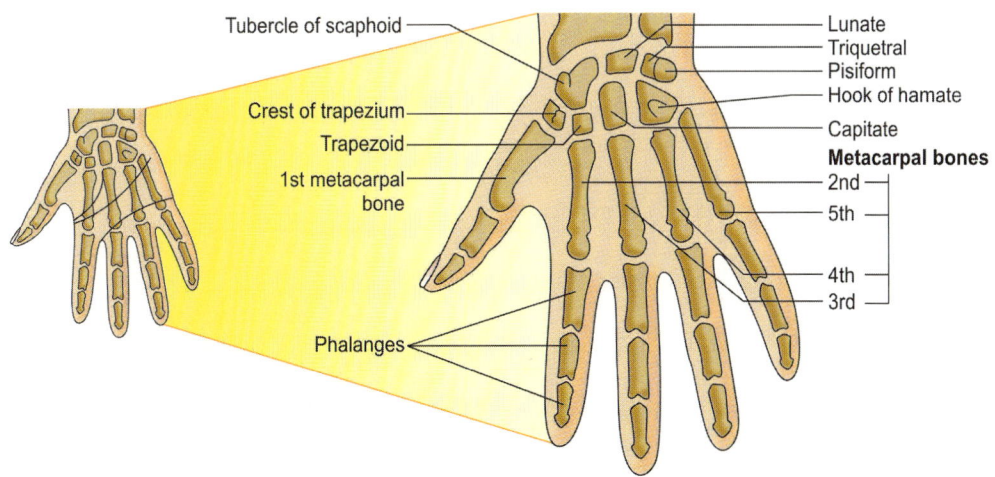

Fig. 9.1: Skeleton of right hand : Palmar aspect

62 | Human Osteology

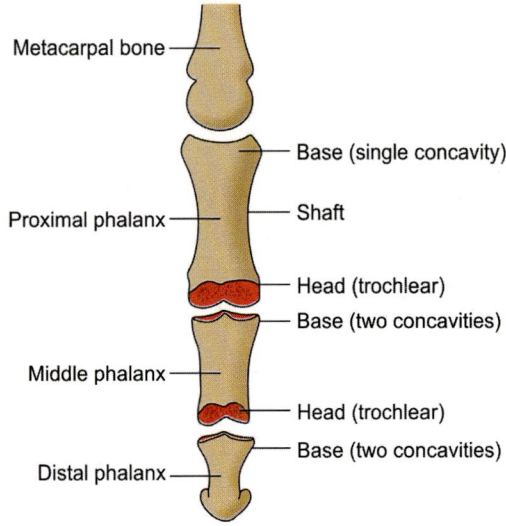

Fig. 9.3: Phalanges

2. Base of proximal phalanx has a concave surface to articulate with the head of metacarpal.
3. Heads of proximal phalanx and middle phalanx are trochlear (pulley like) in nature.
4. Bases of middle and distal phalanges are concave and divided into two parts by a ridge.
5. The distal end of distal phalanx is non-articular and rough.

OSSIFICATION

A. Primary centre

One centre appears for the shaft as follows:
- Proximal phalanx - 10th week of intrauterine life.
- Middle phalanx - 12th week of intrauterine life.
- Distal phalanx - 8th week of intrauterine life.

B. Secondary centre

Only one centre appears for the base of each phalanx

Appearance - 2 years

Fusion - 16 years

APPLIED ANATOMY

1. *Mallet finger* (also called cricket or basket ball finger) is a common condition in which distal phalanx undergoes extreme flexion due to detachment of extensor tendon on its base (Fig. 9.4). It is best treated in a *frog splint* (Fig. 9.5) which keeps the proximal interphalangeal joint in flexion and distal joint in hyperextension so as to repose the avulsed tendon on distal phalanx.
2. Proximal phalanx is surrounded by delicate and complex flexor and extensor tendons. Lumbricals and interossei are inserted into the extensor hood on its dorsum. Damage to these will cause loss of function (Fig. 9.6).
3. *Rotational deformities of the fingers* may pass unnoticed when the finger is extended. However, when flexion occurs the finger deviates to one side or the other and will interfere with the flexion of its neighbour. Normally fingers point towards the thenar eminence during flexion.

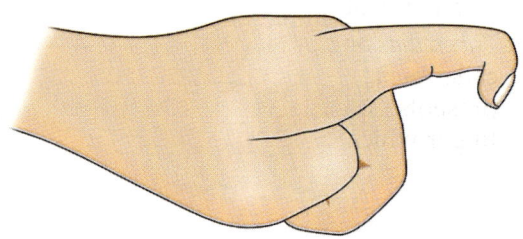

Fig. 9.4: Mallet finger

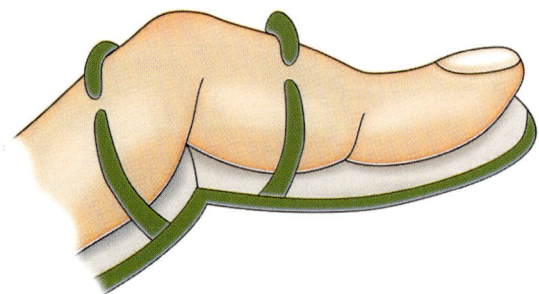

Fig. 9.5: Frog splint

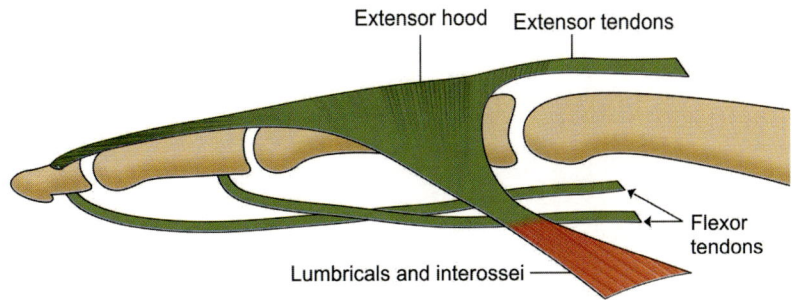

Fig. 9.6: Relations of proximal phalanx

4. An *undisplaced fracture of phalanx* may be satisfactorily treated by strapping of the injured finger to its neighbour. This is called *'buddy strapping'*.
5. *Displaced fracture* of proximal phalanx requires special attention and may require internal fixation.
6. *Fractures of terminal part of distal phalanx* should be ignored and treated as soft tissue injury.
7. *Fractures of phalanges involving interphalangeal joints* need special attention and internal fixation may be required.
8. *Tubercular involvement of proximal phalanx* is called *spina ventosa* (Fig. 9.7). The condition presents "spindle" shaped deformity of the finger which is tender and swollen.

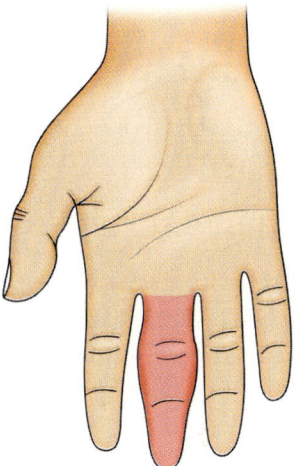

Fig. 9.7: Spina ventosa

CHAPTER
10 The Hip Bone

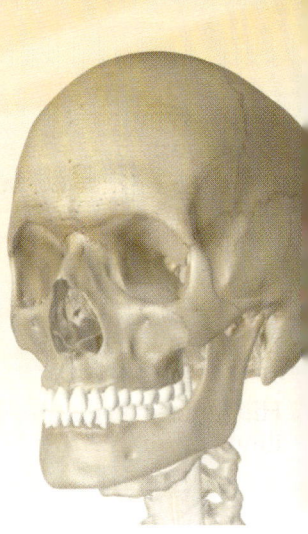

OS INNOMINATUM

Hip bone is also called os innominatum because of its irregular shape and no definite name.

SIDE DETERMINATION (Fig. 10.1)

1. The upper and lower parts of hip bone are expanded while the middle part is constricted.
2. The expanded part with a foramen (*obturator foramen*) is inferior. The other expanded part called *ilium*, is superior.
3. The constriction is marked by a deep hollow (*acetabulum*) which faces laterally.
4. The lower part of hip bone has a thin part (*pubis*) and a thick part (*ischium*). The ischium is relatively posterior while pubis is directed anteriorly.

NORMAL ANATOMICAL POSITION (Fig. 10.2)

1. Pubic tubercle and anterior superior iliac spine lie in the same coronal plane

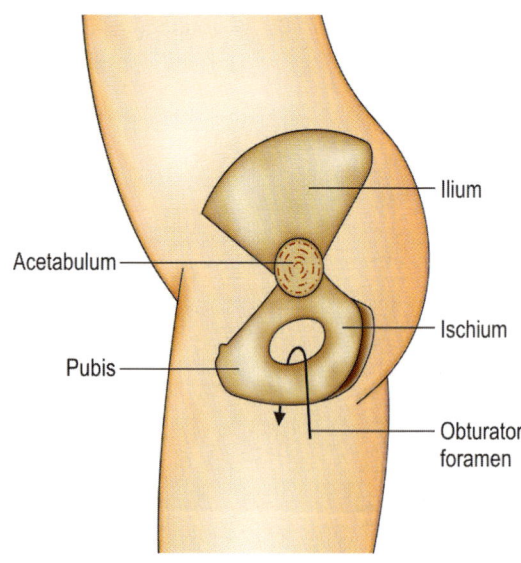

Fig. 10.1: Side determination: Left hip bone

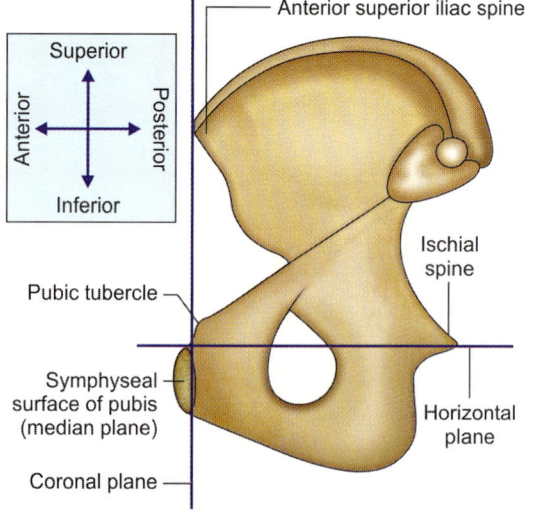

Fig. 10.2: Right hip bone: Medial view (normal anatomical position)

2. The symphyseal surface of pubis lies anteriorly in the median plane.
3. Upper border of pubic symphysis and ischial spine lie in the same horizontal plane.

FEATURES AND ATTACHMENTS
(Figs 10.3, 10.4 and 10.6, 10.7)

Hip bone is made up of three parts known as ilium, ischium and pubis.

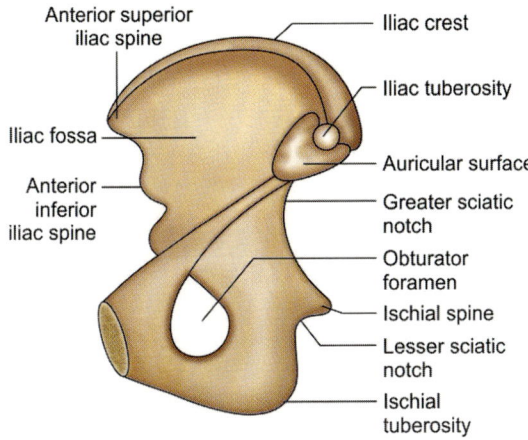

Fig. 10.3: Right hip bone: Medial aspect

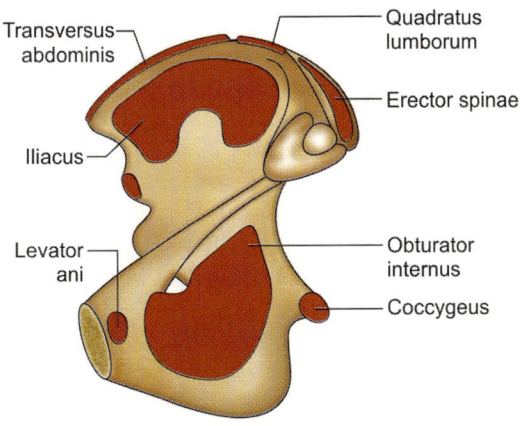

Fig. 10.4: Right hip bone: Medial aspect

I. ILIUM

It forms the upper fan shaped expanded part of the hip bone. It has 2 ends (upper and lower), 3 borders (anterior, posterior and medial) and 2 surfaces (lateral and medial).

A. Ends of ilium

a. Upper end (Fig. 10.5)
1. It is also called *iliac crest*.
2. It is convex upwards in a vertical plane.
3. In the horizontal plane, it is concave inwards anteriorly and convex inwards posteriorly.
4. *Highest point of the iliac crest* is at the level of the interval between 3rd and 4th lumbar spines.
5. *Anterior superior iliac spine* is the anterior end of iliac crest. It receives attachments of *lateral end of inguinal ligament* and *sartorius* which also arises from the upper half of notch below it.
6. *Posterior superior iliac spine* is the posterior end of iliac crest. A dimple 4cm lateral to the second sacral spine marks the posterior superior iliac spine on the body.
7. Morphologically the iliac crest is divided into a *ventral segment* or anterior 2/3rd and a *dorsal segment* or posterior 1/3rd.
8. Ventral segment is divisible into an outer lip an intermediate area and an inner lip.
   i. *Outer lip*
      – *Tubercle of iliac crest* is situated on it 5cm behind the anterior superior iliac spine.
      – *Fascia lata* is attached to its entire extent.
      – *Tensor fasciae latae* originates from it in front of the tubercle of iliac crest.
      – *External oblique muscle* is inserted to its anterior 2/3rd.
      – *Latissimus dorsi* originates from it just behind its highest point.

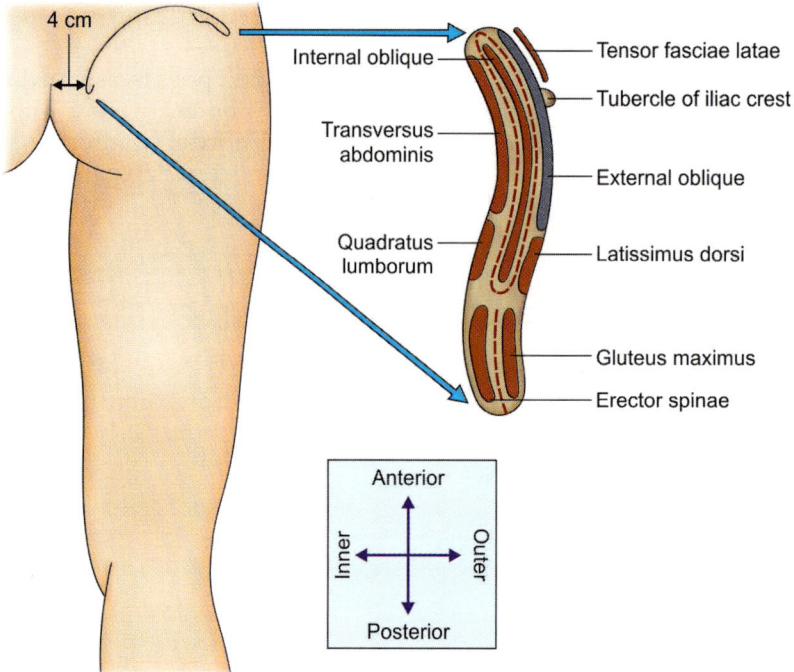

Fig. 10.5: Right iliac crest : Superior view

ii. *Intermediate area*
 − *Internal oblique muscle* arises from its whole extent.
iii. *Inner lip*
 − Its anterior 2/3rd provides attachments to *transversus abdominis, fascia transversalis* and *fascia iliaca*.
 − Its posterior 1/3rd provides attachments to *quadratus lumborum* and *thoracolumbar fascia*.
9. Dorsal segment is divisible into medial (inner) and lateral (outer) slopes.
 i. *Lateral slope:* Gluteus maximus originates from the lateral slope.
 ii. *Medial slope:* Erector spinae muscle originates from its medial slope.
 iii. *Interosseous and dorsal sacroiliac ligaments* are attached to the medial margin of the dorsal segment deep to erector spinae.

b. Lower end
Lower end of ilium reaches acetabulum and forms its upper 2/5th.

B. Borders of ilium

a. Anterior border
1. It extends from anterior superior iliac spine to acetabulum.
2. Its upper half is concave forming a notch. Sartorius originates from upper half of this notch.
3. Its lower half is convex and is called *anterior inferior iliac spine. Straight head of rectus femoris* originates from the upper half of this spine. *Iliofemoral ligament* is attached to the lower half of anterior inferior iliac spine.

b. Posterior border
1. It extends from the posterior superior iliac spine to the upper end of the posterior border of ischium.

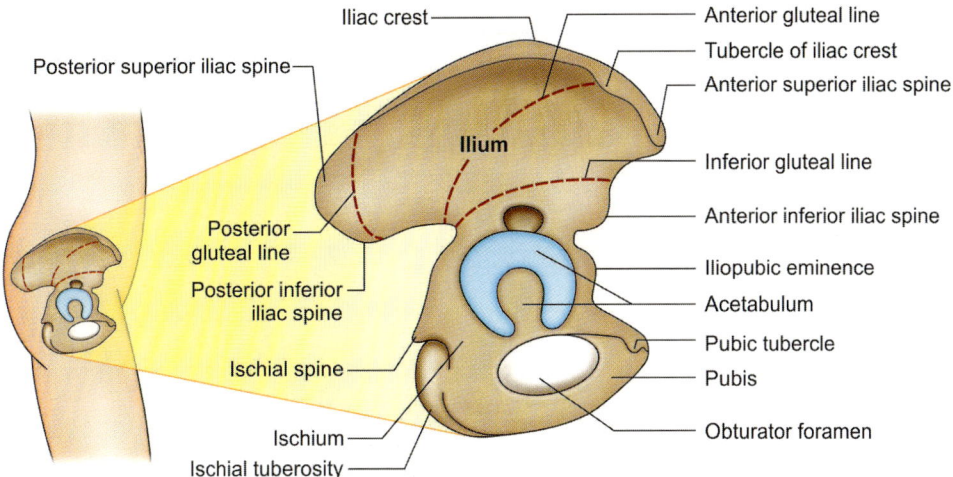

Fig. 10.6: Right hip bone : Lateral aspect

2. Its lower part contributes to the apex, upper margin and upper half of the lower margin of *greater sciatic notch*.
3. Some fibres of *piriformis* originate from upper margin of greater sciatic notch.
4. The junction of greater sciatic notch and upper part of posterior border is marked by *posterior inferior iliac spine*.
5. Posterior border between the two posterior iliac spines receives attachment of *sacrotuberous ligament*.

c. Medial border

1. It extends from the iliac crest to the iliopubic eminence on the inner surface of ilium.
2. This border intervenes between iliac fossa and sacropelvic surface of ilium.
3. Lower part of medial border forms *arcuate line (iliac part of linea terminalis)*.

C. Surfaces of ilium

a. Gluteal surface

1. It is outer surface of ilium.
2. It is convex in front and concave behind.
3. It is divided into 4 areas by 3 gluteal lines from anterior to posterior:

    i. Inferior gluteal line
    ii. Anterior gluteal line
    iii. Posterior gluteal line

Note: *It is important to note that the posterior most line is posterior gluteal line, the middle line is the anterior gluteal line and the anterior most line is inferior gluteal line.*

4. *Gluteus maximus muscle* arises from the area behind the posterior gluteal line.
5. *Gluteus medius muscle* arises from the area between anterior and posterior gluteal lines.
6. *Gluteus minimus muscle* arises from the area between anterior and inferior gluteal lines.
7. *Reflected head of rectus femoris* arises from a groove just above the acetabulum.
8. *Capsule of hip joint* is attached to the acetabular margins.

b. Medial surface

It is divided into iliac fossa and sacropelvic surface by the medial border.

   i. *Iliac fossa*
   1. It is situated on the inner aspect of ilium, in front of medial border.

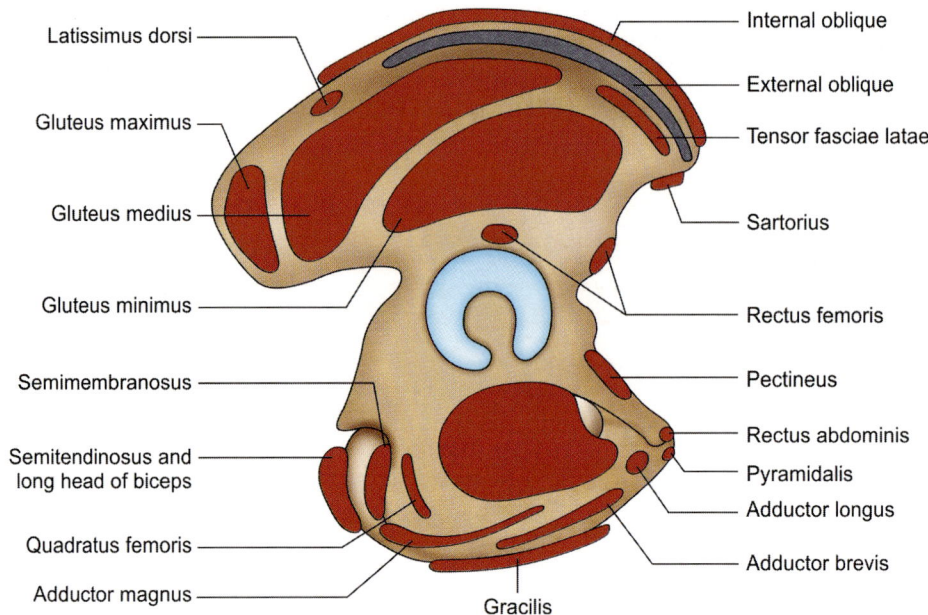

Fig. 10.7: Right hip bone: Lateral aspect

2. It is concave in shape.
3. *Iliacus* arises from its upper 2/3rd

ii. Sacropelvic surface

It is situated behind the medial border, on the inner side of ilium. It has following 3 parts.

1. Iliac tuberosity
   - It is a rough area just below the dorsal segment of iliac crest.
   - *Interosseous sacroiliac ligament* is attached to the greater part of iliac tuberosity.
   - *Dorsal sacroiliac ligament* and *iliolumbar ligament* are also attached to iliac tuberosity.
2. Auricular surface
   - It is situated anteroinferior to iliac tuberosity. It is articular.
   - *Sacroiliac joint* is formed by the articulation of sacrum with the auricular surface.
3. Pelvic surface
   - It is situated anteroinferior to auricular surface.
   - Major part of this surface provides attachment to *obturator internus*.
   - Few fibres of *piriformis* also arise from it.
   - *Preauricular sulcus* is seen on this surface along the upper border of greater sciatic notch. It is deeper in females than males.

II. PUBIS

It is anteroinferior part of hip bone. It forms anterior 1/5th of acetabulum as well as anterior boundary of obturator foramen. Pubis has a body, a superior ramus and an inferior ramus.

A. Body of pubis

It is comprised of pubic crest, pubic tubercle and 3 surfaces (anterior, posterior and medial).

a. Pubic crest

1. It is superior border of body of pubis.
2. *Anterior wall of rectus sheath* and *conjoint tendon* get attached to its anterior margin.

3. *Lateral head of rectus abdominis* and *pyramidalis* arise from its lateral part.
4. *Medial head of rectus abdominis* is related to medial part of pubic crest.

b. Pubic tubercle
1. It is the lateral end of pubic crest.
2. It is an important land-mark in pubic region.
3. It gives attachment to the medial end of *inguinal ligament*.
4. *Spermatic cord* crosses it in males.

c. Surfaces
i. *Anterior surface*
   1. *Adductor longus* originates from the angle between pubic crest and pubic symphysis.
   2. *Gracilis* originates from its lower part and also extends over inferior ramus.
   3. *Adductor brevis* is attached to it lateral to gracilis.
   4. *Obturator externus* is attached to this surface adjacent to obturator foramen.
   5. Adjacent to pubic symphysis, it gives attachment to *ventral pubic ligament*.

ii. *Posterior surface*
   1. This is also called *pelvic surface*.
   2. It is directed upwards and backwards.
   3. It is related to *urinary bladder*.
   4. *Levator ani* and *obturator internus* originate from this surface.

iii. *Symphyseal surface*
   1. This is also called *medial surface*.
   2. Two symphyseal surfaces articulate to form secondary cartilaginous joint called *pubic symphysis*.

B. Superior ramus of pubis

It extends from body of pubis to acetabulum. It is located just above the obturator foramen. It has 3 borders (pectineal line, obturator crest and inferior border) and 3 surfaces (pectineal, pelvic and obturator).

a. Borders
i. *Pectineal line*
   1. This is also called *pecten pubis*.
   2. It extends from pubic tubercle to posterior part of iliopubic eminence.
   3. It receives attachment of *conjoint tendon* near its medial end.
   4. *Lacunar ligament* is attached to its medial end just in front of conjoint tendon.
   5. *Pectineal ligament* is attached to its whole length lateral to lacunar ligament.
   6. *Fascia covering pectineus* is attached to its whole extent.
   7. *Psoas minor muscle,* when present, is attached to pectineal line.

ii. *Obturator crest*
   1. This is also called *anterior border*.
   2. It extends from pubic tubercle to the acetabular notch.

iii. *Inferior border*
   It forms the upper border of *obturator foramen*.

b. Surfaces
i. *Pectineal surface*
   1. It is situated between obturator crest and pectineal line.
   2. It is triangular in shape.
   3. It extends from pubic tubercle to iliopubic eminence.
   4. *Pectineus* arises from the upper part of this surface.

ii. *Pelvic surface*
   1. It is between pectineal line and inferior border of superior ramus.
   2. It is continuous medially with the pelvic surface of the body of pubis.
   3. *Ductus deferens* in males and *round ligament of uterus* in females are related to this surface.

iii. *Obturator surface*
   1. It is situated between obturator crest and inferior border.
   2. *Obturator nerve and vessels* traverse the *obturator groove* seen on this surface.

C. Inferior ramus of pubis
1. It extends from body of pubis to ramus of ischium.
2. It joins the ramus of ischium to form conjoint *ischiopubic ramus*.
   (Attachments to inferior ramus are discussed with ischiopubic ramsus)

III. ISCHIUM

It is the posteroinferior part of hip bone. It contributes to 2/5th of acetabulum. It comprises of a body and a ramus.

A. Body of ischium
It is very thick. It lies below and posterior to the acetabulum. It has 2 ends (upper and lower), 3 borders (anterior, posterior and lateral) and 3 surfaces (femoral, dorsal and pelvic)

a. Ends
   i. *Upper end*
      It forms posteroinferior 2/5th of *acetabulum*.
   ii. *Lower end* (Fig. 10.9)

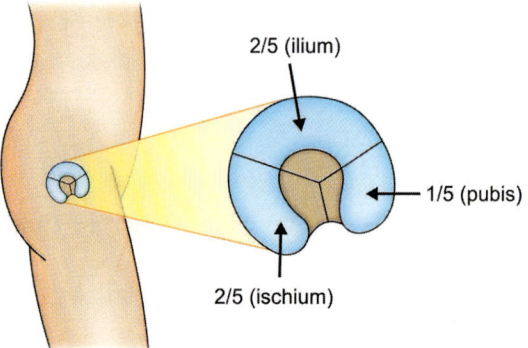

Fig. 10.8: Right acetabulum: Lateral view

1. It forms *ischial tuberosity*.
2. Inferior ramus arises from lower end.
3. Ischial tuberosity is divided by a horizontal ridge into an upper quadrilateral and lower triangular areas.
4. The upper area of ischial tuberosity is divided by a diagonal line into upper lateral and lower medial areas.
5. A longitudinal ridge subdivides the lower triangular area of ischial tuberosity into outer and inner areas.
6. *Semimembranosus* arises from the superolateral part of upper area of ischial tuberosity.

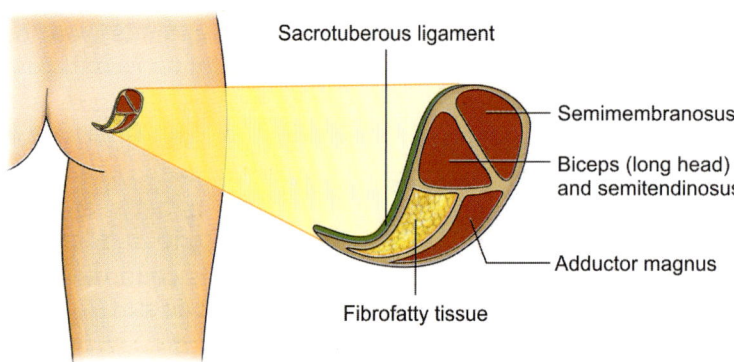

Fig. 10.9: Right ischial tuberosity : Posterior aspect

7. *Semitendinosus* and the *long head of biceps femoris* arise from inferomedial part of upper area of ischial tuberosity.
8. *Adductor magnus* arises from outer part of lower area.
9. Inner part of the lower area is covered by *fibrofatty tissue*. This part supports the body weight while sitting.
10. *Sacrotuberous ligament* is attached to the medial margin of ischial tuberosity.

b. Borders

i. *Anterior border*

It forms posterior part of *obturator foramen*.

ii. *Posterior border*

1. It is continuous with the posterior border of ilium.
2. It ends below at the upper end of ischial tuberosity.
3. It presents a spine called *ischial spine*. *Sacrospinous ligament* is attached to the margins of ischial spine. *Coccygeus and levator ani* also arise from this spine.
4. Ischial spine forms lower boundary of *greater sciatic notch*.
5. Below the ischial spine is *lesser sciatic notch*.
6. Both greater and lesser sciatic notches are converted into foramina by sacrotuberous and sacrospinous ligaments.
7. Structures passing through greater sciatic foramen are:
   - *Piriformis*
   - Superior and inferior gluteal nerves and vessels
   - Nerve to obturator internus
   - Pudendal nerve
   - Internal pudendal vessels
   - Sciatic nerve
   - Posterior cutaneous nerve of thigh
   - Nerve to quadratus femoris
8. Structures related to lesser sciatic foramen are:
   - *Tendon of obturator internus* passes through it.
   - *Superior and inferior gemelli* arise from corresponding margins.
   - *Nerve to obturator internus* enters through it to supply obturator internus.
   - *Pudendal nerve* and *internal pudendal vessels* enter the perineum by passing through it.

Note: To remember structures passing through lesser sciatic foramen you can remember, Never Tell Indian Police,
N = Nerve to obturator internus
T = Tendon of obturator internus
I = Internal pudendal vessels
P = Pudendal nerve

iii. *Lateral border*

It continues with lateral border of ischial tuberosity.

c. Surfaces

i. *Femoral surface*

1. It is situated between anterior and lateral borders.
2. *Obturator externus* orginates from this surface along the obturator foramen.
3. *Quadratus femoris* arises from this surface close to lateral border of upper part of ischial tuberosity.

ii. *Dorsal surface*

1. It continues above with the gluteal surface of ilium.
2. It has 3 parts:
   Upper - convex area adjacent to acetabulum
   Middle – grooved area
   Lower – upper part of ischial tuberosity

3. *Piriformis, sciatic nerve* and *nerve to quadratus femoris* are related to upper convex area.
4. *Obturator internus tendon along with two gemelli* traverses the middle grooved area.
5. *Semitendinosus, long head of biceps* and *semimembranosus* arise from the lower part of dorsal surface.

iii. *Pelvic surface*
1. It is between anterior and posterior borders.
2. *Obturator internus* arises from the greater part of pelvic surface.

B. Ramus of ischium

It arises from the lower part of body and runs forwards, upwards and medially. It meets with the inferior pubic ramus to form ischiopubic ramus.

IV. ISCHIOPUBIC RAMUS

It has two borders (upper and lower) and two surfaces (outer and inner).

A. Borders

a. Upper border
1. It forms lower margin of *obturator foramen*.
2. *Obturator membrane* is attached to it.

b. Lower border
1. It is everted. This feature is more marked in males than females.
2. *Fascia lata* and *membranous layer of superficial fascia (Colles' fascia)* are attached to it.

B. Surfaces

a. Outer surface
1. It is concave
2. Following muscles are attached to it from above downwards:
   i. *Obturator externus*
   ii. *Adductor magnus*
   iii. *Gracilis*

b. Inner surface (Fig. 10.10)
It is convex. It has 2 ridges (upper and lower) and 3 areas (upper, middle and lower) which are meant for following structures:
1. Upper ridge receives attachments of *obturator fascia* and *superior fascia of urogenital diaphragm*.
2. Lower ridge provides attachments to *perineal membrane* and *falciform process of sacrotuberous ligament*.
3. Upper area is meant for attachment of *obturator internus*.

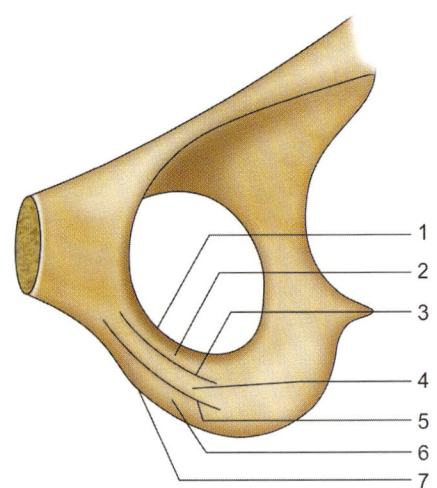

1. Upper border (obturator membrane)
2. Upper area (obturator internus)
3. Upper ridge (obturator fascia and superior fascia of urogenital diaphragm)
4. Middle area (sphincter urethrae and deep transversus perinei)
5. Lower ridge (perineal membrane and falciform process of sacrotuberous ligament)
6. Lower area (crus penis, ischiocavemosus and superficial transversus perinei)
7. Lower border (Colles' fascia and fascia lata)

Fig. 10.10: Inschiopubic ramus of right hip. Inner aspect

4. Middle area receives attachments of *sphincter urethrae* and *deep transversus perinei muscles*.
5. Lower area provides attachments to *crus penis, ischiocavernosus* and *superficial transversus perinei*.

V. ACETABULUM (Fig. 10.8)

1. Literal meaning of acetabulum is vinegar cup.
2. It is a cup shaped deep concavity facing laterally and anteroinferiorly.
3. All the three parts of hip bone contribute to it as follows:
   Pubis-its anterior 1/5th
   Ischium-little more than its posterior 2/5th
   Ilium-little less than its superior 2/5th.
4. Its margin is deficient inferiorly to form *acetabular notch*. *Transverse acetabular ligament* bridges this gap to form *acetabular foramen*.
5. Margin of acetabulum provides attachment to *labrum acetabulare* which bridges the acetabular notch as *transverse acetabular ligament*.
6. It has a horse-shoe shaped articular surface (*lunate surface*) and nonarticular central *acetabular fossa*. Lunate surface is covered by hyaline cartilage while acetabular fossa lodges a pad of fat.

VI. OBTURATOR FORAMEN

1. It is the gap in the lower part of hip bone.
2. It is situated between pubis and ischium.
3. *Obturator membrane* is attached to its margins. The membrane bridges the *obturator groove* to convert it into *obturator canal* which transmits *obturator nerve and vessels*.

OSSIFICATION

A. Primary centres

3 primary centres appear:
1 for ilium - appears during 2nd month of intrauterine life.
1 for ischium - appears during 3rd month of intrauterine life.
1 for pubis - appears during 4th month of intrauterine life.

The ramus of ischium and inferior ramus of pubis fuse during 7th year.

At birth most of the bone is ossified except for 3 cartilaginous parts which are:
a. Whole of iliac crest.
b. 'Y' shaped cartilage of acetabulum.
c. A strip along inferior margin of hip bone.

B. Secondary centres

There are 5 secondary centres:
 2 for iliac crest
 2 for 'Y' shaped acetabular cartilage
 1 for ischial tuberosity

Appearance: Puberty

Fusion

1. Ossification of acetabulum is completed by 17 years.
2. Ossification of rest of the bone is completed by 20–25 years.

SEXUAL DIMORPHISM

Table 10.1: Sexual dimorphism in hip bone

Features	Female	Male
1. Greater sciatic notch	Wider (90°)	Narrower (<90°)
2. Ischial spine	Not inverted	Inverted
3. Ischiopubic ramus	Not everted	Everted
4. Obturator foramen	Triangular	Oval
5. Acetabular diameter	Less than 5cm	More than 5cm.
6. Distance between pubic tubercle and acetabular margin.	Greater than acetabular diameter.	Equal or less than acetabular diameter.

APPLIED ANATOMY

See "**The Bony Pelvis**" in Chapter 11.

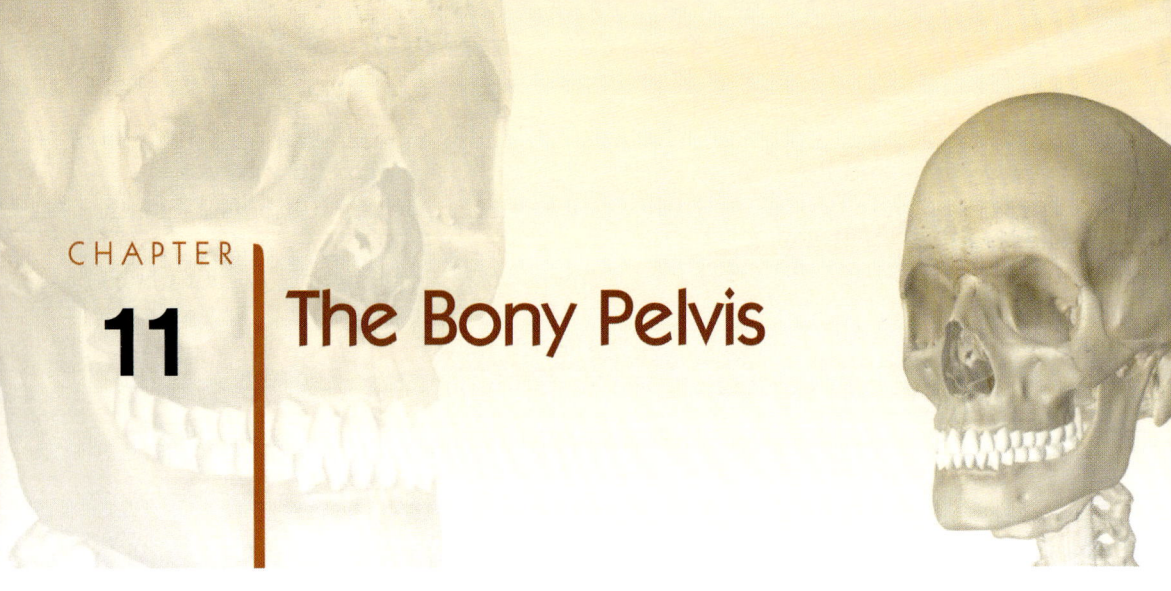

CHAPTER 11
The Bony Pelvis

TERMINOLOGY

Pelvis is a Latin word which means 'a basin'. Following are the similarities between the pelvis and basin (Fig. 11.1).
1. Back or posterior wall is wide
2. Front or anterior wall is narrow
3. Walls are sloping
4. Inlet is above
5. Outlet is below

PELVIC GIRDLE

It is a bony ring below the fifth lumbar vertebra and between femoral heads. Four bones participate in the formation of pelvic girdle. These are two hip bones, one sacrum and one coccyx.

These four bones articulate with each other to form two synovial (sacroiliac) and two symphyseal (pubic and sacrococcygeal) joints.

DIVISIONS OF PELVIS

The plane of pelvic inlet divides the bony pelvis into two parts:
   I. Part above the pelvic inlet is called pelvis major or greater pelvis or false pelvis.
  II. Part below the pelvic inlet is called pelvis minor or lesser pelvis or true pelvis or obstetric pelvis.

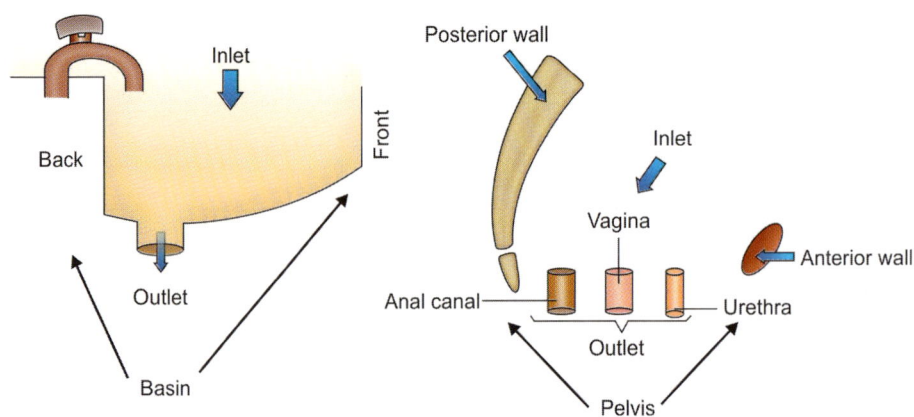

Fig. 11.1: Comparing pelvis with basin

DIVISIONS OF LESSER PELVIS (Fig. 11.2)

For the sake of description the lesser pelvis is divided into three parts:
  I. Inlet
  II. Outlet
  III. Cavity

ANATOMICAL POSITION

1. Pubic symphysis lies in midsagittal plane.
2. Anterior superior iliac spines and pubic tubercles lie in the same coronal plane.

BOUNDARIES OF PELVIC INLET (Fig. 11.3)

I. Bony contributions (pelvic brim)
  A. Sacral contributions
   a. Sacral promontory
   b. Ala of sacrum
  B. Contributions by hip bone (*linea terminalis*)
   a. Iliac part–*Arcuate line*
   b. Pubic part–(i) *Pecten pubis*; (ii) *Pubic crest*

Note: *Pelvic brim and pelvic inlet are synonyms for obstetricians.*

II. Articular contributions
  A. Anteriorly in the midline – *Pubic symphysis*
  B. Posterolateral – *Sacroiliac joints*

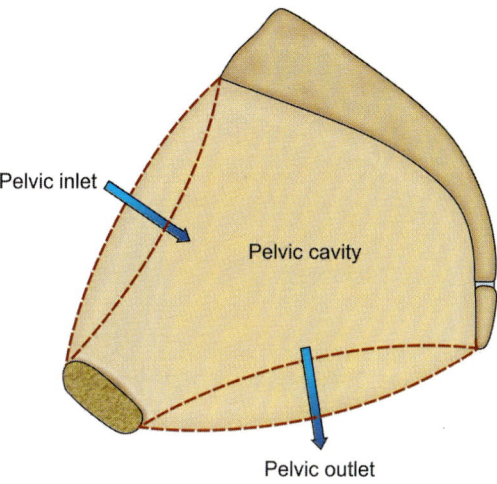

Fig. 11.2: Subdivisions of lesser pelvis

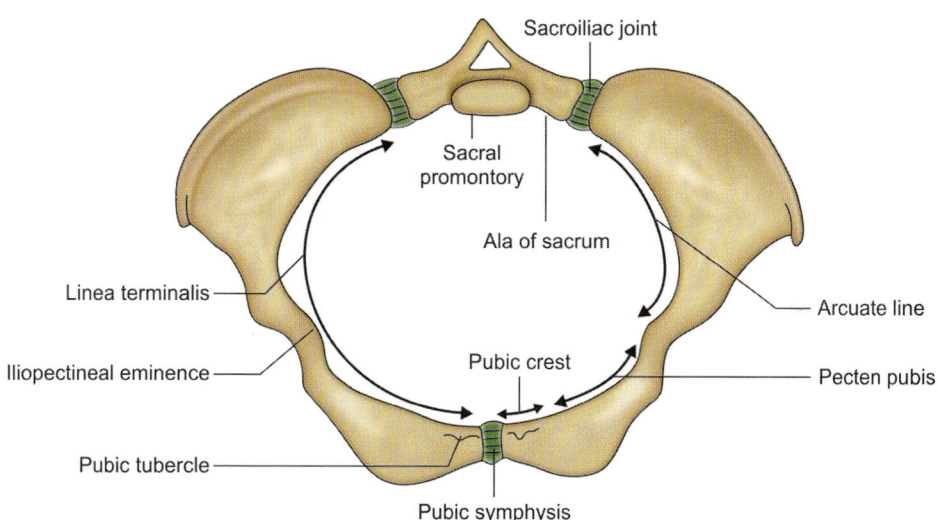

Fig. 11.3: Boundaries of pelvic inlet

BOUNDARIES OF PELVIC OUTLET (Fig. 11.4)

Anteriorly – Lower border of pubic symphysis
Posteriorly – Tip of coccyx
On each side – Half of the pubic arch
– Ischiopubic ramus
– Ischial tuberosity
– Sacrotuberous ligament

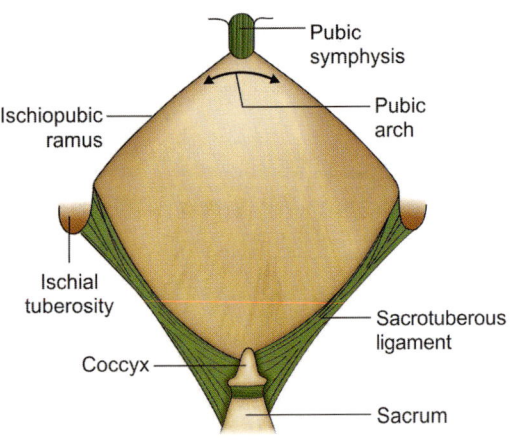

Fig. 11.4: Boundaries of pelvic outlet

Note: *Obstetricians ignore coccyx due to its mobility. Therefore 'obstetrical outlet' is bounded posteriorly by tip of sacrum. Tip of coccyx forms the posterior boundary of 'anatomical outlet'.*

BOUNDARIES OF PELVIC CAVITY (Fig. 11.5)

Anteriorly- Pelvic surfaces of
 - Pubic symphysis
 - Body of pubis
 - Pubic rami
Posteriorly- Pelvic surfaces of
 - Sacrum
 - Coccyx
Laterally - Pelvic surfaces of - Ilium
 - Ischium

Note: *To simplify the boundaries, one can remember that pelvic cavity is bounded by pelvic surfaces of all the three components of hip bone i.e. ilium, pubis and ischium and pelvic surfaces of sacrum and coccyx.*

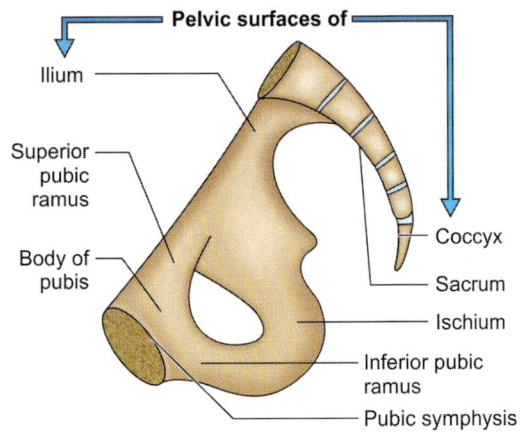

Fig. 11.5: Boundaries of pelvic cavity

PUBIC ARCH AND SUBPUBIC ANGLE (Fig. 11.6)

The inferior margins of pubic symphysis and adjacent inferior pubic rami together form pubic arch. Angulation between margins of pubic arch is called subpubic angle. In gynecoid pelvis the subpubic angle is more than 90° and is called Norman type. In android pelvis this angle is acute, i.e. less than 90° and is also called Gothic type.

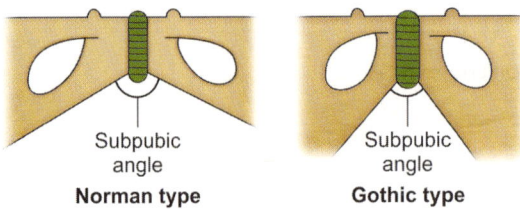

Fig. 11.6: Pubic arch and subpubic angle

FUNCTIONS OF PELVIS

1. Locomotion.
2. Weight transmission.

3. Provides areas for the attachments of muscles.
4. Protection of pelvic viscera.
5. Plays important role in parturition (birth of baby).

AXES OF PELVIS (Fig. 11.7)

I. Axis of inlet
It is perpendicular to the plane of pelvic inlet and passes through its centre. On projection it passes through umbilicus and middle of coccyx.

II. Axis of outlet
It passes through centre of anteroposterior axis of outlet. It is also perpendicular to this axis and is directed downwards and slightly backwards. When projected upwards, it reaches the sacral promontory.

III. Axis of pelvic cavity
It is a curved line following the curvature of pelvic surfaces of sacrum and coccyx. It is perpendicular to innumerable planes of pelvis between planes of inlet and outlet.

PELVIC SEGMENTS (Fig. 11.8)

The widest transverse diameter divides the pelvic brim into anterior segment (forepelvis) and posterior segment (hindpelvis). The hindpelvis is important clinically because of being more variable in shape and capacity.

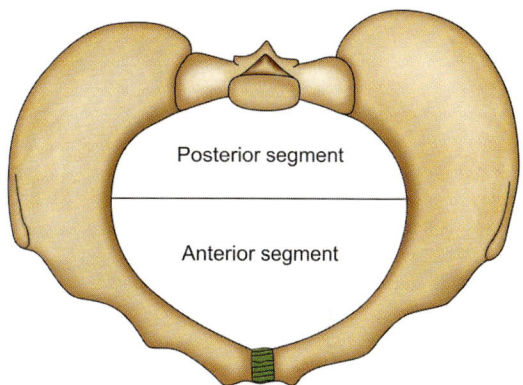

Fig. 11.8: Pelvic segments

POSTERIOR SAGITTAL DIAMETER OF KLEIN (Fig. 11.9)

It extends from middle of bituberous diameter to the tip of sacrum. The diameter is of clinical significance. In cases of android pelvic, the foetal head is pushed backwards. If the said diameter is inadequate, there will be difficulty in delivery.

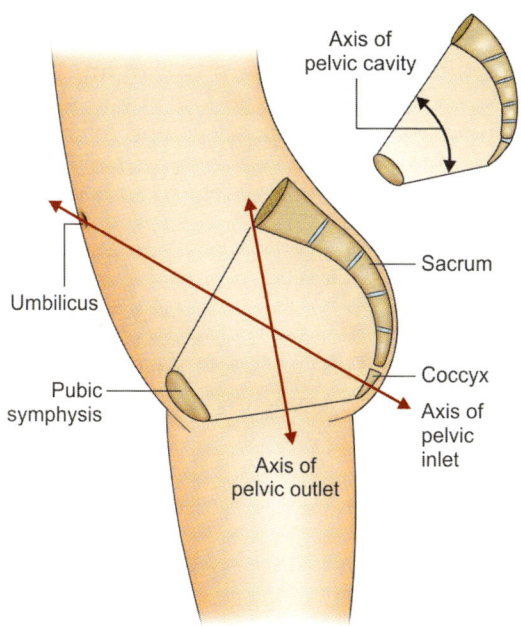

Fig. 11.7: Axes of pelvis

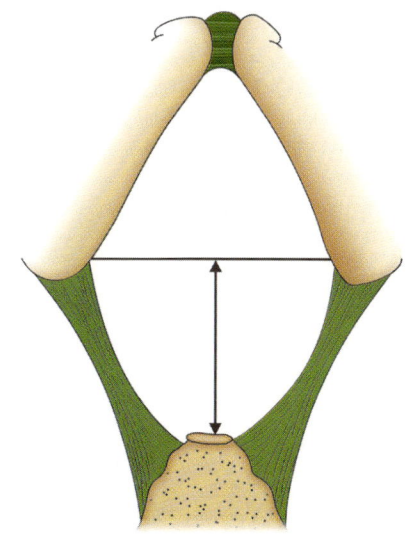

Fig. 11.9: Posterior sagittal diameter of Klein

PELVIC INCLINATION (Fig. 11.10)

The plane of pelvic inlet forms an angle of 550° with the horizontal plane. The plane of pelvic outlet forms an angle of approximately 15° with the same.

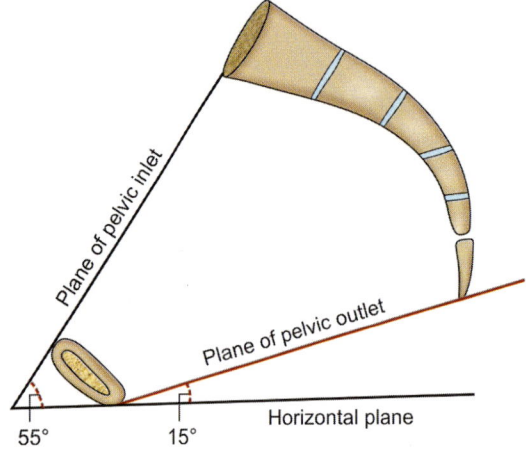

Fig. 11.10: Pelvic inclination

PLANES OF PELVIC DIMENSIONS

I. Plane of greatest pelvic dimensions

It is an imaginary plane passing through middle of pubic symphysis and junction of 2nd and 3rd sacral vertebrae.

II. Plane of least pelvic dimensions or narrow pelvic plane

It is an imaginary plane passing through the lower border of pubic symphysis, the ischial spines and the tip of sacrum.

CONJUGATE DIAMETERS (Fig. 11.11)

I. External conjugate

It is the distance between upper border of pubic symphysis and tip of 1st sacral spine.

II. True conjugate

This is also called anteroposterior diameter of inlet. It is the distance between middle of sacral promontory and superior border of pubic symphysis.

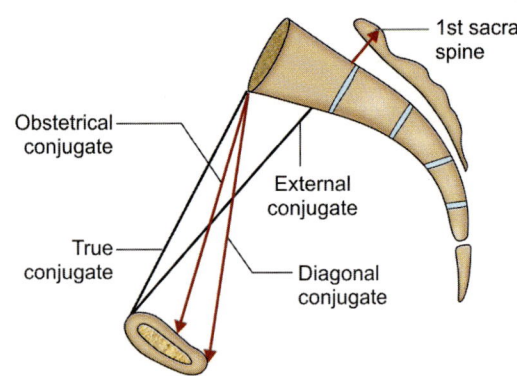

Fig. 11.11: Conjugate diameters

III. Diagonal conjugate

It is the distance between middle of sacral promontory and inferior border of pubic symphysis. It is important clinically because it is an indirect assessment of anteroposterior diameter of pelvic inlet and can be roughly measured by per vaginal (P/V) examination.

IV. Obstetrical conjugate

It is the shortest distance between the pelvic surface of pubic symphysis and sacral promontory.

LEAST DIAMETER OF PELVIS

It is the distance between two ischial spines.

TYPES OF PELVIS (Fig. 11.12)

Four types of female pelvis have been described.

I. Gynaecoid/gynecoid type
1. It is typical female pelvis.
2. It is observed in 42% females.
3. It is spacious and roomy and therefore suitable for easy passage of baby during delivery.

II. Android type
1. It is typical male type of pelvis found in females.
2. It is observed in 32% females.

The Bony Pelvis

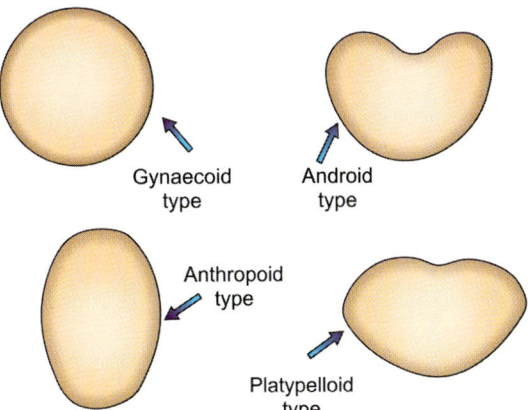

Fig. 11.12: Shapes of inlets in four types of female bony pelvis

3. Its inlet is heart shaped.
4. It may result into obstructed labour.

III. Anthropoid type
1. Its inlet is compressed from sides.
2. It is found in 23% females.
3. Such pelvis will obstruct the smooth delivery of foetus.

IV. Platypelloid type
1. Its inlet is anteroposteriorly compressed.
2. It is rare type of pelvis observed in 2% females only.
3. This type of pelvis also poses difficulty in delivery.

DIAMETERS OF PELVIS
(Figs 11.13 and 11.14)

Three diameters i.e. anteroposterior, oblique and transverse, are considered at each of the three levels, i.e. inlet, cavity and outlet. The details are as follows:

I. Inlet of pelvis
A. Anteroposterior diameter
It extends from middle of sacral promontory to upper margin of pubic symphysis.

B. Oblique diameter
It extends from upper end of sacroiliac joint of one side to iliopectineal eminence of the opposite side.

C. Transverse diameter
It is the greatest width of inlet i.e., maximum transverse diameter.

II. Cavity of pelvis
A. Anteroposterior diameter
It extends from middle of pubic symphysis to middle of body of 3rd sacral vertebra.

B. Oblique diameter
It is the distance between the lower end of sacroiliac joint of one side to the middle of obturator membrane of opposite side.

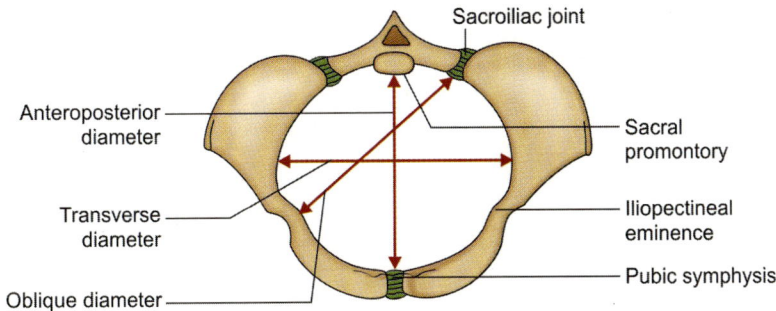

Fig. 11.13: Diameters of inlet of pelvis

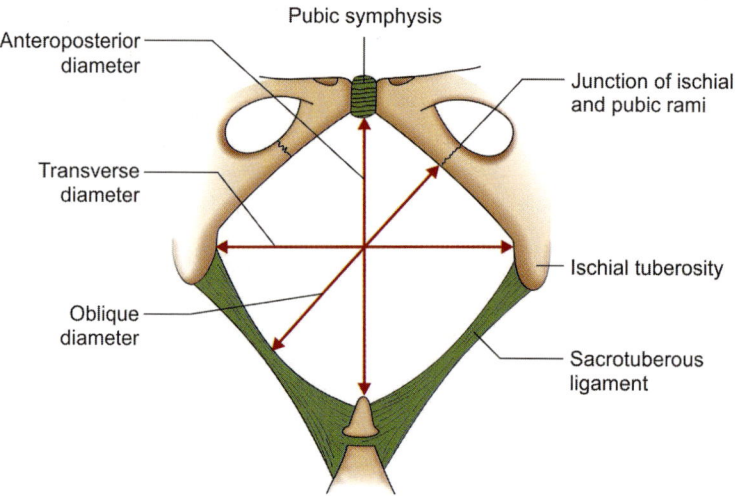

Fig. 11.14: Diameters of outlet of pelvis

C. Transverse diameter
It is the greatest width of the cavity.

III. Outlet of pelvis
A. Anteroposterior diameter
It extends between tip of coccyx to the lower border of pubic symphsysis.

B. Oblique diameter
It is the distance between the middle of sacrotuberous ligament of one side and junction of ischial and pubic rami of opposite side.

C. Transverse diameter
It is the distance between inner margins of two ischial tuberosities.

Table. 11.1: Approximate measurements (cm) of different pelvic diameters

Diameters	Inlet	Cavity	Outlet
Anteroposterior diameter	11	12	13
Oblique diameter	12	12	12
Transverse diameter	13	12	11

SEX DIFFERENCES IN ADULT PELVIS

Table. 11.2: Sex differences in adult pelvis

Features	Male	Female
1. General structure	Thick and heavy	Thin and light
2. Markings for muscular attachments	Very prominent	Less prominent
3. False pelvis	Deep	Shallow
4. Pelvic inlet	Heart shaped	Circular or oval
5. Sacral promontory	More prominent	More flat
6. Pubic tubercles	Closer	Wider apart
7. Cavity	Narrower and deeper	Wider and shallower
8. Sacrum evenly curved	Narrower, longer and sharply forwards in its lower part	Wider, shorter and bends

Contd.

The Bony Pelvis

Table. 11.2: Sex differences in adult pelvis (Contd.)

Features	Male	Female
9. Sciatic notch	Narrower	Wider
10. Ischial spine	Projected inwards	Projected outwards
11. Ischial tuberosity	Inverted	Everted
12. Subpupic angle	More acute (angle, <90°)	Wider (angle, 90° or >90°)
13. Ischiopubic rami	More everted	Less everted
14. Obturator foramen	Oval	Triangular
15. Preauricular sulcus	Less prominent	More prominent
16. At the sacral base, ratio between transverse width of facet for 5th lumbar vertebra and that of entire base	1 or <1:2	>1 : 2
17. Acetabulum	Larger	Smaller
18. If the distance between anterior rim of acetabulum and pubic symphysis is '1', then the diameter of acetabulum is	1	> 1
19. Sacral index i.e. Breadth of sacrum × 100/ Length of sacrum	Lesser	Greater
20. Pelvic outlet	Comparatively smaller	Comparatively larger

APPLIED ANATOMY

1. Diameters of the pelvic inlet in females are very important due to obstetrical reasons.
2. Interspinous diameter (least pelvic diameter) can be estimated by palpating sacrospinous ligament through vagina. The length of this ligament is equal to the half the interspinous diameter.
3. Per vaginal examination and radiographs are two best known methods to judge the adequacy of pelvic canal in females for child birth. These methods will provide an idea about prominence of sacral promontory and ischial spines, sacral concavity and subpubic arch.
4. The anteroposterior diameter of foetal head prefers the widest diameter of pelvis during childbirth. Therefore during fixation of head the foetal occiput faces twards right or left, i.e. the anteroposterior diameter of foetal head lies transversely at inlet (both 13 cm). At the outlet the

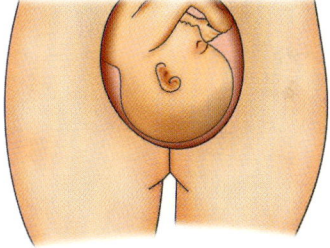

Fixation of head

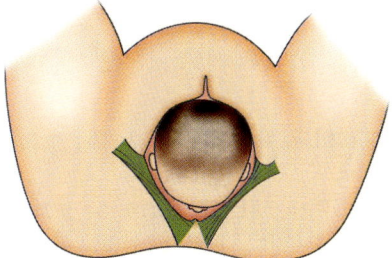

Foetal head at outlet

Fig. 11.15: Rotations of head during child birth

foetal head rotates for about 90° so that the occiput usually faces anteriorly and the anteroposterior diameters of both foetal head and outlet correspond to each other (both 13 cm) (Fig. 11.15).

5. The pelvis is very strong and usually a direct violence of high velocity is required to fracture it.
6. Lateral part of hip is strongest.
7. Weak areas of pelvis are:
   a – Upper part (ala) of ilium
   b – Sacroiliac region
   c – Pubic rami
8. Pelvis is like a ring. When fractured, this ring tends to break at two places. If only one fracture is visible, one should consider the possibility of disruption of a sacroiliac joint.
9. Fracture of pelvis can be classified as,
   a. *Stable fracture* with intact pelvic ring (Fig. 11.16).

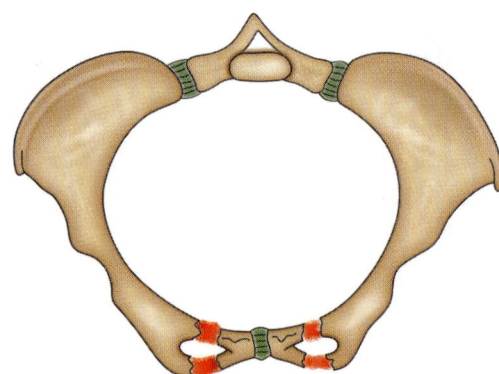

Fig. 11.17: Straddle fracture

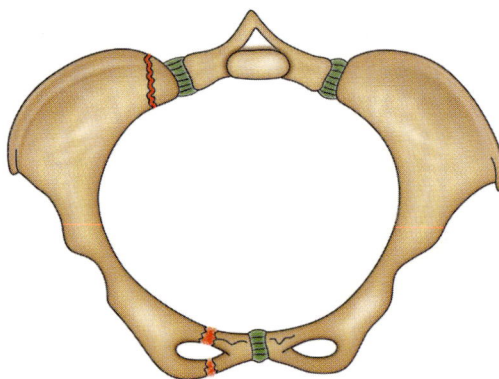

Fig. 11.18: Malgaigne's fracture

   iii. *Bucket handle fracture*: Fracture of ala of sacrum on one side and pubis on the other side (Fig. 11.19).

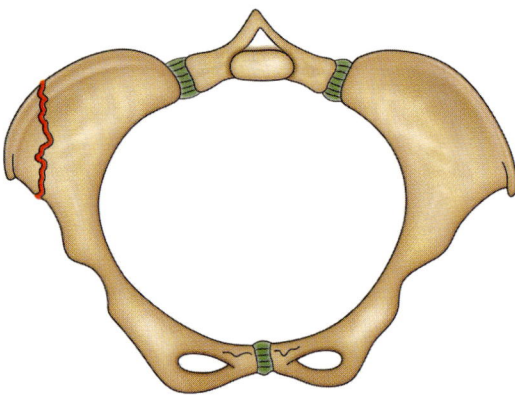

Fig. 11.16: Stable fracture of pelvis

   b. *Unstable fracture* with disrupted pelvic ring.
      i. Bilateral fracture of pelvic ring (*Straddle fracture*) (Fig. 11.17).
      ii. *Malgaigne's fracture*: Fracture of pubic rami and ala of sacrum on the same side (Fig. 11.18).

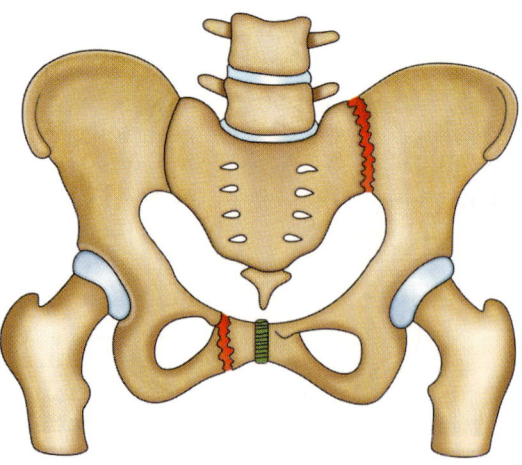

Fig. 11.19: Bucket handle fracture

c. *Complicated fracture* with visceral damage.
10. The bladder and urethra are most vulnerable viscera during pelvic fracture.
11. When the head of femur is pushed medially (*central dislocation of hip*) it causes fracture of acetabulum (Fig. 11.20).

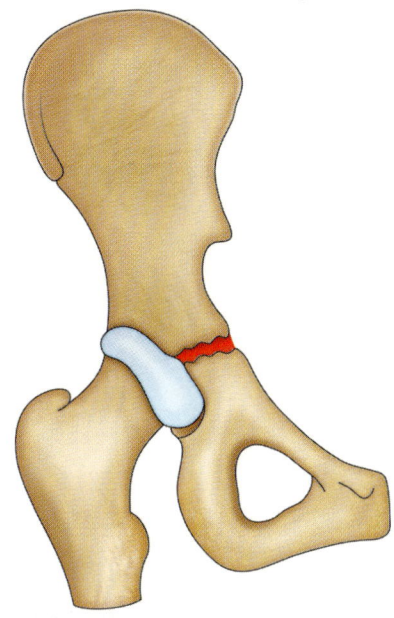

Fig. 11.20: Central dislocation of hip

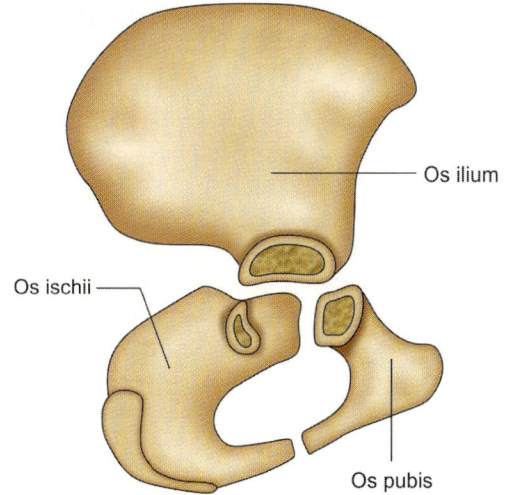

Fig. 11.21: Fracture of acetabulum at the junctions of its three components

12. The acetabulum will be fractured into its three components if the injury occurs in a person under 17 years of age (Fig. 11.21).
13. Acetabulum is a deep socket for the head of femur and therefore dislocation of hip is commonly associated with acetabular fracture.
14. "Wandering" *acetabulum* is a complication of the tuberculosis of the hip. It is due to partial absorption of acetabulum and femoral head leading to dislocation (Fig. 11.22).

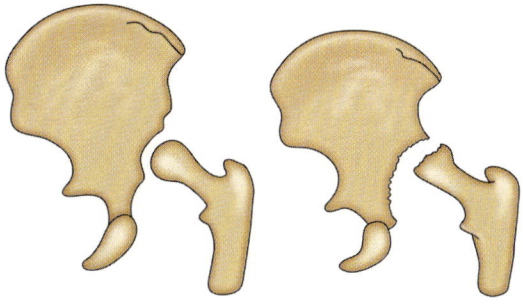

Fig. 11.22: Hip joint: (a) Normal; (b) Wandering acetabulum

15. *Trendelenburg's sign* (Fig. 11.23)
   Normally when a patient is asked to lift one of his legs, the pelvis is also lifted on the same side simultaneously due to strong action of abductors (gluteus medius and gluteus minimus) on weight bearing side. If the pelvis sags instead of going up on the unsupported side, Trendelenburg's sign is considered to be positive. Any deficiency in the power (weak gluteal muscles), fulcrum (diseased hip) and levers (deformity of upper femur) will result into a positive sign.
16. Sometimes patient masks the deformity at hip by tilting the pelvis. In case of adduction deformity the patient lifts the pelvis on the same side. This masks the adduction. To detect such tilting of pelvis one should square the pelvis by moving the affected limb into further adduction or measure the apparent lengths of lower limbs (apparent length is measured from

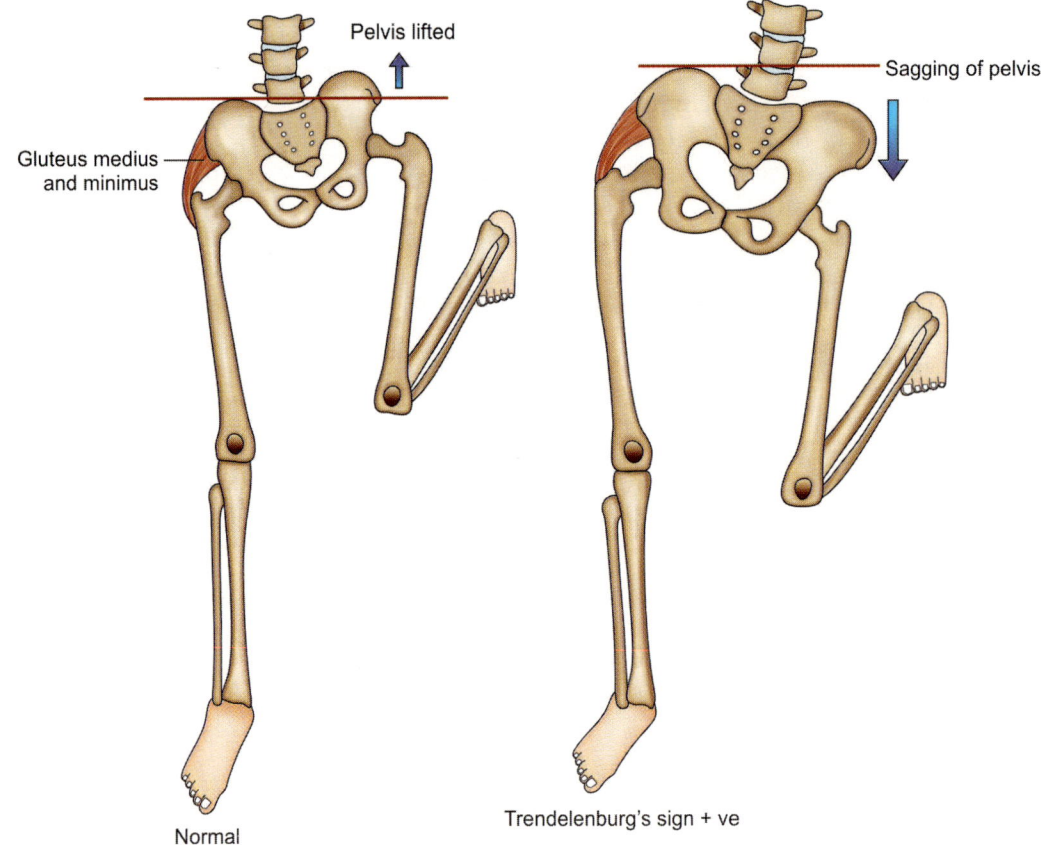

Fig. 11.23: Trendelenburg's sign

umbilicus to medial malleolus). Adduction causes apparent shortening and the abduction causes apparent lengthening of lower limb (Fig. 11.24).

17. Pelvis should always be fixed by holding it with hand before measuring the hip movements.
18. *Osteoarthritis* of hip may complicate and involve acetabulum of hip bone.
19. Sacroiliac joints may be involved in case of *seronegative polyarthritis*.
20. *Ankylosing spondylitis* commences in sacroiliac joints and progresses to spine (vertebral column).
21. *Still's disease* is seronegative polyarthritis occurring in children in which the sacroiliac joints are commonly involved.
22. The pelvis is one of the areas of active bone marrow and therefore prone to *myeloma* (*myelomatosis*), one of the malignant tumours of bone (Fig. 11.25).
23. *Secondary malignant tumours* of bone are more common than primary malignant tumours. Pelvis is one of the common bony site for secondary carcinoma.
24. *Eosinophilic granuloma* is another tumour of bone which favours pelvis.
25. Frank *dysplasia of the hip with deficient acetabulum* is one of the factors leading to congenital dislocation of the hip (Fig. 11.26).
26. Fragmentation and flattening of epiphysis are common in *Perthes' disease*. Early acetabular involvement, though rare may also be noticed (Fig. 11.27).

The Bony Pelvis | 85

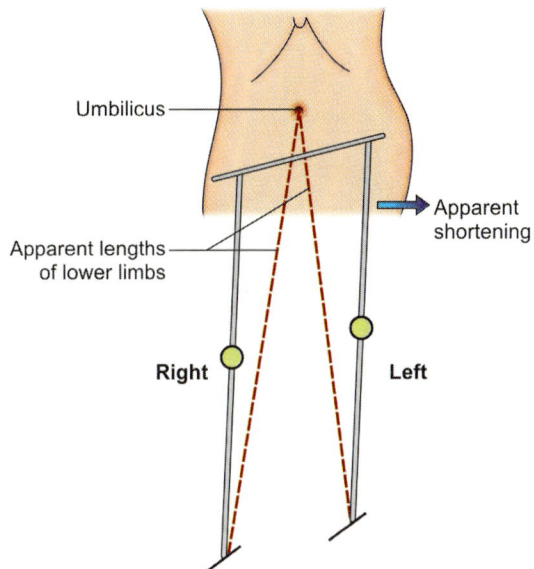

Fig. 11.24: Adduction deformity causing apparent shortening of left lower limb

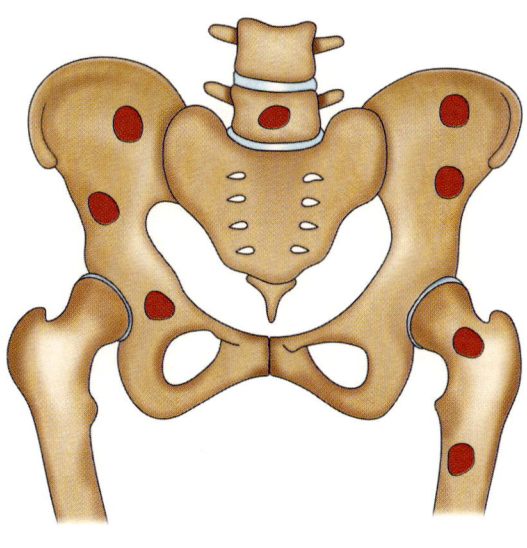

Fig. 11.25: Myeloma (myelomatosis) or secondary carcinoma

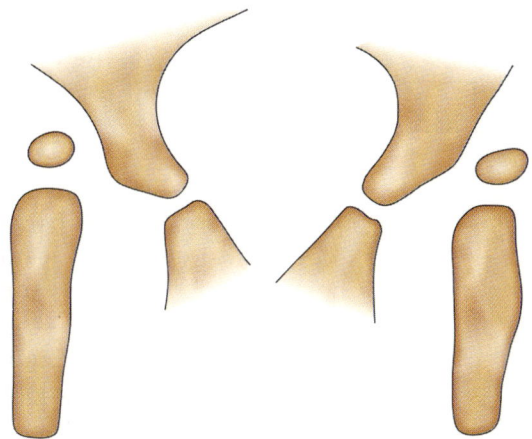

Fig. 11.26: Radiographic appearance of congenital dislocation of hip

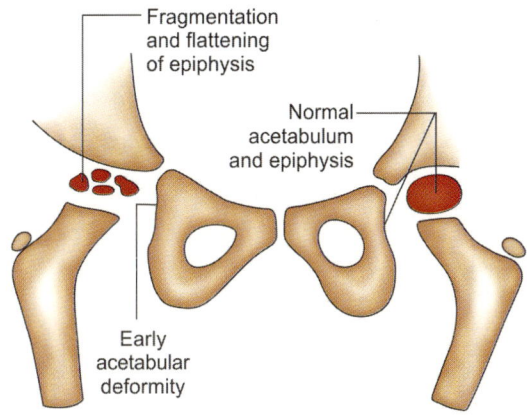

Fig. 11.27: Radiological findings of Perthes' disease

27. Sacroiliac joint may be involved in inflammation (*sacroiliitis*), *trauma of pelvis* and *pregnancy* or *labour*. Such involvements present as *backache*.

28. *Coccydynia* refer to any condition causing pain in the region of coccyx.

29. In cases of *total hip replacement* an artificial acetabulum is added in the region of hip in addition to artificial head, whereas in partial hip replacement only an artificial head is fixed in the region (Fig. 11.28).

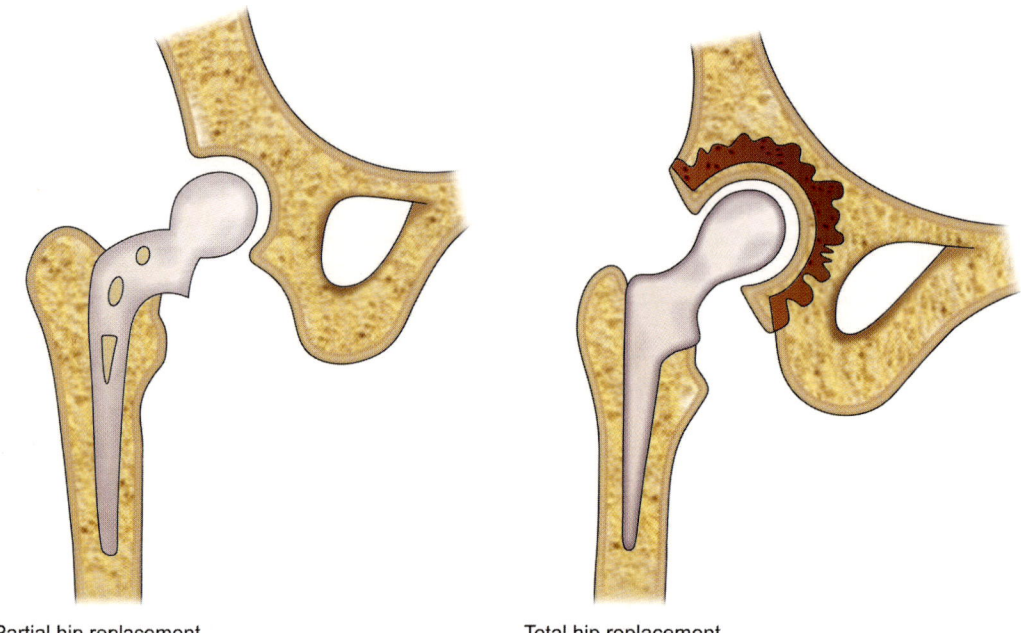

Partial hip replacement   Total hip replacement

Fig. 11.28: Hip replacement

30. Iliac crest is the ideal site for *bone graft harvesting*.
31. *Sprinter's fracture*: It is an avulsion fracture of the the anterosuperior or anteroinferior iliac spine caused by violent muscular action.

CHAPTER 12

The Femur

TERMINOLOGY

Femur is a Latin word means thigh. It is named so because it belongs to thigh.

PECULIARITIES

1. Femur is the strongest and longest bone of the body.
2. Femur constitutes more than one-quarter of the height of the individual.

SIDE DETERMINATION

1. Femur is a vertical bone.
2. Rounded head is located at the upper end.
3. Head is directed medially.
4. Convexity of shaft is directed forwards.

ANATOMICAL POSITION
(Figs 12.1 and 12.2)

1. Keep the bone vertically in such a way so that head faces upwards, medially and slightly forwards.

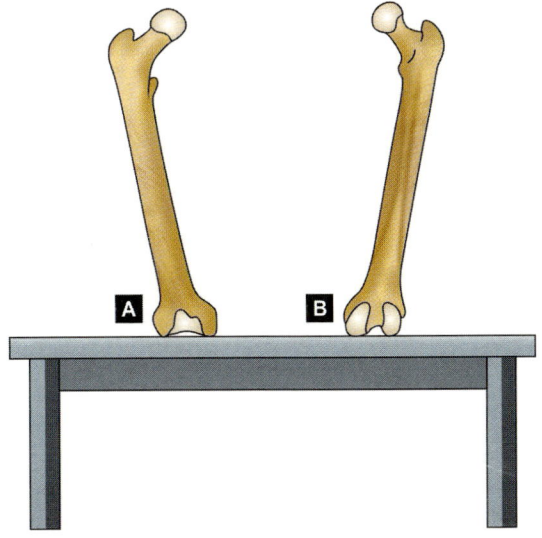

Fig. 12.1: Right femur held vertically on a table. (A) Front view; (B) Posterior view

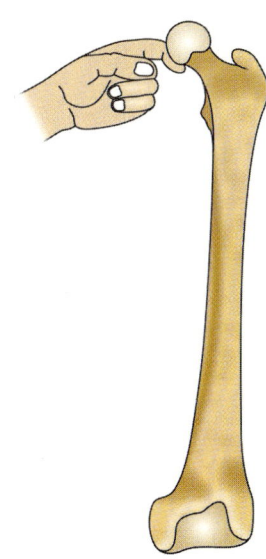

Fig. 12.2: Balancing the femur with index finger

> **Note:** *Remember the femur helps the body in pushing forwards, i.e. propulsion, therefore the head is directed forwards.*

2. The long axis of shaft is directed downwards and medially.

> **Note:** *To achieve this keep the lower end of femur on a table in such a way that the inferior surfaces of both the condyles touch the table. This can also be achieved by balancing the neck on your index finger.*

ANGLE OF FEMORAL TORSION (Fig. 12.3)

The vertical plane passing through the long axis of head and neck does not lie in coronal plane due to forward bending of head and neck in normal anatomical position. The long axis of the lower end of femur runs transversely in coronal plane. The angle between aforementioned planes at the two ends of femur is called torsion of femur. It is approximately 15°.

FEATURES AND ATTACHMENTS (Figs 12.4 and 12.6 to 12.8)

Femur has an upper end, a shaft and a lower end.

I. UPPER END

It includes head, neck, greater trochanter and lesser trochanter. The junction of neck with the shaft is marked anteriorly by intertrochanteric line and posteriorly by intertrochanteric crest.

A. Head

1. It forms more than half of a sphere.
2. It articulates with hip bone at acetabulum to form *hip joint*.
3. *Fovea capitis* is a roughened pit just below and behind the centre of head. *Ligament of head of femur (ligamentum teres)* is attached to fovea and carries acetabular

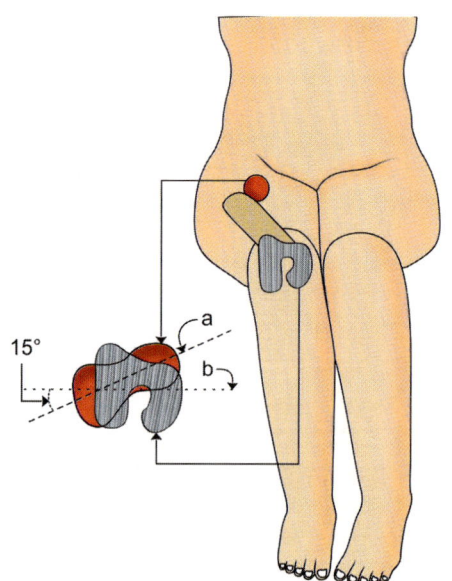

Fig. 12.3: Torsion of femur. (a) Long axis of upper end; (b) Long axis of lower end

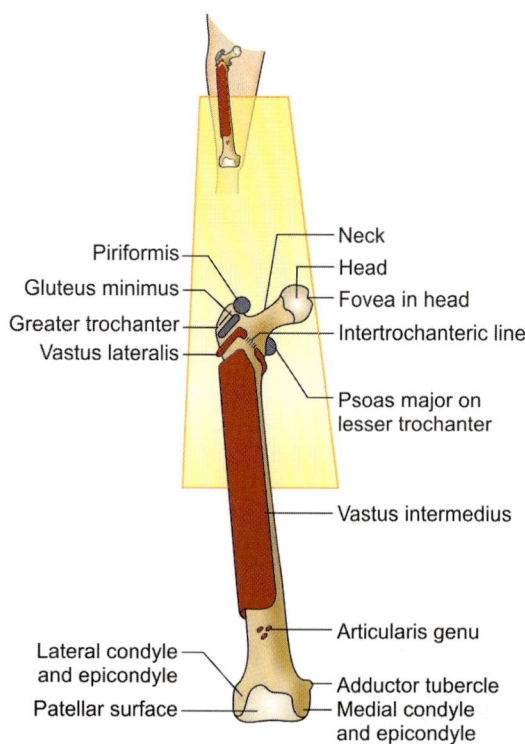

Fig. 12.4: Right femur. Anterior aspect

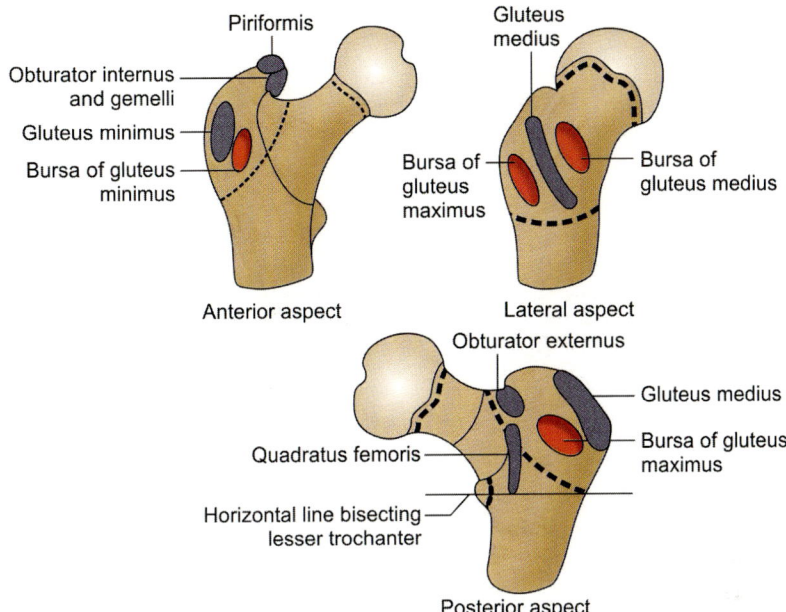

Fig. 12.5: Relations and attachments of greater trochanter of right side. Continuous lines, capsular attachments; Dotted lines, epiphyseal lines

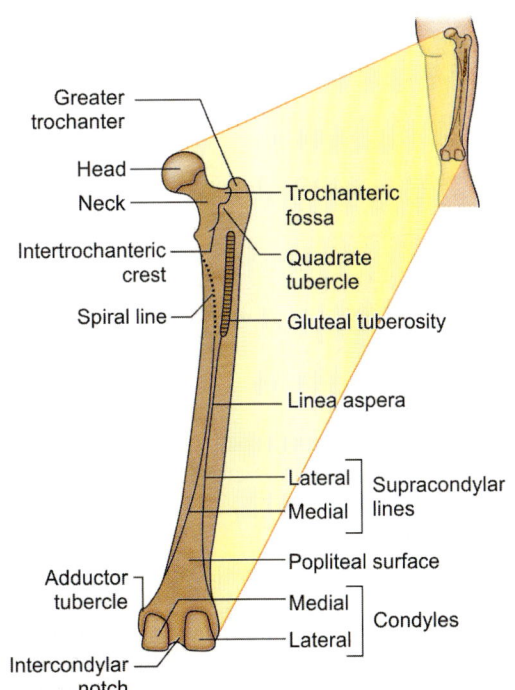

Fig. 12.6: Right femur : Posterior aspect

branches of obturator and medial circumflex femoral arteries.

B. Neck

1. It connects head with shaft.
2. It is 5cm long.
3. Neck-shaft angle is the angle between lower border of neck and medial border of shaft. It is about 125° in adult male. It is less in female and short femora.
4. Neck has two borders (upper and lower) and two surfaces (anterior and posterior).
   a. *Upper border*
      It meets the shaft near greater trochanter.
   b. *Lower border*
      It meets the shaft near lesser trochanter.
   c. *Anterior surface*
      1. It is completely intracapsular.
      2. It meets the shaft at intertrochanteric line.
      3. *Cervical fossa of Allen*

Human Osteology

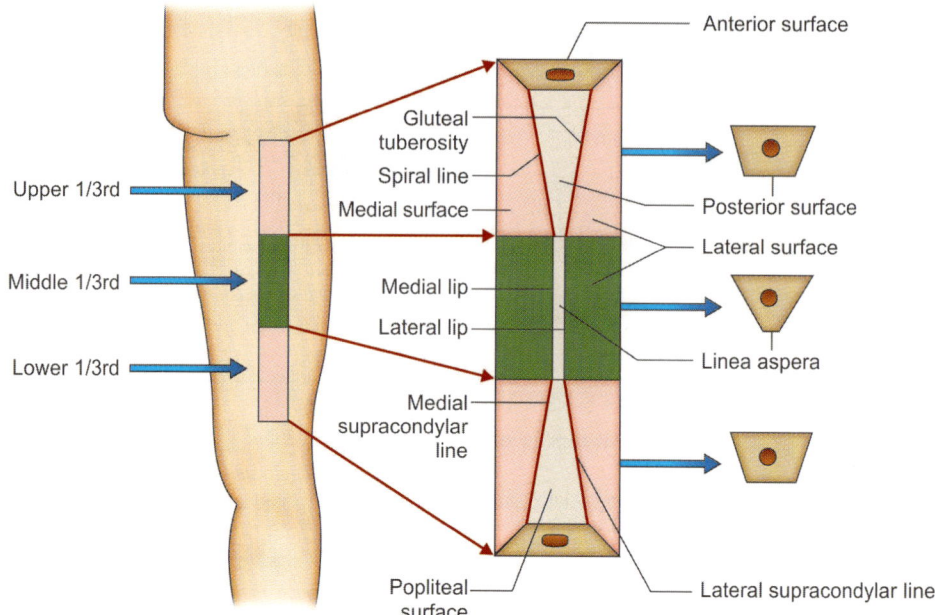

Fig. 12.7: General features of right femoral shaft: Posterior aspect

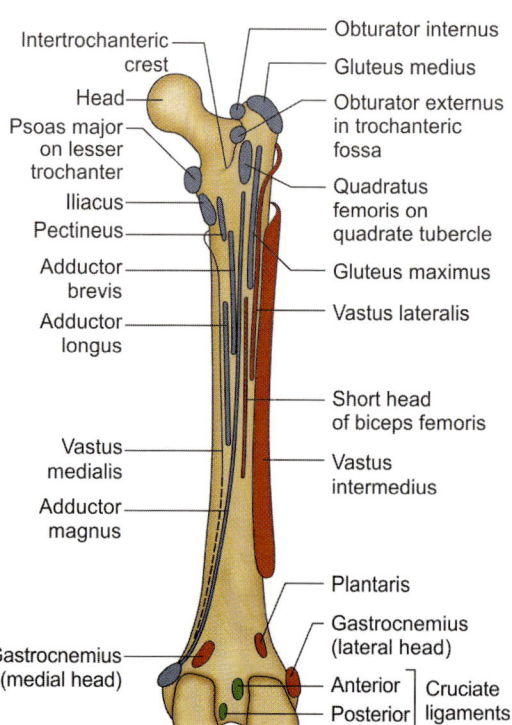

Fig. 12.8: Right femur : Posterior aspect

It is a small depression on the anterior surface of femoral neck near articular margin.

d. Posterior surface
1. It meets the shaft at intertrochanteric crest.
2. Its medial half is intracapsular.

C. Greater trochanter (Fig. 12.5)

Lateral aspect of femur continues up as greater trochanter. It has one border (upper) and three surfaces (anterior, medial and lateral).

a. Upper border

Its posterior part is inturned called *apex*. Apex receives attachment of *piriformis*.

b. Anterior surface

It is divided into lateral and medial areas.
  i. Lateral area has a ridge for attachment of *gluteus minimus*.
  ii. Medial area is related to a bursa under cover of gluteus minimus called as *trochanteric bursa* of *gluteus minimus*.

c. Medial surface

It is divided into lower and upper parts.

i. Lower part is marked by a depression (*trochanteric fossa*) for *obturator externus*.

ii. Upper part is marked by an impression for insertion of *obturator internus, superior gemellus* and *inferior gemellus*.

> **Note:** Remember people of International fame need GUARDS for protection, i.e. INTER or Obturator Internus is accompanied by G or Gemelli. Also remember that trochanteric fossa is like guest house and it is the external examiner, i.e. Obturator Externus, who is kept inside the guest house.

d. Lateral surface

It has a ridge, which runs downwards and forwards and two areas in relation to it.

i. Ridge

This is meant for the attachment of *gluteus medius*.

ii. Area anterior to ridge

It is covered by gluteus medius. A bursa between this muscle and area is called *trochanteric bursa of gluteus medius*.

iii. Area posterior to ridge

This is related to another bursa. Since this area is covered by gluteus maximus, the bursa is named as *bursa of gluteus maximus*.

D. Lesser trochanter

1. It is a conical projection directed medially.
2. It has an apex for the attachment of *psoas major*.
3. *Iliacus* is attached to its front.

> **Note:** Because of close association of iliacus and psoas major the two are considered together as iliopsoas getting attached to lesser trochanter.

4. Its posterior surface is separated from upper horizontal fibres of *adductor magnus* by a *bursa*.

E. Intertrochanteric line

1. It marks the junction of neck and shaft anteriorly.
2. It continues downwards below the lesser trochanter and on the posterior aspect of femur as *spiral line*.
3. Following structures are attached to it:
   i. *Capsule of hip joint*.
   ii. *Iliofemoral ligament*
   iii. *Vastus lateralis* to its upper end
   iv. *Vastus medialis* to its lower end

F. Intertrochanteric crest

1. It marks the junction of neck with the shaft posteriorly.
2. It connects greater trochanter with the lesser trochanter.
3. Quadrate tubercle

   It is a rounded tubercle above the middle of this crest. *Quadratus femoris* is attached to this tubercle and further downwards upto a line which bisects the lesser trochanter.

II. SHAFT

It is cylindrical in shape, convex forwards and narrowest in the middle.

A. General features of shaft

For describing borders and surfaces, the shaft is divided into upper 3rd, middle 3rd and lower 3rd.

a. Middle 1/3rd of shaft

It has 3 borders and 3 surfaces.

i. Borders

1. Medial border
2. Lateral border
3. Posterior border

   It is most prominent. It is also called *linea aspera*. It has distinct medial and lateral lips.

ii. Surfaces

1. Anterior surface
2. Medial surface
3. Lateral surface

b. **Upper 1/3rd of shaft**

Medial lip of linea aspera continues upwards as *spiral line*. The lateral lip of linea aspera continues upwards as *gluteal tuberosity*. Spiral line and gluteal tuberosity diverge from each other to enclose a triangular posterior surface. Upper 1/3rd of shaft therefore has got four borders and four surfaces.

i. Borders
1. Medial border
2. Lateral border
3. Spiral line
4. Gluteal tuberosity

It is a broad rough ridge along the lateral limit of posterior surface. Sometime there is a linear elevation along the gluteal tuberosity called as *crista glutei*. If a conical projection is present in the gluteal tuberosity, it is called as *third trochanter*. Third trochanter is present in 20% of Indian femora and is twice more common in females.

ii. Surfaces
1. Anterior surface
2. Medial surface
3. Lateral surface
4. Posterior surface.

c. **Lower 1/3rd of shaft**

Medial lip of linea aspera continues downwards as *medial supracondylar line*. Lateral lip of linea aspera continues downwards as *lateral supracondylar line*. Medial and lateral supracondylar lines diverge from each other to enclose an additional triangular surface called as *popliteal surface*. Lower 1/3rd of shaft therefore has got four borders and four surfaces.

i. Borders
1. Medial border
2. Lateral border
3. Medial supracondylar line
4. Lateral supracondylar line

ii. Surfaces
1. Anterior surface
2. Medial surface
3. Lateral surface
4. Popliteal surface

Note: *Remember that the intertrochanteric line, spiral line, medial lip of linea aspera and medial supracondylar line form a continuous line from above downwards. Similarly the gluteal tuberosity, lateral lip of linea aspera and lateral supracondylar line form another continuous line.*

B. Attachments to the shaft

Shaft of femur receives attachments of muscles and intermuscular septa.

a. **Attachments of muscles**

i. *Gastrocnemius*

Medial head arises from popliteal surface just above the medial condyle. Lateral head arises mainly from the upper part of lateral surface of lateral condyle but also extends over the lower end of lateral supracondylar line.

ii. *Plantaris*

It originates from the lower end of lateral supracondylar line just above the lateral head of gastrocnemius.

iii. *Vastus intermedius*

It arises from the upper 3/4th of anterior and lateral surfaces.

iv. *Articularis genu*

It arises from lower 1/4th of anterior surface.

v. *Vastus lateralis*

It arises from:
1. Upper part of intertrochanteric line
2. Anterior and inferior borders of greater trochanter
3. Lateral lip of gluteal tuberosity
4. Upper half of lateral lip of linea aspera

vi. *Vastus medialis*

It arises from:
1. Lower part of intertrochanteric line
2. Spiral line
3. Medial lip of linea aspera
4. Upper 1/4th of medial supracondylar line

vii. *Gluteus maximus*

Deeper part of its lower half is inserted into the gluteal tuberosity.

viii. *Adductor longus*

It is inserted into the medial lip of linea aspera.

ix. *Pectineus*

It is inserted into a line extending from lesser trochanter to upper end of linea aspera.

x. *Adductor brevis*

It is inserted into a line extending from the area lateral to lower part of pectineus to middle of linea aspera.

xi. *Adductor magnus*

It is attached to a line extending from the lower end of quadratus femoris to adductor tubercle. Specifically it is attached to:
1. Medial margin of gluteal tuberosity
2. Linea aspera
3. Medial supracondylar line
4. Adductor tubercle

xii. *Short head of biceps femoris*

It arises from:
1. Lateral lip of linea aspera
2. Upper 2/3rd of lateral supracondylar line

b. Attachments of intermuscular septa (Fig. 12.9)

1. Medial intermuscular septum is attached to the medial lip of linea aspera.
2. Lateral intermuscular septum is attached to the lateral lip of linea aspera.

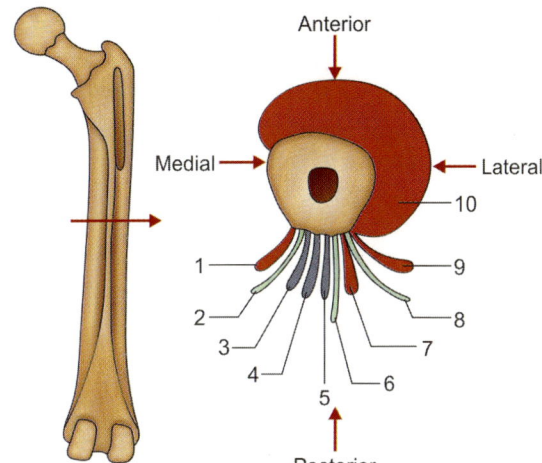

Fig. 12.9: Attachments to linea aspera (cross sectional view): (1) Vastus medialis; (2) Medial intermuscular septum; (3) Adductor longus; (4) Adductor brevis; (5) Adductor magnus; (6) Posterior intermuscular septum; (7) Biceps femoris (short head); (8) Lateral intermuscular septum; (9) Vastus lateralis; (10) Vastus intermedius

3. Posterior intermuscular septum is attached to linea aspera just medial to attachment of short head of biceps femoris.

Note: *To remember the attachments of muscles to linea aspera remember the rhyme "I Love Bindu, Miss Bindu Loves Me, i.e. from lateral to medial these are I, L, B, M, B, L, M, which stand for vastus Intermedius, vastus Lateralis, short head of Biceps femoris, adductor Magnus, adductor Brevis, adductor Longus and vastus Medialis respectively.*

III. LOWER END

It includes two condyles (medial and lateral), a deep space between the two condyles posteriorly (intercondylar fossa or notch) and articular surfaces (patellar and tibial).

A. Medial condyle

It possesses 5 surfaces:

a. Medial surface

1. Its most prominent point is *medial epicondyle for medial collateral ligament*.
2. Above and behind the medial epicondyle is *adductor tubercle*, for *ischial fibres of adductor magnus*.

b. Lateral surface

It forms medial boundary of *intercondylar fossa*.

c. Anterior surface

It forms part of the *patellar articular surface*.

d. Posterior surface

It articulates with tibia during full flexion of knee joint.

e. Inferior surface

It articulates with medial condyle of tibia during extension of knee.

B. Lateral condyle

It presents 5 surfaces:

a. Lateral surface

1. An elevation on this surface is called *lateral epicondyle*. This is meant for attachment of *fibular collateral ligament of knee joint*.
2. *Smooth impression* above and behind the lateral epicondyle gives origin to *lateral head of gastrocnemius*.
3. A *groove* below and behind the lateral epicondyle provides attachment to *popliteus* in its anterior part. Tendon of popliteus occupies the posterior part of groove during full flexion at the knee joint.

b. Medial surface

It forms lateral boundary of *intercondylar fossa*.

c. Anterior surface

It forms part of the *patellar articular surface*.

d. Posterior surface

It articulates with lateral condyle of tibia during full flexion at knee joint.

e. Inferior surface

It articulates with lateral tibial condyle during full extension at knee.

C. Intercondylar fossa (notch)

1. It separates posterior and inferior parts of two condyles.
2. It is limited by patellar articular surface anteriorly and *intercondylar line* posteriorly.
3. It is intracapsular but mostly extrasynovial.
4. *Anterior cruciate ligament* is attached to the posterior part of the medial surface of lateral condyle.
5. *Posterior cruciate ligament* is attached to the anterior part of the lateral surface of medial condyle.

> **Note:** *To remember the attachments of cruciate ligaments one should remember LAMP in which L = Lateral condyle, A = Anterior cruciate ligament, M = Medial condyle and P = Posterior cruciate ligament, i.e. Lateral condyle receives Anterior and Medial condyle receives Posterior cruciate ligaments respectively.*

6. *Capsular ligament* is attached to the intercondylar line.

D. Articular surfaces

a. Patellar articular surface

1. It covers the anterior surfaces of both the condyles.
2. It extends higher on the lateral condyle.
3. It has a vertical groove in its middle.
4. Two grooves separate this surface from tibial articular surfaces. These grooves are related to anterior end of respective meniscus during full extension of the knee.

b. Tibial articular surfaces

1. These cover the inferior and posterior surfaces of both the condyles.
2. These articulate with the condyles of tibia.
3. These are separated from each other by intercondylar fossa.

CAPSULAR ATTACHMENTS (Fig. 12.10)

I. Upper end

Capsule is attached:
A. Anteriorly to intertrochanteric line.
B. Posteriorly to middle of neck so that the medial half of posterior surface of neck becomes intracapsular.

II. Lower end

Capsule is attached:
A. Posteriorly to intercondylar line and articular margins.
B. Laterally and medially to a line 1 cm above the articular margins (groove for popliteus is intracapsular).
C. Anteriorly it is deficient for communication between *suprapatellar bursa* and knee joint cavity.

SEX DIFFERENCES

Table 12.1: Features differentiating male and female femur bones

Features	Male	Female
1. General	Larger, stronger and heavier	Smaller, weaker and lighter
2. Muscular markings	More prominent	Less prominent
3. Neck-shaft angle	Relatively more	Relatively less
4. Obliquity of shaft	Relatively less	Relatively more
5. Radiogram	Less translucent	More translucent

OSSIFICATION

A. Primary centre

One centre appears for shaft at 8th week of intrauterine life.

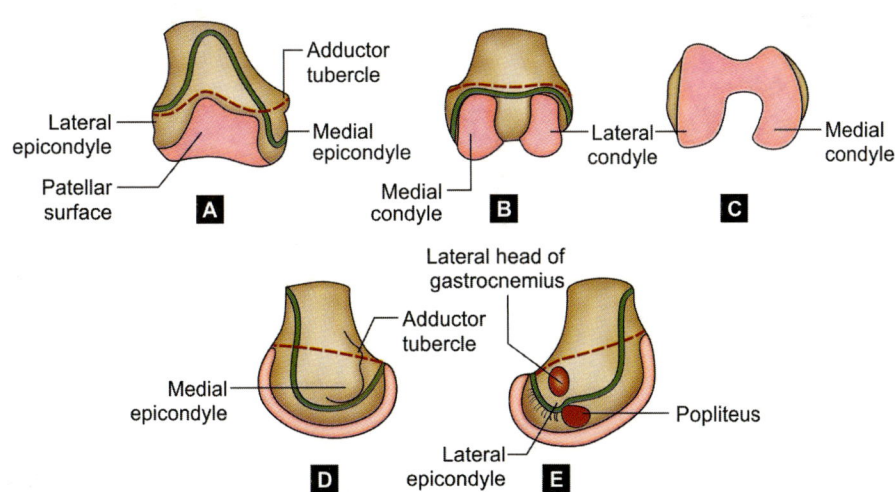

Fig. 12.10: Lower end of right femur. (A) Anterior aspect; (B) Posterior aspect; (C) Inferior aspect; (D) Medial aspect; (E) Lateral aspect. Continuous lines, capsular attachments; Dotted lines, epiphyseal lines

B. Secondary centres

4 in all, 3 for upper end and one for lower end.

a. Upper end

Appearance

  – Head ....1 year
  – Greater trochanter.....3 years
  – Lesser trochanter.....13 years

Fusion

There will be three epiphyses which fuse with shaft separately at 18th year.

b. Lower end

Appearance

9 Months of intrauterine life (i.e. day of birth)

Fusion

20 years

APPLIED ANATOMY

1. *Common sites of fracture:* In young age group (below 16 years) the common site of fracture is shaft. In old age (above 60 years) the commonest site of fracture is femoral neck (Fig. 12.11).

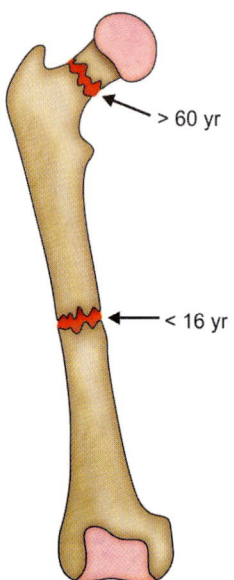

Fig. 12.11: Common sites of fracture in femur

2. *Medicolegal importance:* Since the centre for the lower end of femur appears just before birth (9 months of IUL), its presence proves the viability of baby and therefore is of great medicolegal importance.
3. The neck shaft angle of femur is usually reduced (<125°) if the disease involves its head and neck. This is called *coxa vara*. If the angle is >135°, the condition is called *coxa valga* (Fig. 12.12).

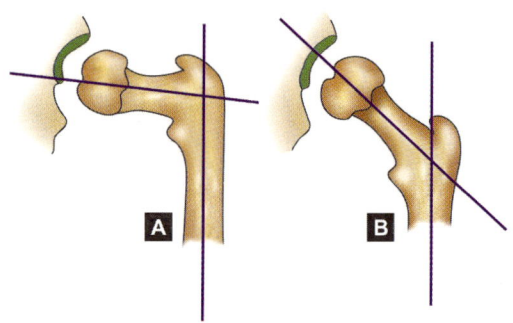

Fig. 12.12: Neck shaft angle of femur: (A) Coxa vara (<125°); (B) Coxa valga (>135°)

4. Since powerful muscles tend to cause shortening or angulation of fracture, traction is indicated in fracture of femur.
5. The head of femur receives blood supply from lateral side through vessels running with retinacula. Therefore in case of fracture of neck of femur these vessels are invariably damaged leading to *avascular necorsis of head* (Fig. 12.13).

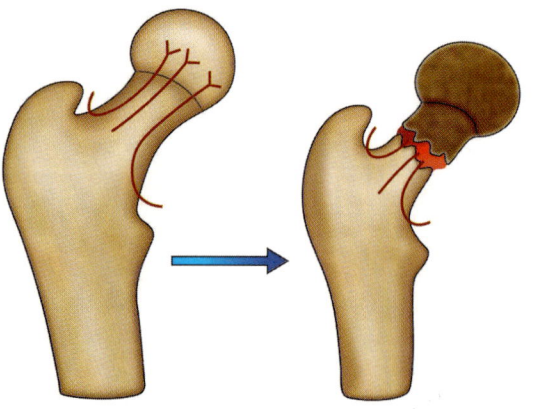

Fig. 12.13: Fracture of femoral neck leading to avascular necrosis

6. *Fracture of femoral neck* is more common in older women than in men because their bones become markedly weakened owing to postmenopausal osteoporosis.
7. In cases of *fracture of femoral neck*, the usual deformity observed is shortening and lateral rotation of the injured lower limb. Lateral rotation results from the change in the axis of the limb due to separation of body and head of femur. Strong adductors which are normally medial rotators, become lateral rotators after fracture of neck of femur. Shortening of lower limb results from the superior pull (spasm) of muscles connecting the femur to hip bone (Fig. 12.14).

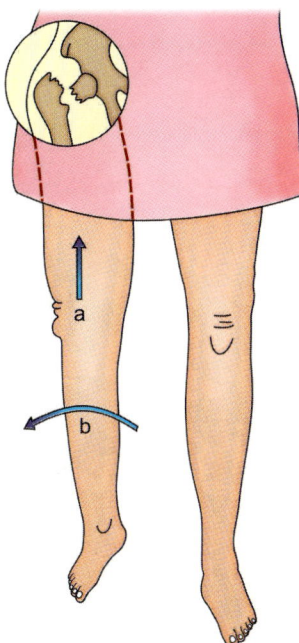

Fig. 12.14: Fracture of neck of right femur. (a) Upward pull; (b) Lateral rotation

8. *Dislocation of the hip joint* is uncommon owing to the stability of this articulation. But the traumatic dislocations of the hip joint may occur during automobile accidents when the hip is flexed and thigh is medially rotated. This is called a *dashboard injury of hip*. A backward thrust leads to posterior dislocation and therefore injury of sciatic nerve. This makes the posterior dislocation, the most common type of hip dislocation.
9. In case of *supracondylar fracture* of the femur, the gastrocnemius tends to pull backwards the distal fragment. Therefore immobilization of the fracture with the knee in flexion is desirable (Fig. 12.15).

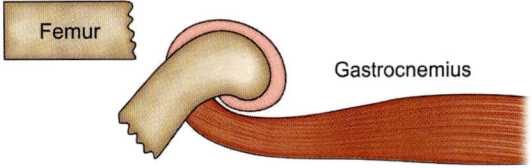

Fig. 12.15: Supracondylar fracture of femur (distal segment is pulled backwards by gastrocnemius)

10. The treatment of fracture of femoral neck depends on whether the fracture is intracapsular or extracapsular. *Extracapsular fractures* do not damage the blood supply to the femoral head and therefore the problem of avascular necrosis and non-union does not arise.
11. Classification of fractures of neck of femur:
    a. **Anatomical classification (Fig. 12.16):**
        a. *Subcapital*: At the junction of head and neck.

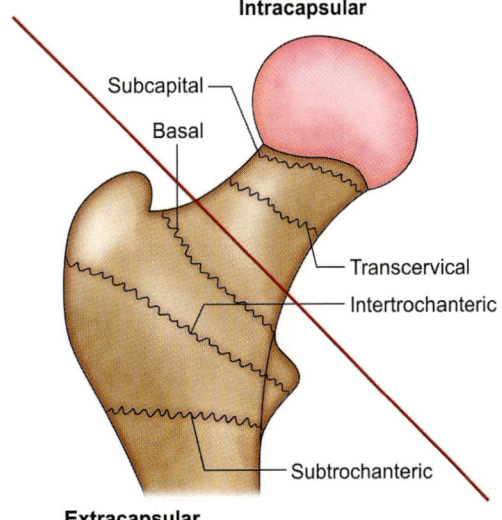

Fig. 12.16: Sites of fractures of the femoral neck

b. *Transcervical*: Through middle 3rd of neck.
c. *Basal*: At the junction of neck and shaft.

b. **Garden classification (Fig. 12.17):**
   a. *Grade I* : Incomplete fracture with one cortex intact.
   b. *Grade II*: Complete fracture with no displacement.
   c. *Grade III*: Complete fracture with partial displacement.
   d. *Grade IV*: Complete fracture with displacement and rotation.

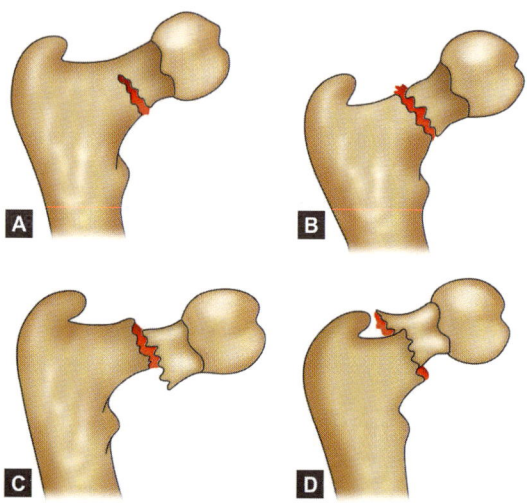

Fig. 12.17: Garden classification of fractures of neck of femur. (A) Grade I; (B) Grade II; (C) Grade III; (D) Grade IV

12. Classification of trochanteric fractures:
    a. **Anatomical classification (Fig. 12.18):**
       a. *Cervicotrochanteric*.

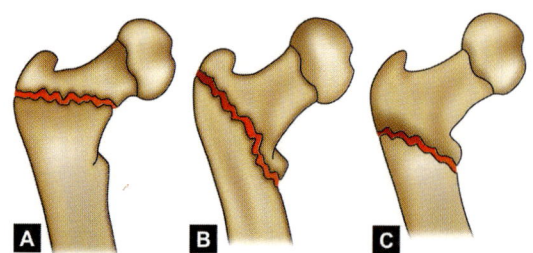

Fig. 12.18: Anatomical classification of trochanteric fractures. (A) Cervicotrochanteric; (B) Intertrochanteric; (C) Subtrochanteric

b. *Intertrochanteric*.
c. *Subtrochanteric*.

b. **Boyd and Griffin classification (Fig. 12.19):**
   a. *Type 1* : Trochanteric fracture without displacement.
   b. *Type 2* : Trochanteric fracture with displacement of proximal segment.
   c. *Type 3* : Trochanteric fracture with displacement of proximal segment in association with vertical break in shaft.
   d. *Type 4* : Multiple fractures at the level of lesser trochanter.

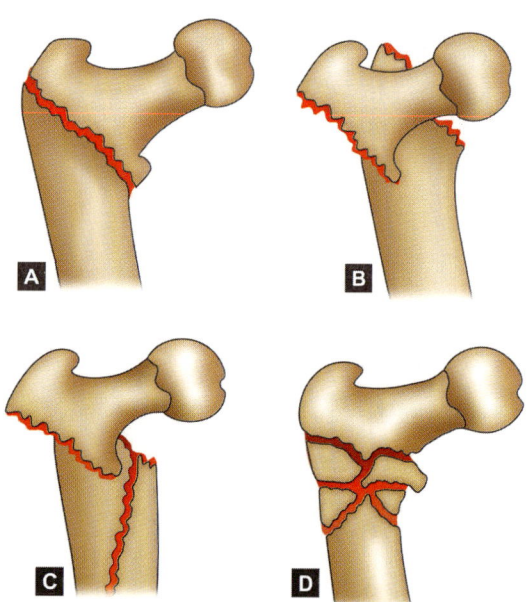

Fig. 12.19: Boyd and Griffin classification of trochanteric fractures. (A) Type 1; (B) Type 2; (C) Type 3; (D) Type 4

c. **Mechanical classification (Fig. 12.20):**
   a. *Stable fracture*: The abductors and adductors create the force of compression at fracture line.
   b. *Unstable fracture*: Abductors pull the proximal segment laterally while adductors pull the distal segment medially.

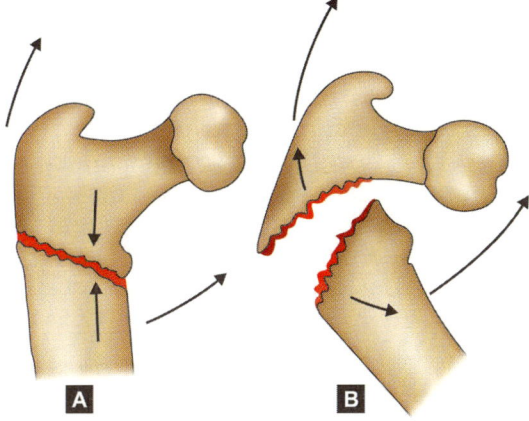

Fig. 12.20: Mechanical classification of trochanteric fractures: (A) Stable fracture; (B) Unstable fracture

13. Muscle forces acting across the shaft of femur play a very important role in displacement of segments of fractured femur shaft. Different muscles affect different segments of femur as follows (Fig. 12.21):

Segment of femur shaft	Muscles affecting displacement
1. Proximal 3rd	Flexors and abductors of hip
2. Middle 3rd	Adductors of thigh
3. Distal 3rd	Gastrocnemius (flexes distal segment)

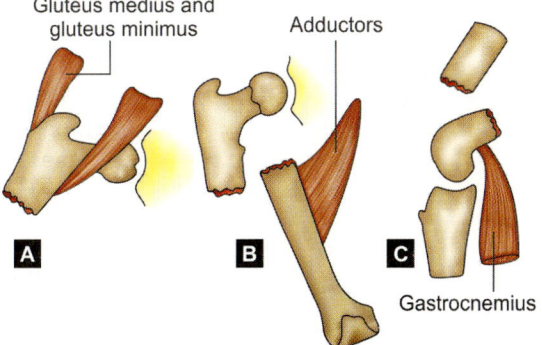

Fig. 12.21: Muscles affecting displacement of fractured femoral shaf: (A) Proximal 3rd fracture; (B) Middle 3rd fracture; (C) Distal 3rd fracture

14. In *'T' fracture* at lower end of femur, supracondylar fracture is associated with a vertical fracture between the two condyles. Rarely only one condyle is involved called as *'condylar fracture'* (Fig. 12.22).

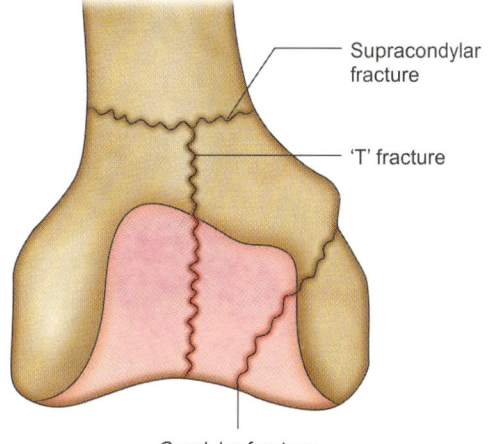

Fig. 12.22: Fractures at lower end of femur

15. *Osteochondritis dissecans* is a condition in childhood in which an osteochondral fragment of bone (usually in the lateral aspect of medial condyle of femur) becomes avascular, loosens and drops away to form a loose body. The condition

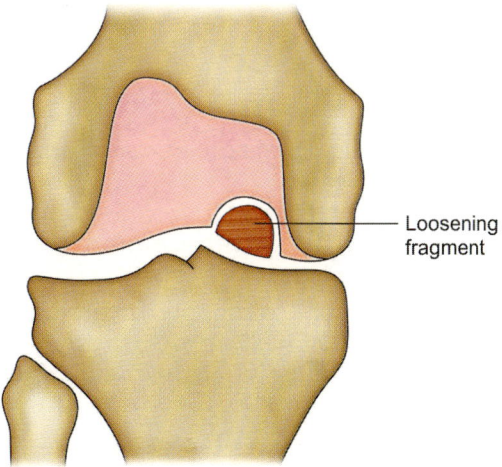

Fig. 12.23: Osteochondritis dissecans of knee

is easily diagnosed radiologically (Fig. 12.23).

16. Lower end of femur is one of the common sites of *osteomyelitis*. Infection usually occurs in the metaphysis of the bone. Supplying the adjacent epiphyseal plate are arcades of capillaries and it is thought that slowing of blood flow in these capillaries allows circulating organisms to settle.

17. Typical radiological appearances greatly help in diagnosis of *tumours* (Fig. 12.24).

21. *Osteosarcoma* presents an interesting radiological appearance. The tumour shows areas of osteosclerosis in the metaphysis. Radiologically osteosarcoma is *osteosclerotic* or *osteolytic type*. *Osteosclerotic variety* is more common. Tumour bursts on the surface to appear as soft tissue mass, which in turn stimulates periosteum to form new bone leading to formation of a triangular region deep to periosteum called as *Codman's triangle* (Fig. 12.25).

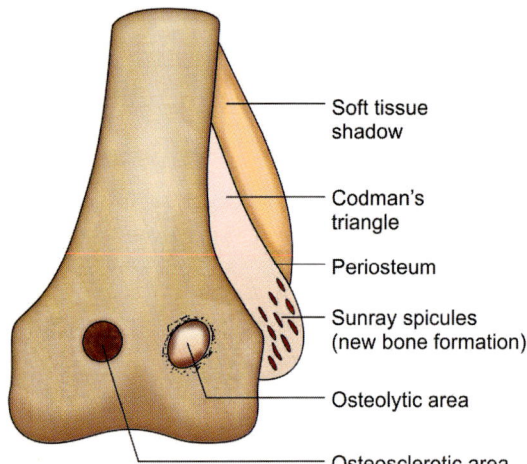

Fig. 12.25: Radiological appearance of osteosarcoma of the distal femur

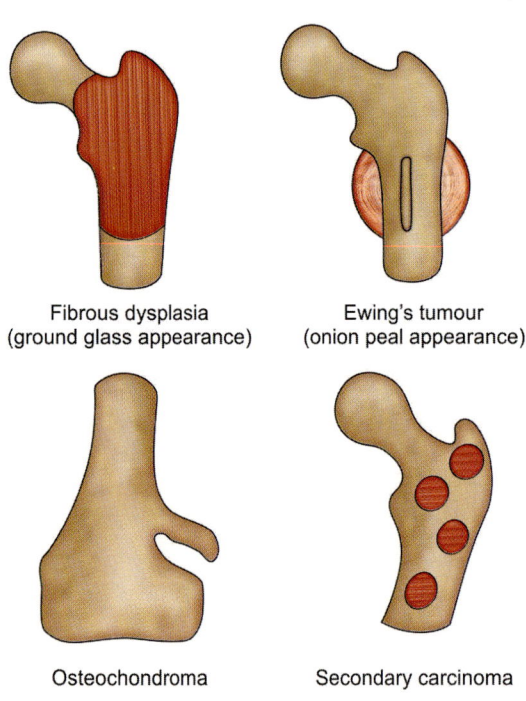

Fig. 12.24: Radiological appearances of some of the tumours of femur

18. Femur is the most common site of tumours of bones.
19. Bone tumours commonly involving the femur are *osteoclastoma, osteosarcoma, myeloma, Ewing's sarcoma* and *fibrous displasia*.
20. Most common site of *osteoclastoma* is the lower end of femur.

22. Recently femur has gained additional importance due to its surgical involvements during operations for *hip and knee replacements*.
23. Flexion, adduction, and internal rotation is the characteristic posture in *posterior dislocation of hip*.
24. Injury to the popliteal artery in fracture of lower end of femur is often due to distal segment pressing the artery.
25. **Klein's line:** It is a line along upper border of neck of femur in AP view of hip X-ray. Normally it passes through upper one third of head of femur. In case of slipped capital femoral epiphysis this line passes above the head of femur (Fig. 12.26).

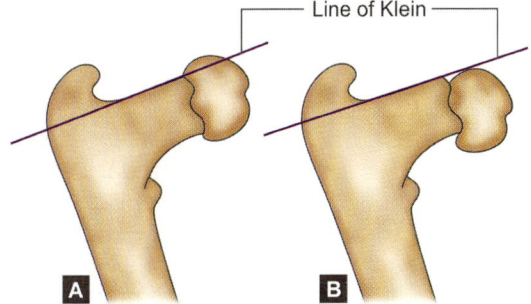

Fig. 12.26: Line of klein. (A) Normal; (B) Slipped capital femoral epiphysis, +ve Trethowan's sign i.e. line of Klein fails to intersect the epiphysis

26. **Pauwels' classification of fracture neck femur (Fig. 12.27):** This classification is based on the angle between fracture line and horizontal line. These are of three types:
    a. Type I : 30°
    b. Type II : 50°
    c. Type III: 70°

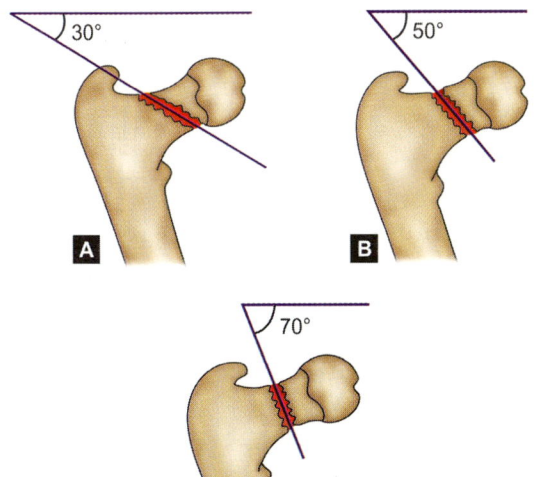

Fig. 12.27: Pauwels' classification of fracture neck femur. (A) Type I; (B) Type II; (C) Type III

27. Normally in a radiograph of hip, AP view, inferior margin of femoral neck and inferior border of superior ramus of pubis form a continuous curved line. This line is called *Shenton's line* (Fig. 12.28). This line is broken in case of *fracture neck femur* and *congenital dislocation of hip*.

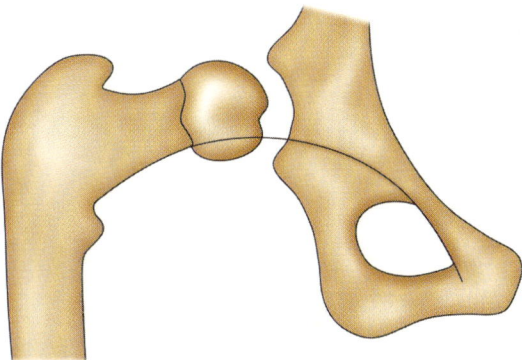

Fig. 12.28: Shenton's line

28. Differences between fracture neck femur and trochanteric fracture.

Features	Fracture neck femur	Trochanteric fracture
1. Age	After 50 years	After 60 years
2. Sex	Male	Female
3. Injury	Trivial	Significant
4. Pain	Mild	Severe
5. Swelling	Nil	Present
6. Tenderness	In Scarpa's triangle	On greater trochanter
7. External rotation	Less than 45°	More than 45°
8. Shortening	Less than 1 inch	More than 1 inch
9. Complication	Nonunion	Malunion

CHAPTER
13

The Patella

Patella is a Latin word which means 'little plate'. It is also named as, knee cap.

PECULIARITIES

1. Patella is a sesamoid bone developing in the tendon of quadriceps.
2. It is the largest sesamoid bone in the body.
3. It is situated in front of lower end of femur about 1 cm above the knee joint line.
4. It participates in the formation of knee joint.
5. It improves the leverage of quadriceps femoris by increasing the angulation of the line of pull of leg.
6. It lacks periosteum therefore patellectomy (removal of patella) is often a choice of treatment for fracture of patella as there is no chance for regeneration. Removal of patella does not hamper the movements at knee.

SIDE DETERMINATION (Fig. 13.1)

1. Patella is triangular in shape. Its base faces upwards while apex is downwards. Margins or borders are medial and lateral.
2. It has anterior and posterior surfaces. Posterior surface is marked by smooth articular surface.

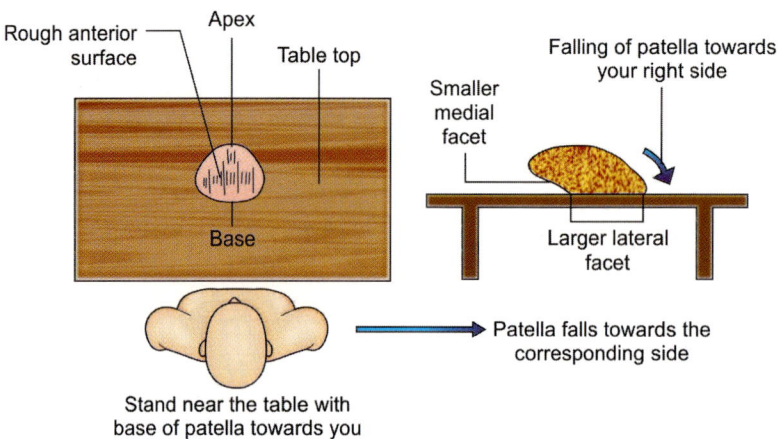

Fig. 13.1: Determination of side of patella by simple method

3. Articular surface is divided by a vertical ridge into medial and lateral parts. Lateral part is larger.

> **Note:** *Remember 'L' stands for Lateral area as well as Large and therefore Lateral area is Larger. Observe another very interesting phenomenon. Keep the articular surface of patella on the flat table top in such a way that its base is directed towards you and apex is directed away from you. Now observe the tilt of patella. The patella will always tilt towards the side to which it belongs.*

FEATURES AND ATTACHMENTS

Patella has an apex, three borders (superior, lateral and medial) and two surfaces (anterior and posterior).

I. Apex

Ligamentum patellae is attached to the margins of apex and lower part of the rough portion of posterior surface.

II. Borders

A. Superior border
1. It is also called *base*.
2. *Rectus femoris* is attached to its anterior part.
3. *Vastus intermedius* is attached to its posterior part.

B. Lateral border
Expansion of tendon of vastus lateralis (*lateral patellar retinaculum*) is attached to it.

C. Medial border
1. Expansion of tendon of vastus medialis (*medial patellar retinaculum*) is attached to it.
2. *Muscular fibres of vastus medialis* get attached directly to the medial border behind the medial patellar retinaculum.

III. Surfaces

A. Anterior surface (Fig. 13.2)
1. It is rough and convex.

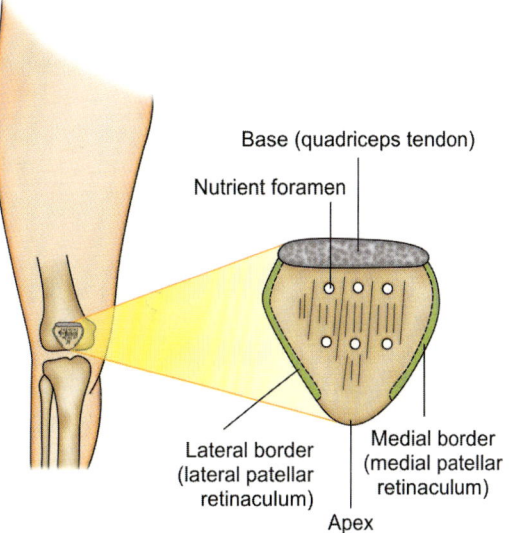

Fig. 13.2: Right patella: Anterior aspect

2. *Prepatellar bursa* intervenes between skin and anterior surface.
3. It is perforated by nutrient vessels.
4. It is covered by an *expansion from the quadriceps tendon*.

B. Posterior surface (Fig. 13.3)
1. Its lower 1/4th is rough and non-articular while upper 3/4th is smooth and articular.
2. Nonarticular part is divided into two areas:

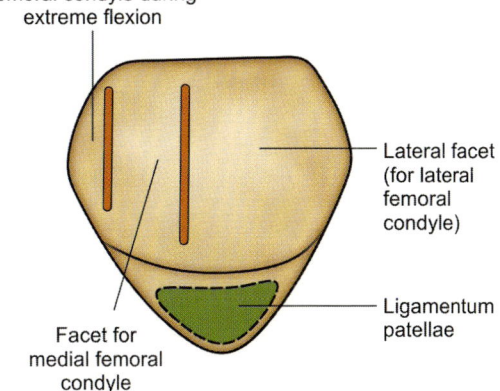

Fig. 13.3: Right patella : Posterior aspect

a. **Lower area** provides attachment to *ligamentum patellae*.
   b. **Upper area** is related to *infrapatellar pad of fat*.
3. A vertical ridge divides the articular area into a larger lateral area and a smaller medial area. The ridge itself occupies the groove in the patellar surface of femoral lower end in the extended position of knee. The larger lateral area lies in contact with the lateral femoral condyle in all positions of knee.
4. Medial area is separated from medial strip by another vertical ridge. Medial femoral condyle is related to the medial area during extension of knee and the medial strip during full flexion at knee (Fig. 13.4).

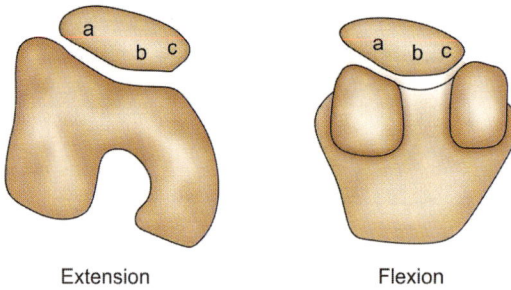

Fig. 13.4: Relations of right femoral condyles with patella in different positions at knee. (a) Lateral area; (b) Medial area; (c) Medial strip

OSSIFICATION

1. Several centres appear during 3–6 years.
2. Ossification of patella is completed at puberty.

APPLIED ANATOMY

1. There is a tendency in patella to displace laterally due to an oblique upward pull by the quadriceps (Fig. 13.5).
   There are three factors which counter this tendency to stabilize the patella.
   a. **Bony factor**
      Lateral femoral condyle projects more forwards than medial condyle (Fig. 13.6).

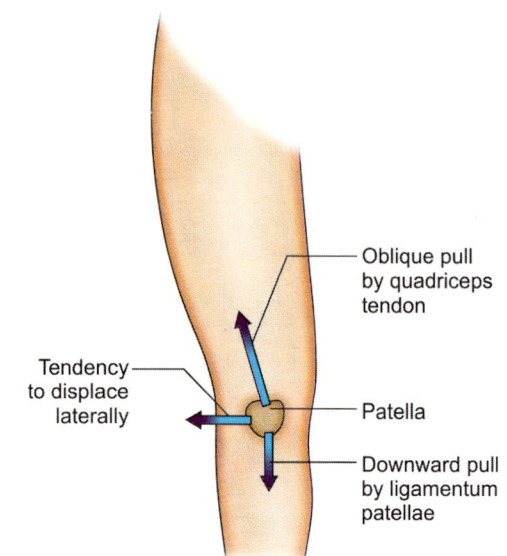

Fig. 13.5: Tendency of patella to displace laterally

   b. **Muscular factor**
      Muscle fibres of vastus medialis get attached directly to the medial border of patella. These fibres are called *vastus medialis obliquus* (Fig. 13.6).

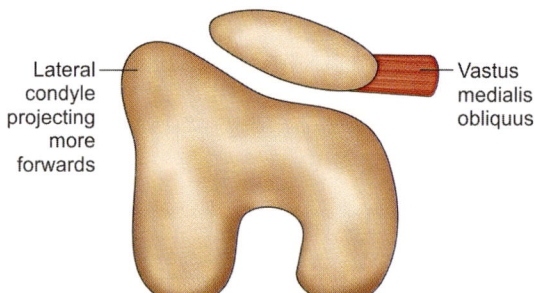

Fig. 13.6: Inferior view of right femoral condyles and patella

   c. **Ligamentous factor**
      Medial patellar retinaculum exerts a medial pull on patella.
2. Abnormal ossification centres in patella may give rise to one or two separate pieces of bone. Such patellae are called *bipartite* or *tripartite* respectively. This condition should not be confused with fracture of patella as the former is bilateral and symmetrical, with smooth margins (Fig. 13.7).

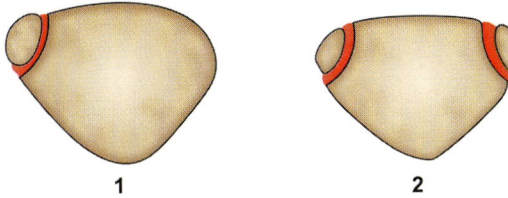

Fig. 13.7: Bipartite (1) and tripartite (2) patellae

3. **Chondromalacia patellae (Runner's knee)**
   In this case there is soreness and aching around and deep to patella. It occurs as a result of softening and fibrillation of the articular cartilage.
4. **Fractures of patella (Figs 13.8 and 13.9)**
   a. A direct blow fractures the patella into multiple pieces (*comminuted fracture*).
   b. Sudden and forceful contraction of quadriceps causes a *transverse fracture of patella*. It can be;
      i. *Undisplaced*
      ii. *Displaced*
   c. *Avulsion fracture*: It can be;
      i. At proximal pole
      ii. At distal pole
5. **Knee jerk**
   In this test patellar tendon is tapped and contraction of quadriceps is felt or seen.

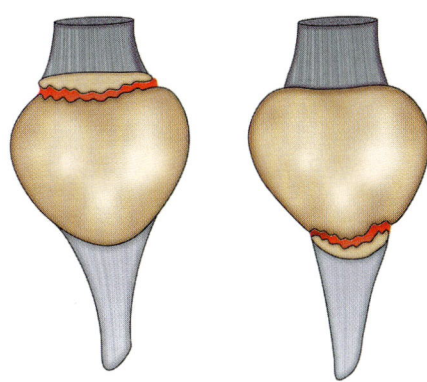

Fig. 13.9: Avulsion fractures of patella

Afferent impulses travel in femoral nerve to reach the spinal segments $L_{2, 3, 4}$. Efferent impulses reach the quadriceps through femoral nerve again.

6. Fractured segments of patella do not show displacement in radiograph if the quadriceps expansions and patellar retinacula remain intact.
7. The patella can be removed with little disability. Procedure is called *Patellectomy*. It can be total or partial.
8. **Recurrent dislocation of patella** is usually due to underlying abnormality, e.g. small or high patella and underdeveloped lateral condyle. High riding patella is called *patella aeta*.
9. **Extensor lag:** This is the inability of the patient to perform the last 5° to 10° of extension at knee. This is observed in patients undergone patellectomy (Fig. 13.10).

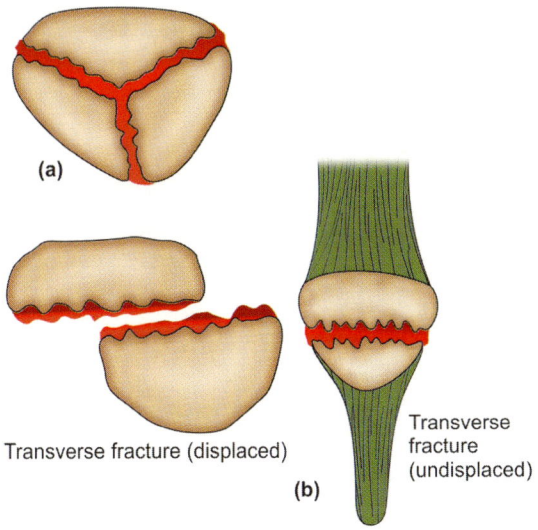

Fig. 13.8: Comminuted (a) and transverse (b) fractures of patella

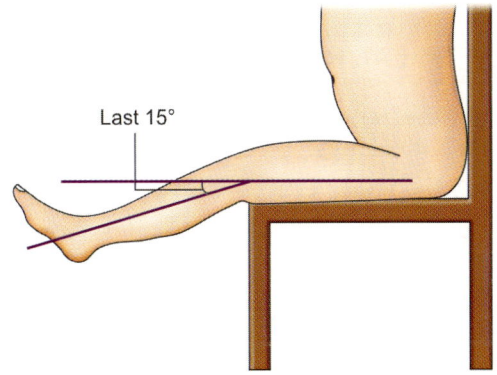

Fig. 13.10: Extensor lag at knee

CHAPTER 14
The Tibia

TERMINOLOGY

Tibia is also called *'shin-bone'*

PECULIARITIES

1. Tibia is the 2nd largest bone of body.
2. It is homologous with radius of forearm.
3. It is main weight bearing bone of leg in standing posture.

SIDE DETERMINATION

1. The broader end is the upper end of tibia.
2. A downward projection (*medial malleolus*) from the lower end is medial in position.
3. Keep the most prominent border of shaft anteriorly.

ANATOMICAL POSITION (Fig. 14.1)

1. Hold the bone in the hand of same side to which it belongs.
2. Keep the bone vertical.
3. *Tibial plateau* (superior surface of the upper end of tibia) lies in horizontal plane.

FEATURES AND ATTACHMENTS

Tibia consists of an upper end, a shaft and a lower end.

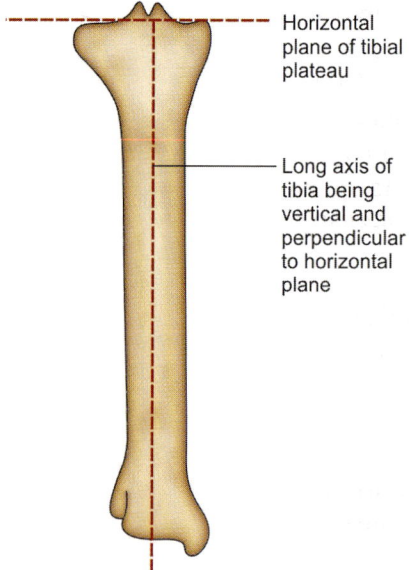

Fig. 14.1: Normal anatomical position of tibia

I. UPPER END (Fig. 14.2)

It has two condyles (medial and lateral), an intercondylar area and tibial tuberosity.

A. Medial condyle

It is comprised of 4 surfaces.

a. Superior surface

1. It is articular.
2. It is oval in shape with long axis directed anteroposteriorly.

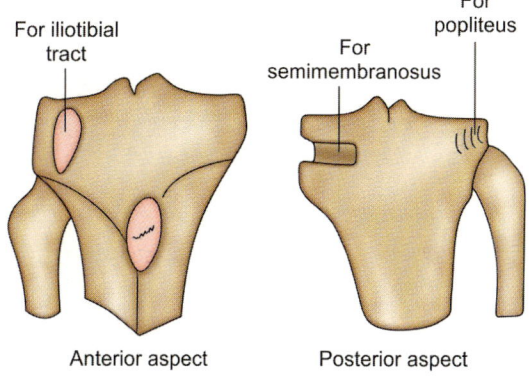

Fig. 14.2: Upper end of right tibia

3. Its central part is concave to articulate with the convex medial femoral condyle.
4. Its peripheral part is flattened for the *medial meniscus*.
5. Its lateral border extends over the *medial intercondylar tubercle*.
6. Its margins receive attachment of *capsular ligament of knee*.

b. Posterior surface

It is deeply grooved for the attachment of *tendon of semimembranosus*.

c. Anterior surface

d. Medial surface

Anterior and medial surfaces receive the attachment of *medial patellar retinaculum*.

B. Lateral condyle

Like medial condyle, lateral condyle also has 4 surfaces.

a. Superior surface

1. It is articular.
2. It is circular in shape.
3. Its central part is concave to articulate with the convex lateral femoral condyle.
4. Its peripheral part is flattened for the *lateral meniscus*.
5. Its medial border extends over the *lateral intercondylar tubercle*.

6. Its margins provide attachment to the *capsular ligament*.

b. Posterior surface

1. Inferolaterally, this surface shows a circular smooth articular facet for head of fibula.
2. Between the articular facet for fibula and margin of superior surface there is a shallow groove for tendon of popliteus.

c. Anterior surface

It has *flat triangular facet for the attachment of iliotibial tract*.

d. Lateral surface

Anterior and lateral surfaces receive attachment of *lateral patellar retinaculum*.

C. Intercondylar area (Fig. 14.3)

1. It is the roughened area between the superior articular surfaces of two tibial condyles.
2. The middle of intercondylar area is marked by an elevation called *intercondylar eminence* which is formed by two small tubercles called *medial* and *lateral intercondylar tubercles*.

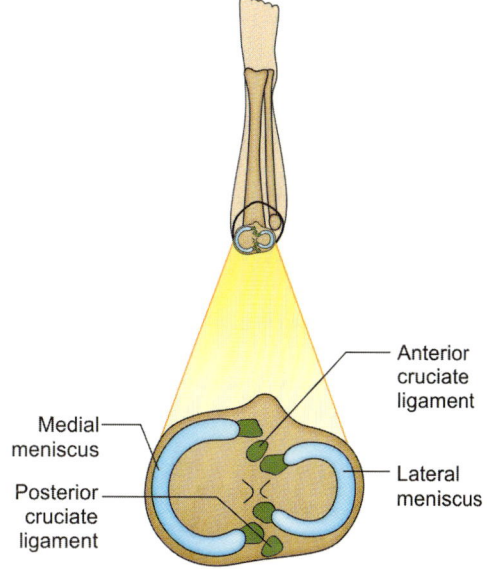

Fig. 14.3: Proximal articular surface of right tibia

3. Intercondylar eminence divides the intercondylar area into two parts.
   i. *Anterior intercondylar area.*
   ii. Posterior intercondylar area.
4. From before backwards, the intercondylar area provides attachments to following 6 structures, of which 3 are located in its anterior part and 3 in its posterior part:
   i. Anterior horn of medial meniscus.
   ii. Anterior cruciate ligament.
   iii. Anterior horn of lateral meniscus.
   iv. Posterior horn of lateral meniscus.
   v. Posterior horn of medial meniscus.
   vi. Posterior cruciate ligament.

Note: *To remember the sequence remember the rhyme "Medical College Lucknow, Lucknow Medical College. Also remember that both the Lucknow are together in the middle adjacent to intercondylar eminence.*

D. Tibial tuberosity

1. It is located on the anterior aspect and marks the upper end of anterior border of shaft.
2. It is divided into upper smooth and lower rough part.
3. *Ligamentum patellae* is attached to upper smooth part.
4. Lower rough part is related to subcutaneous *infrapatellar bursa* which separates it from the skin.
5. Epiphyseal line at the upper end of tibia passes between the smooth and rough parts of the tibial tuberosity

II. SHAFT (Figs 14.4 and 14.6 to 14.10)

It has 3 borders (anterior, medial and lateral) and 3 surfaces (lateral, medial and posterior).

A. Borders

a. Anterior border

1. It is sharpest.
2. It extends from tibial tuberosity to anterior border of medial malleolus.
3. It is also called *shin*.
4. It is subcutaneous.
5. *Deep fascia* of leg is attached to it.
6. *Superior extensor retinaculum* of ankle is attached to its lower part.

b. Medial border

1. It extends from medial condyle to the posterior border of medial malleolus.
2. *Soleal line* (a roughened ridge on the posterior surface) joins the medial border at the junction of its upper 1/3rd with the lower 2/3rd.
3. Medial border above the soleal line receives attachment of *fascia covering the popliteus.*
4. Below the soleal line medial border provides attachments to (Fig. 14.5):
   i. *Deep fascia of leg.*
   ii. *Soleus in its upper part.*
   iii. *Deep transverse fascia.*

c. Lateral (interosseous) border

1. It extends from lateral condyle to the anterior border of fibular notch.
2. *Interosseous membrane* is attached to it.
3. *Anterior tibiofibular ligament* is attached to the lower end of lateral border.

B. Surfaces

a. Lateral surface

1. It is between anterior and interosseous borders.
2. Its upper 2/3rd receives attachment of *tibialis anterior.*
3. Its lower 1/3rd is crossed by following structures from medial to lateral.
   i. *Tibialis anterior.*
   ii. *Extensor hallucis longus.*
   iii. *Anterior tibial artery.*
   iv. *Deep peroneal nerve.*
   v. *Extensor digitorum longus.*
   vi. *Peroneus tertius.*
4. *Superior extensor retinaculum* covers the lower part of the lateral surface.

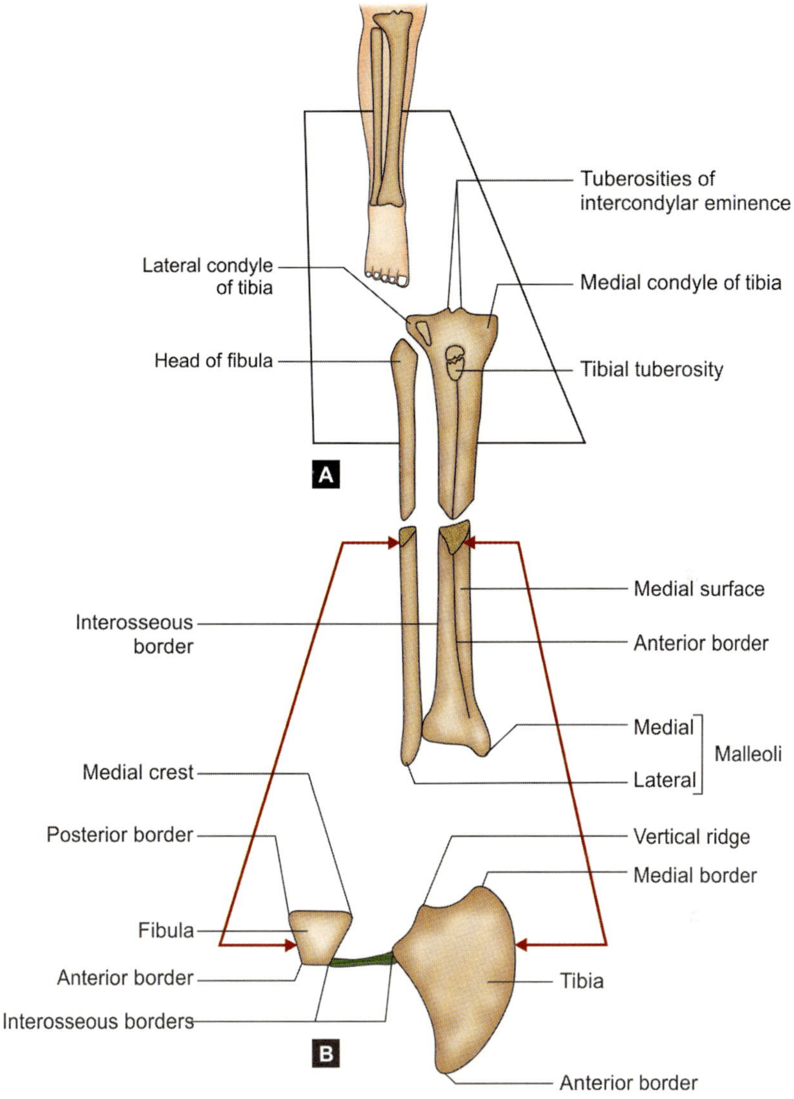

Fig. 14.4: Tibia and fibula. (A) Anterior aspect; (B) Cross section

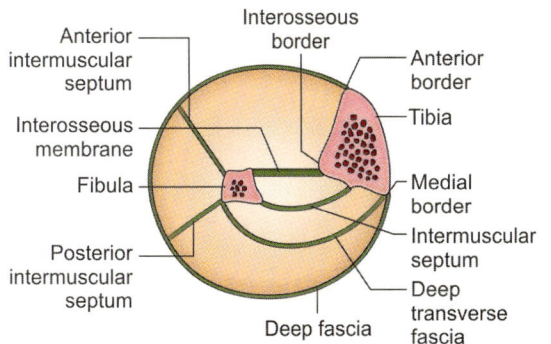

Fig. 14.5: Osseofascial compartments of leg

b. Medial surface

1. It is between anterior and medial borders.
2. It is mostly subcutaneous.
3. Its upper part receives attachments of following structures from before backwards:
    i. *Sartorius*
    ii. *Gracilis*
    iii. *Semitendinosus*
    iv. *Tibial collateral ligament*

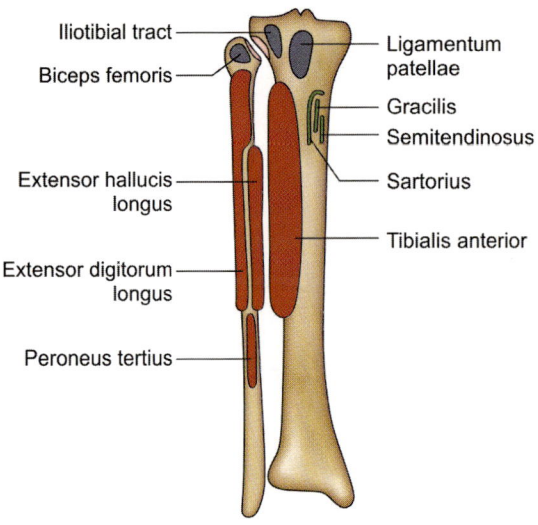

Fig. 14.6: Right tibia and fibula: Anterior aspect

Note: *To remember the names of three muscles attached to the upper part of medial surface of tibia, one can remember "General between two Sergeants".*

4. *Great saphenous vein* is related to lower 1/3rd of medial surface.

c. Posterior surface

1. It is between medial and lateral borders.
2. There is a roughened ridge extending from fibular facet to the junction of upper and middle 3rd of the medial border. This is named as *soleal line*. This line gives attachments to following structures from above downwards (Fig. 14.9):
    i. *Fascia covering popliteus.*
    ii. *Fascia covering soleus.*
    iii. *Soleus (origin).*
    iv. *Deep transverse fascia.*

    The *tendinous arch* for origin of soleus is attached to a tubercle at the upper end of soleal line.
3. A triangular area above the soleal line provides attachment to *popliteus*.

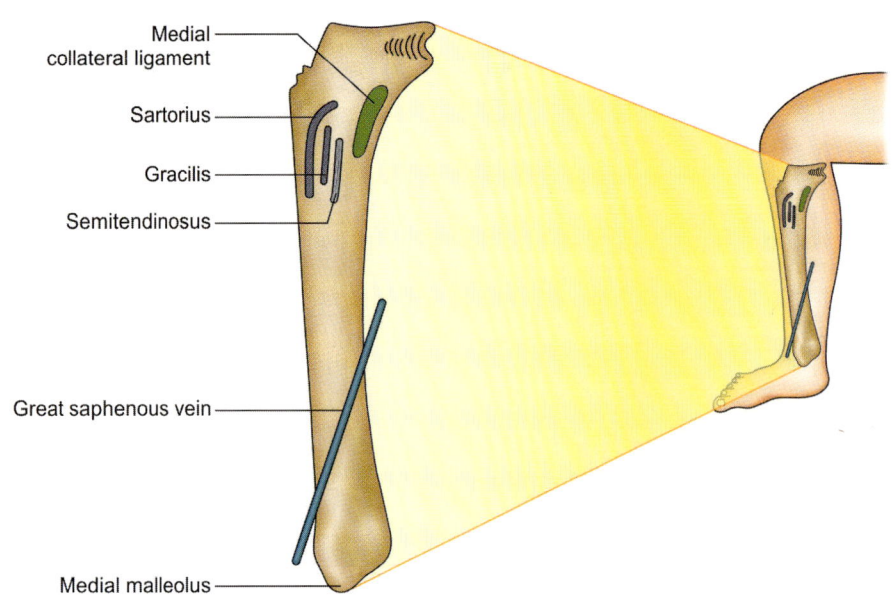

Fig. 14.7: Right tibia : Medial aspect

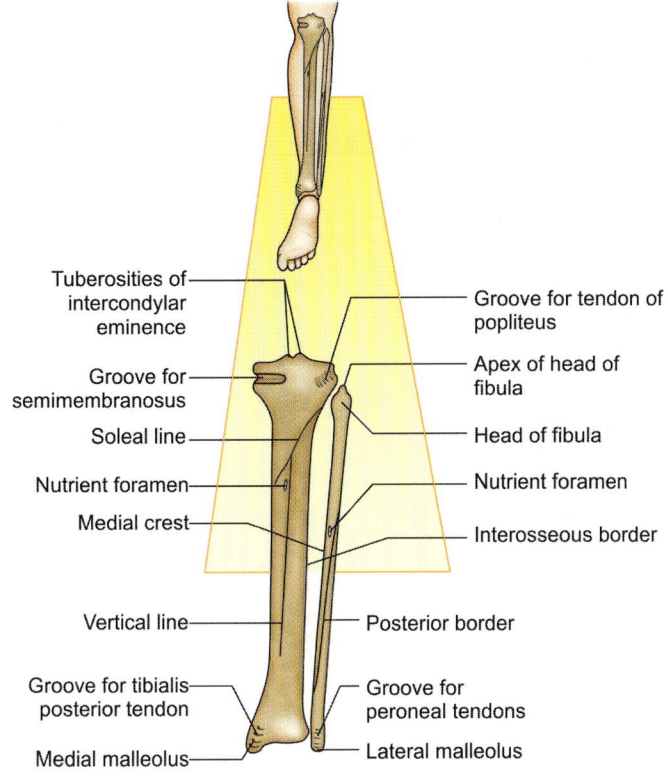

Fig. 14.8: Right tibia and fibula: Posterior aspect

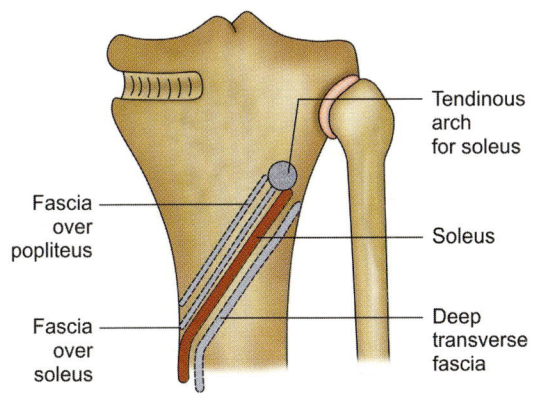

Fig. 14.9: Attachments to soleal line

4. The area below the soleal line is divided into a medial and a lateral parts by a vertical line which itself receives attachment of *fascia covering the tibialis posterior*.

5. *Nutrient foramen* is situated at the upper end of vertical line. Nutrient canal is directed downwards i.e. away from the knee. Thus the upper end is the growing end of bone. *Nutrient artery*, a branch of posterior tibial artery, is the largest nutrient artery of the body.
6. *Flexor digitorum longus* is attached to the medial area below the soleal line.
7. *Tibialis posterior* is attached to the lateral area below the soleal line.
8. Lower 1/4th of the posterior surface is related to following structures from medial to lateral:
   i. Tibialis posterior.
   ii. Posterior tibial vessels.
   iii. Tibial nerve.
   iv. Flexor hallucis longus.

Human Osteology

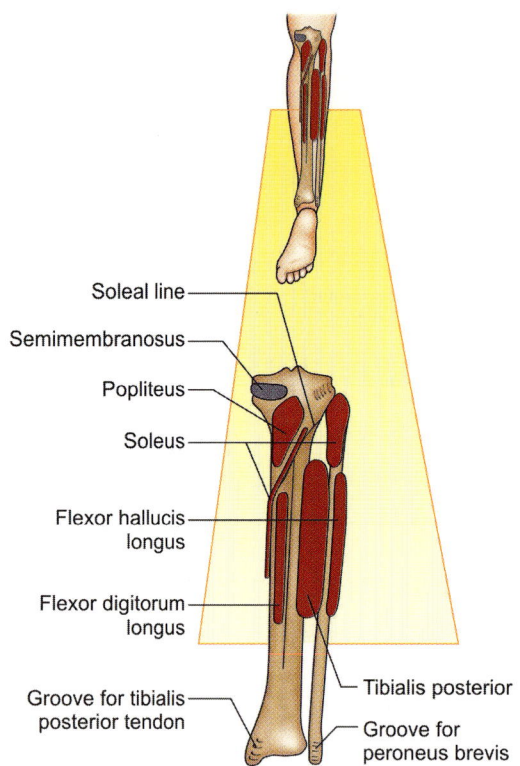

Fig. 14.10: Right tibia and fibula: Posterior aspect

Note: *Flexor digitorum longus tendon is separated from the bone by tendon of tibialis posterior.*

III. LOWER END

It has 5 surfaces (anterior, posterior, medial, lateral and inferior) and a downward projection from the medial part called medial malleolus.

A. Surfaces

a. Anterior surface

1. It extends beyond inferior surface.
2. It is separated from the inferior surface by a groove.
3. This groove receives attachment of anterior part of *capsule of ankle joint*.
4. Anterior surface above the groove is related to following structures from medial to lateral:

   i. *Tibialis anterior.*
   ii. *Extensor hallucis longus.*
   iii. *Anterior tibial artery.*
   iv. *Deep peroneal nerve.*
   v. *Extensor digitorum longus.*
   vi. *Peroneus tertius.*

Note: *For remembering this sequence remember the rhyme "The Himalayas Are Not Dry Plateaus.*

b. Posterior surface

1. Its lower margin receives attachment of posterior part of *capsule of ankle joint*.
2. Area above the lower margin is related to following structures from medial to lateral:

   i. *Tibialis posterior.*
   ii. *Flexor digitorum longus.*
   iii. *Posterior tibial artery.*
   iv. *Tibial nerve.*
   v. *Flexor hallucis longus.*

Note: *For remembering this sequence remember the rhyme "The Doctors Are Not Hunters".*

c. Medial surface

1. It is subcutaneous.
2. It continues downwards as medial surface of medial malleolus.

d. Lateral surface

1. It forms the *fibular notch*.
2. Its anterior and posterior margins provide attachments to *anterior and posterior tibiofibular ligaments* respectively.
3. *Interosseous tibiofibular ligament* is attached to its upper rough part between anterior and posterior tibiofibular ligaments.
4. Its lower 4 mm is smooth and related to an upward prolongation of synovial membrane of talocrural (ankle) joint.

e. Inferior surface

1. It articulates with superior articular surface of talus to form *talocrural (ankle) joint*.

2. Medially it continues as the articular surface of medial malleolus.

B. Medial malleolus
It has 4 surfaces (anterior, posterior, medial and lateral) and an inferior border.

a. Anterior surface
Capsular ligament of ankle joint is attached to it.

b. Posterior surface
1. It is grooved by *tendon of tibialis posterior*.
2. Medial margin of groove gives attachment to the *flexor retinaculum*.

c. Medial surface
It is subcutaneous.

d. Lateral surface
It has a comma shaped facet for articulation with the malleolar facet on the medial surface of talus.

e. Inferior border
It provides attachment to capsular ligament and *deltoid ligament* of the ankle joint.

CAPSULAR ATTACHMENTS (Fig. 14.11)

At the upper end, capsule is attached to the margins of tibial plateau medially, laterally and posteriorly. Anteriorly the capsule blends with patellar retinacula and is indirectly attached to anterior surfaces of tibial condyles.

At the lower end the capsule is attached to the margins of articular surfaces except laterally where it shifts over the lower end of fibula.

OSSIFICATION

A. Primary centre
One centre appears for the shaft at the age of 8th week of intrauterine life.

B. Secondary centres
Two in all, one for upper end and one for lower end.

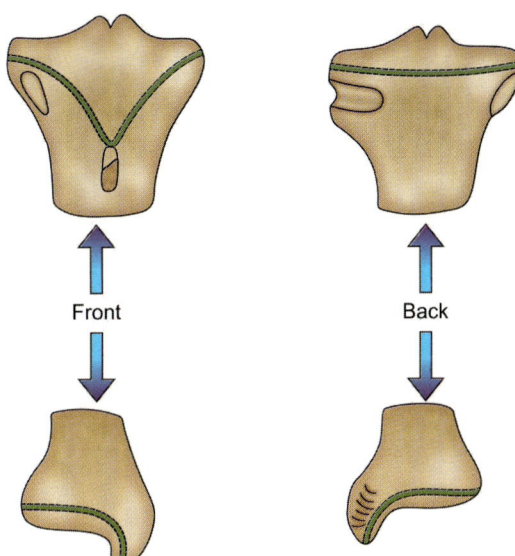

Fig. 14.11: Capsular attachments of right tibia

a. Upper end
Appearance : At birth
Fusion : 20 years

b. Lower end
Appearance : 2 years
Fusion : 18 years

APPLIED ANATOMY

1. *Osteomyelitis* commonly involves upper end of tibia. The knee joint is usually spared from simultaneous involvement as the metaphysis is extracapsular (Fig. 14.12).
2. Since the shaft of tibia is unprotected medially throughout its course and is relatively slender at the junction of upper 2/3rd with the lower 1/3rd, this bone is said to be one of the most common long bones to be fractured. Due to same reason it usually suffers compound injury.
3. If the nutrient canal is involved during fracture of tibia, it predisposes to nonunion due to damage of nutrient artery.

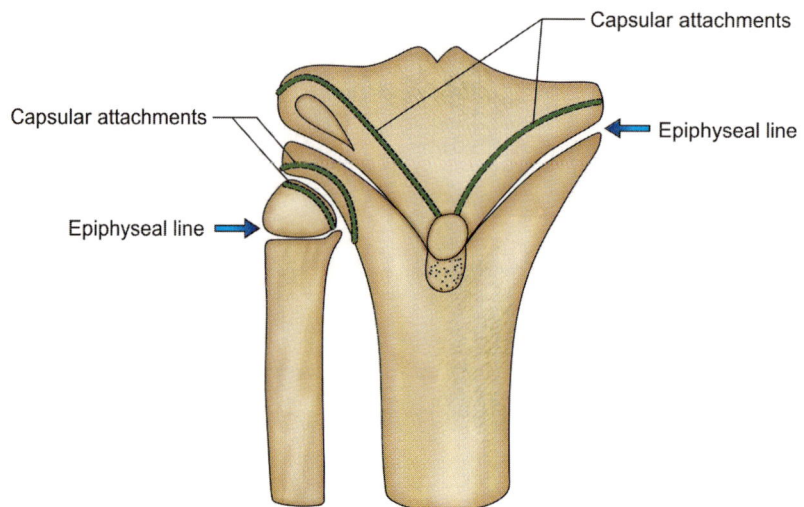

Fig. 14.12: Interrelationship of capsular attachments and epiphyseal lines at the upper ends of right tibia and fibula: Anterior aspect

4. The junction of lower 1/3rd of the shaft with middle 1/3rd is narrowest and therefore the commonest site for fracture.
5. *Rickets* (a disease of infancy and childhood because of 'Ca' deficiency in the body) particularly shows its effect on the tibia which bends due to inadequate calcification leading to bow legs. This effect is maximum at the narrowest site, i.e. junction of middle 3rd with the lower 3rd.
6. *Spiral fracture* of tibia is due to rotatory force applied on it when the foot is firmly applied on the ground, a situation commonly faced by football players. Again the site of fracture is the junction of middle 3rd and lower 3rd.
7. Fracture of tibia may also be due to direct blow e.g. a direct strike by the bumper of a car. Such fractures are rightly called as "bumper fractures". It is a fracture of tibial condyles (Fig. 14.13).
8. Lower third of tibial shaft is bare as there is no attachment of muscle or tendon, and the blood supply is relatively low. Fracture in this region therefore may show delayed union or nonunion.

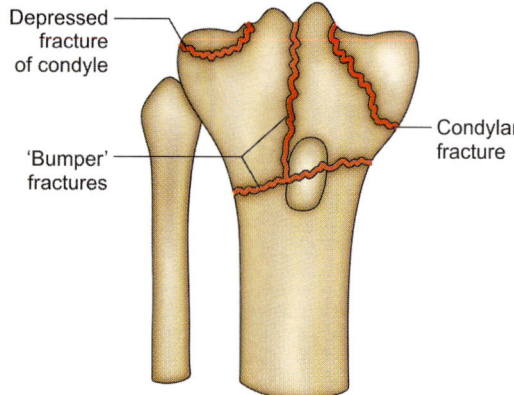

Fig. 14.13: Some common fractures at the upper end of tibia

9. Due to extensive subcutaneous surface of tibia it is easily accessible for examination as well as obtaining bone for grafting.
10. Some of the common fractures in the region of ankle involving lower end of tibia are as follows:
    a. External rotation injuries **(Fig. 14.14)**
    Truely speaking it is an inversion injury. Since inversion is associated with external rotation of talus, such

injuries are also called external rotation injuries.

Depending upon the severity of injury, following is the order of fractures:

i. Fracture of lateral malleolus.
ii. Fracture of medial malleolus.
iii. Fracture of posterior margin of articular surface of tibia i.e. third malleolus.

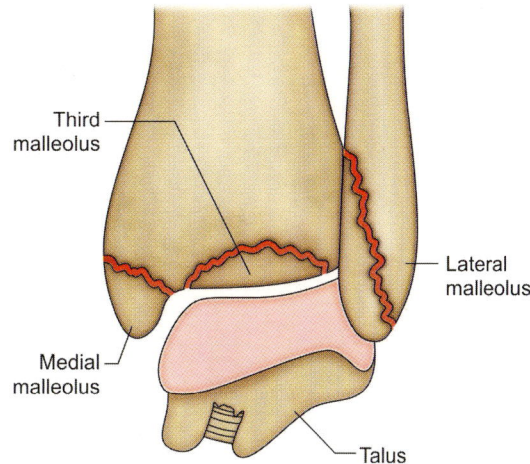

Fig. 14.15: Cotton's (Trimalleolar fracture) due to external rotation injuries

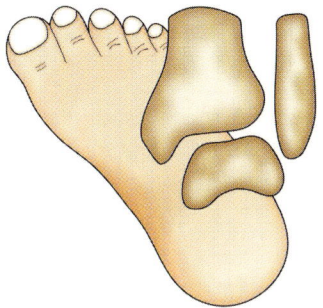

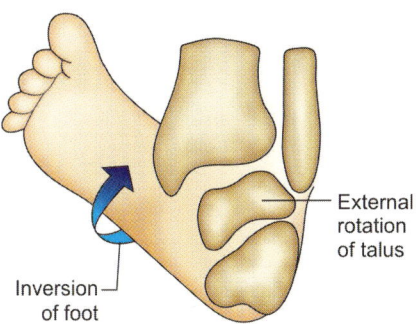

Fig. 14.14: External rotation injuries

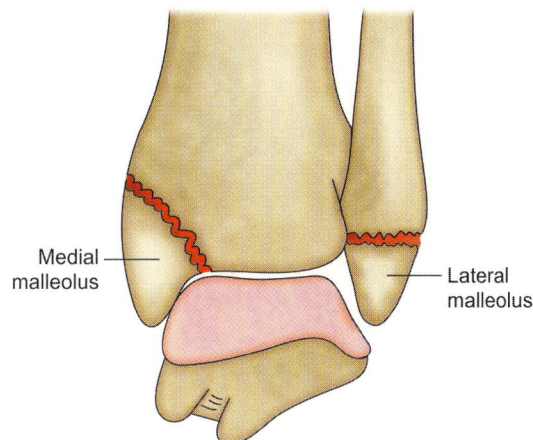

Fig. 14.16: Pott's fracture (Bimalleolar fracture) due to adduction injuries

When fractures occur at all the above mentioned 3 sites, then this is named as trimalleolar fracture or Cotton's fracture (Fig. 14.15). Bimalleolar fracture is Pott's fracture (Fig. 14.16).

b. Adduction injuries

In this case the foot is fixed and talus moves medially knocking off the medial malleolus and pulling off the lateral malleolus (Fig. 14.16).

c. Abduction injuries

In this case again the foot is fixed and talus moves laterally breaking both the malleoli in such a way that the fractures are horizontal at the level of joint (Fig. 14.17).

d. Vertical compression fracture

In this case the talus pushes the lower end of tibia upwards leading to fracture of articular surface (Fig. 14.18).

11. *Paget's disease* particularly involves skull and tibia where bones become more spongy, broader and weaker. Bending

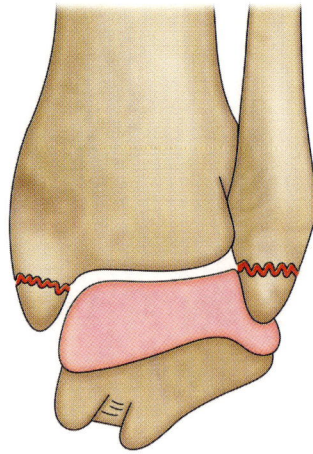

Fig. 14.17: Pott's fracture (Bimalleolar fracture) due to abduction injuries

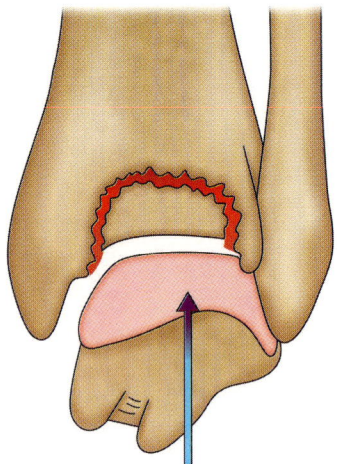

Vertical force from below

Fig. 14.18: Vertical compression fracture

and pathological fractures are common in tibia.

12. Following tumours of bone preferentially involve the bones in the region of knee and therefore upper end of tibia.

   i. *Osteoclastoma.*
   ii. *Osteosarcoma.*
   iii. *Synovial sarcoma.*
   iv. *Chondrosarcoma.*

13. *Genu valgum* (knock knee) and *genu varum* (bow legs):

   In some diseases like *rickets* or *Blount's disease*, the tibia bends abnormally to produce deformities. *Genu valgum* is outward curving of tibia and *genu varum* is inward curving of tibia (Fig. 14.19).

14. Pain in the shin may occur due to over exertion, *stress fracture* and *anterior tibial compartment syndrome.*

15. *Paratrooper's fracture:* It is a fracture of posterior articular margin of tibia with or without malleolar fracture.

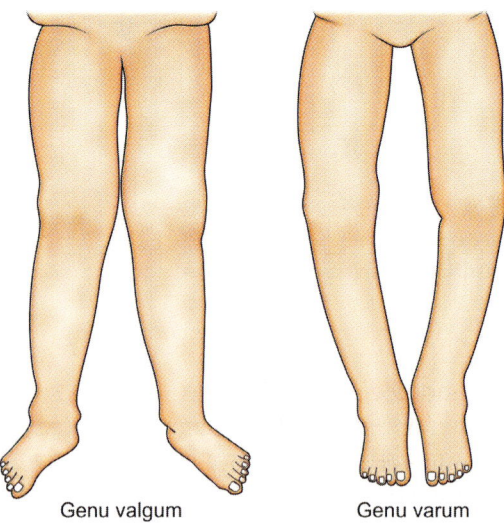

Genu valgum   Genu varum

Fig. 14.19: Genu valgum and varum deformities

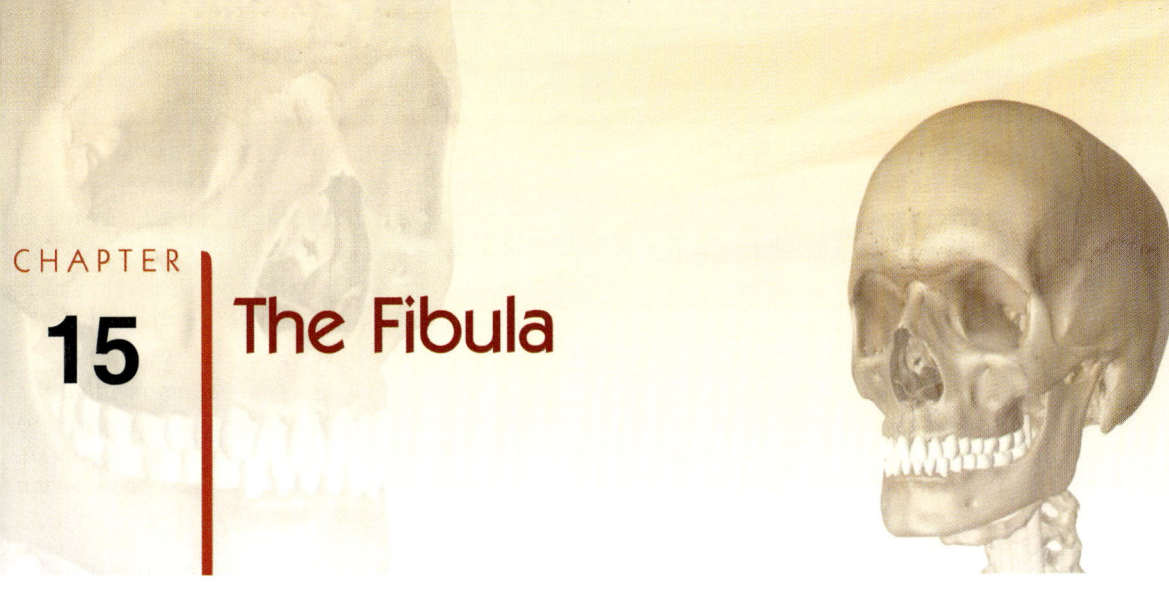

CHAPTER 15
The Fibula

TERMINOLOGY

Fibula is a Latin word which means 'pin'. It is rightly named so because it is a long pin like bone.

PECULIARITIES

1. It is the lateral bone of leg.
2. It is homologous with ulna.
3. It is smaller of the two bones of leg.
4. Although fibula does not take part in transmission of body weight, it is very important for stability of ankle joint.

SIDE DETERMINATION (Fig. 15.1)

1. Rounded end of bone is called head which is always superior.
2. The lower end is relatively flattened. It is marked by a triangular articular facet which faces medially.
3. A depression (*malleolar fossa*) at the lower end is posterior to triangular articular facet.

Note: *Proper placement of malleolar fossa will help you in determining the side of fibula. Keep the fibula on the lateral side of leg in such a way that malleolar fossa faces downwards, backwards and medially.*

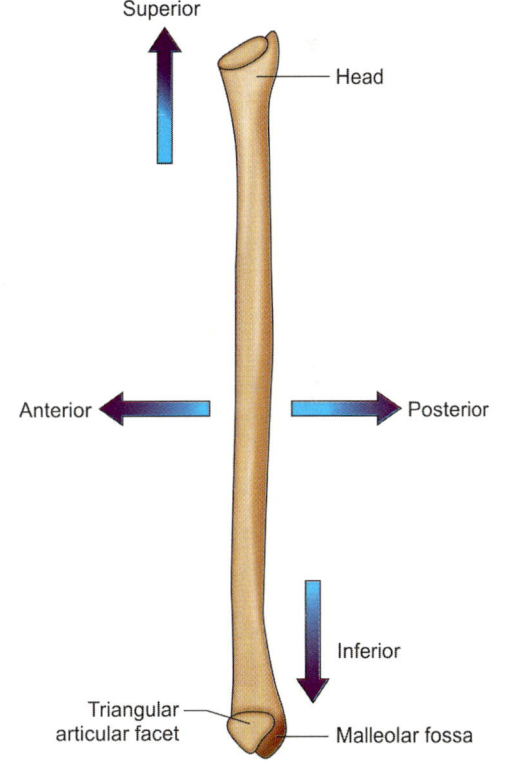

Fig. 15.1: Right fibula: Medial aspect

NORMAL ANATOMICAL POSITION

Hold the bone vertically with the hand of corresponding side keeping in the mind the direction of malleolar fossa.

FEATURES AND ATTACHMENTS
(Figs 15.2 and 15.4 to 15.8)

Fibula has an upper end, a shaft and a lower end.

I. UPPER END (Fig. 15.3)

1. It is also called *head* of fibula.
2. Its superior surface bears a circular articular facet which faces superiorly and antero- medially. It articulates with lateral condyle of tibia to form *superior tibiofibular* joint. Its margin provides attachment to capsule of this joint.
3. *Styloid process* is an upward projection from the posterolateral aspect of the head.
4. Front of styloid process provides attachment to the *fibular callateral ligament*.
5. Areas anterior, lateral and posterior to attachment of fibular callateral ligament

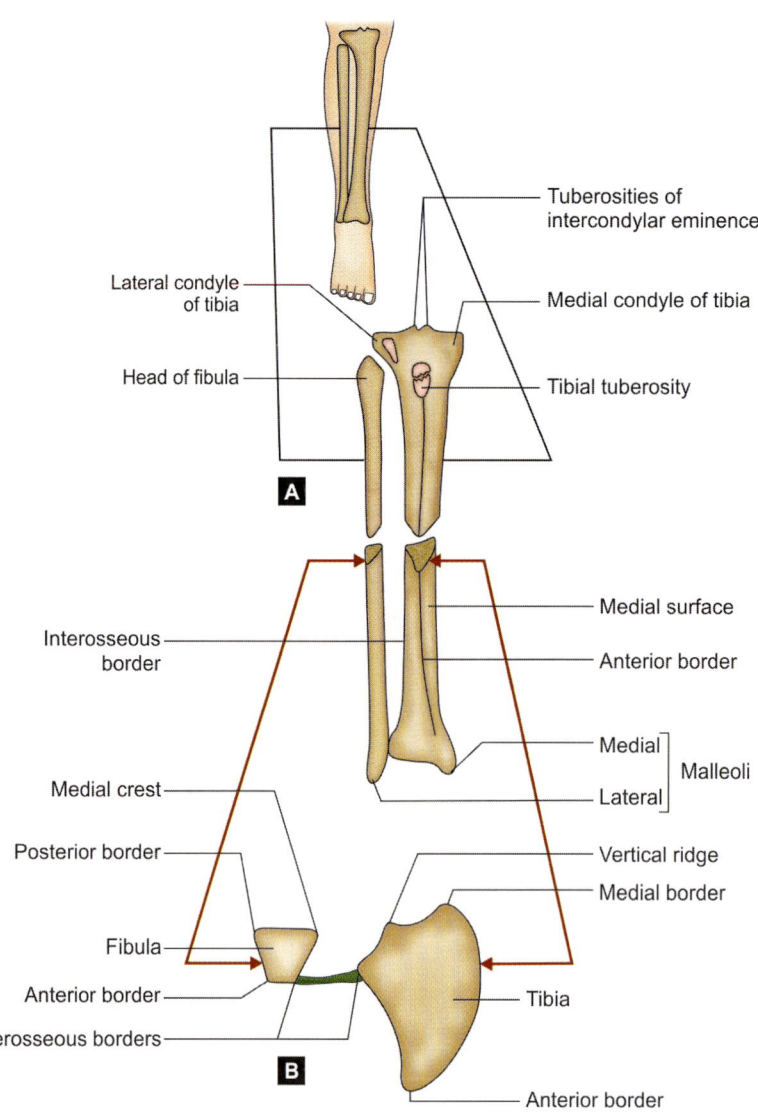

Fig. 15.2: Right tibia and fibula. (A) Anterior aspect; (B) Cross section

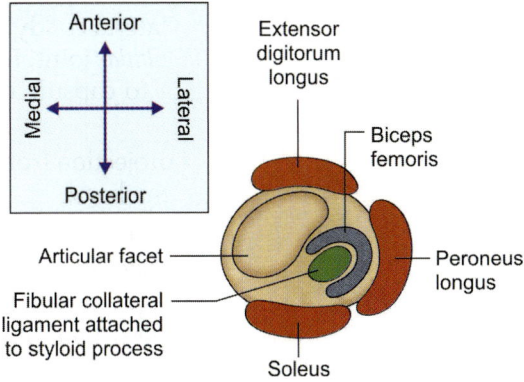

Fig. 15.3: Head of right fibula: Superior aspect

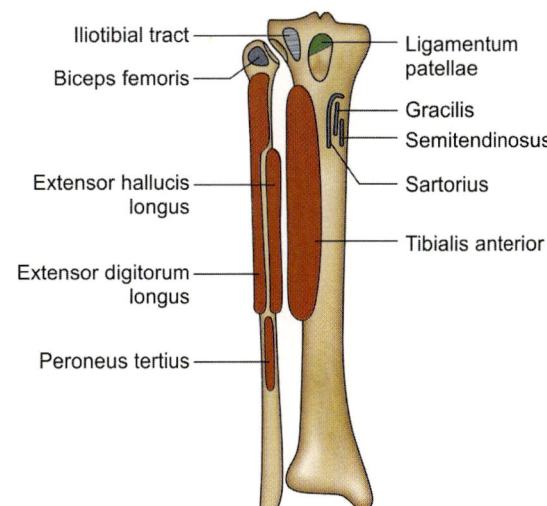

Fig. 15.5: Right tibia and fibula: Anterior aspect

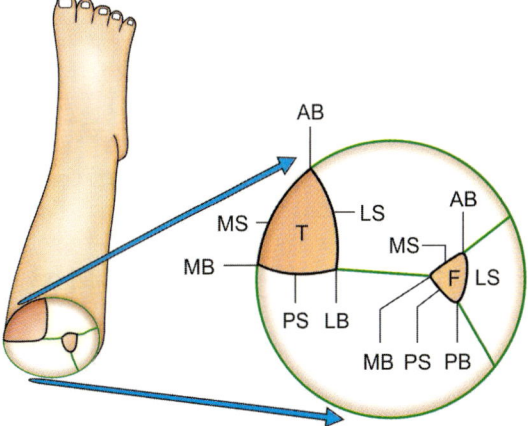

Fig. 15.4: Cross sectional views of tibia and fibula. (T) Tibia; (F) Fibula; (AB) Anterior border; (MB) Medial border, (PB) Posterior border; (LB) Lateral border; (MS) Medial surface; (LS) Lateral surface; (PS) Posterior surface

form a 'C' shaped attachment of *biceps femoris*.

6. *Extensor digitorum longus, peroneus longus* and *soleus* are attached to anterior, lateral and posterior surfaces of head respectively.
7. *Common peroneal nerve* is related to posterolateral aspect of neck (lower limit of head) of fibula.

II. SHAFT

It has 3 borders (anterior, posterior and medial) and 3 surfaces (medial, lateral and posterior).

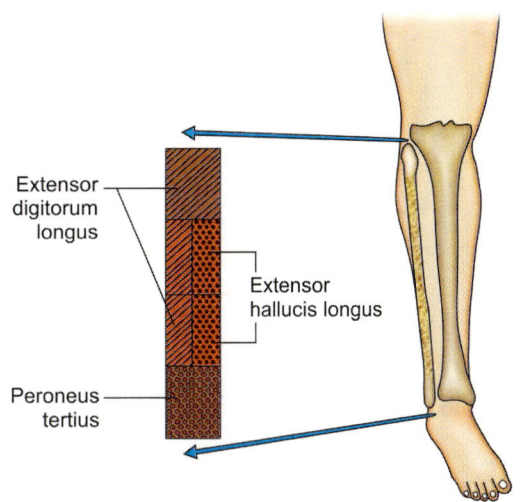

Fig. 15.6: Muscular attachments to the medial surface of right fibula

A. Borders

a. Anterior border

1. Anterior intermuscular septum of leg is attached to the upper 3/4th of anterior border.
2. Inferiorly it splits to enclose a triangular area which continues with lateral surface of lateral malleolus.
3. *Superior extensor retinaculum* is attached to the anterior margin of the triangular area.

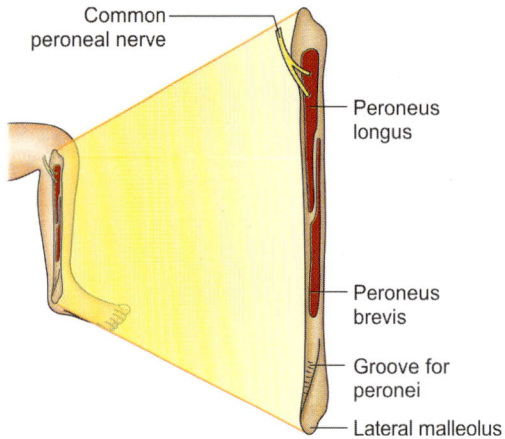

Fig. 15.7: Right fibula : Lateral aspect

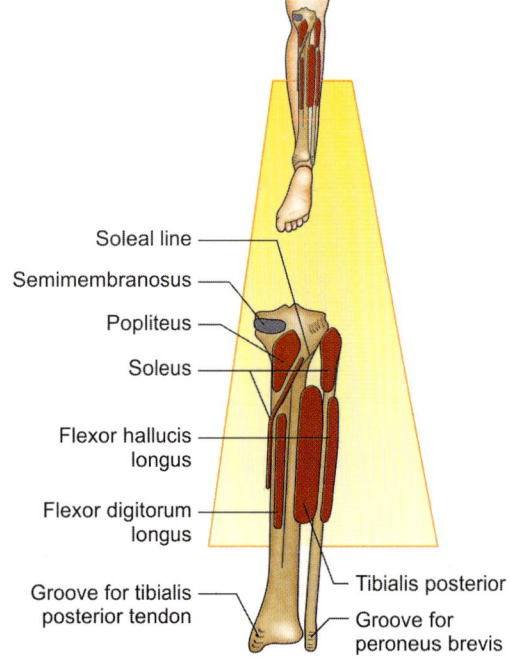

Fig. 15.8: Right tibia and fibula : Posterior aspect

4. *Superior peroneal retinaculum* is attached to the posterior margin of the triangular area.

b. Posterior border

1. It extends from the posterior aspect of head to the medial margin of groove on the back of lower end of fibula.

2. *Posterior intermuscular septum* of leg is attached to its upper 3/4th.

c. Medial (interosseous) border

1. It lies close and just medial to the anterior border.
2. Inferiorly it ends at the upper end of the roughened area for the interosseous ligament.
3. *Interosseous membrane* is attached to it except at the upper end where a gap between tibia and fibula transmits the *anterior tibial vessels*.

B. Surfaces

a. Medial surface

1. It is between anterior and medial borders.
2. It is very narrow.
3. *Extensor digitorum longus* is attached to the whole of its upper fourth and anterior half of its middle 2/4th.
4. *Extensor hallucis longus* is attached to the posterior half of the middle 2/4th.
5. Its lower 1/4th receives attachment of *peroneus tertius*.

b. Lateral surface

1. It is between anterior and posterior borders.
2. *Peroneus longus* is attached to its upper 1/3rd and posterior half of the middle 1/3rd.
3. *Peroneus brevis* is attached to its lower 1/3rd and the anterior half of its middle 1/3rd.

c. Posterior surface

1. It is between medial (interosseous) border and the posterior border.
2. Its upper 2/3rd is divided into medial and lateral areas by a sharp vertical ridge termed as *medial crest*.
3. Fascia covering the tibialis posterior is attached to the medial crest.
4. Lower part of the posterior surface presents a rough triangular area whose

anterior margin, intermediate area and posterior margin provide attachments to *anterior tibiofibular, interosseous tibiofibular* and *posterior tibiofibular ligaments* respectively.

5. Medial area (grooved surface between medial crest and medial border) gives origin to *tibialis posterior*.
6. Upper 1/4th of the lateral area gives origin to *soleus*.
7. Lower 3/4th of the lateral area gives origin to *flexor hallucis longus*.
8. *Peroneal artery* descends in relation to medial crest.
9. *Nutrient artery*, a branch of peroneal artery, enters the nutrient foramen present just above the middle of the posterior surface.
10. Nutrient canal is directed downwards and therefore the upper end of fibula is growing end.

III. LOWER END (LATERAL MALLEOLUS) (Fig. 15.9)

Lateral malleolus is 0.5 cm lower than the medial malleolus.

> **Note:** *Remember that in case of bones of forearm, the styloid process of radius is lower than the styloid process of ulna. Therefore it can be said that the lateral bones of both, forearm and leg project more downwards than the medial bones*
>
> Lateral malleolus has four surfaces (medial, lateral, anterior and posterior) and an inferior border.

A. Surfaces

a. Medial surface

1. It bears a triangular articular surface anteriorly which articulates with talus.
2. More posteriorly there is *malleolar fossa*.
3. *Posterior tibiofibular ligament* is attached to the upper part of malleolar fossa.
4. Lower part of malleolar fossa receives attachment of *posterior talofibular ligament*.

b. Lateral surface

It is subcutaneous.

c. Anterior surface

It gives attachment to *anterior talofibular ligament*.

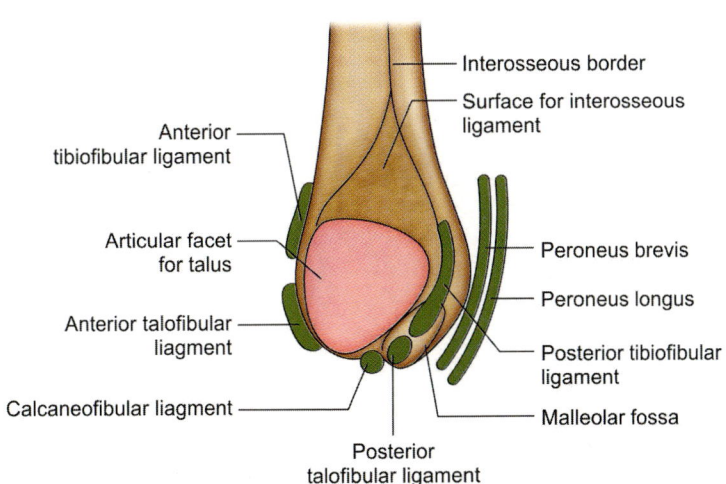

Fig. 15.9: Lower end of right fibula: Medial aspect

d. Posterior surface

1. It has a groove for *tendons of peroneus longus and peroneus brevis*. The former is more superficial.

> **Note:** *Imagine brevis as a child and longus as an adult, because a child has to be protected that is why it is deep in the groove.*

2. Lateral border of the groove gives attachment to *superior peroneal retinaculum*.

B. Inferior border

It presents a notch to which is attached *calcaneofibular ligament*.

OSSIFICATION

A. Primary centre

One centre appears for the shaft of fibula at 8th week of intrauterine life.

B. Secondary centres

Two in all, one for upper end and one for lower end.

a. Upper end

Appearance : 4 years
Fusion with shaft : 20 years

b. Lower end

Appearance : 2 years
Fusion with shaft : 18 years

> **Note:** *To remember the ossification of fibula, one can number the upper end as 420 and lower end as 218, i.e. times of appearance for upper end and lower end are 4 and 2 years respectively while fusion take place at 20 and 18 years respectively. Upper end is 420 in another sense also because it defies the law of ossification which states that the centre that appears first fuses last but in case of upper end of fibula, the centre appears late and fuses late as compared to lower end.*

APPLIED ANATOMY

1. Fibula is the common source of bone for *grafting* as it does not take part in weight transmission.
2. An injury to neck of fibula is most likely to injure the *common peroneal nerve*.
3. Position of nutrient foramen of fibula is important clinically. When obtaining a graft surgically, the periosteum and nutrient artery are generally removed with the piece of bone so that the graft will remain alive when transplanted to another site.
4. Isolated fracture of fibula is uncommon. However it can occur due to direct injury.
5. Both tibia and fibula are the sites for *stress fractures*. These usually occur in athletes who are undergoing training over long distances.
6. In cases of severe external rotation injuries, there is *Pott's fracture* which involves both the malleoli (bimalleolar fracture). In more severe cases 3rd malleolus may also be involved leading to trimalleolar fracture (Cotton's fracture) (Fig. 15.10).
7. In cases of *adduction injuries* the foot is fixed and the talus moves medially with great force knocking the medial malleolus and pulling off the lateral malleolus (Fig. 15.11).
8. In case of *abduction injuries* the foot is fixed and the talus tilts forcefully in the lateral direction breaking both the malleoli (Fig. 15.12).
9. Most commonly involved ligament in ankle sprain is the anterior talofibular ligament.
10. **Dupuytren's fracture** (Fig. 15.13)
    It includes the following:
    i. Fracture of medial malleolus (A) and distal fibula (B)

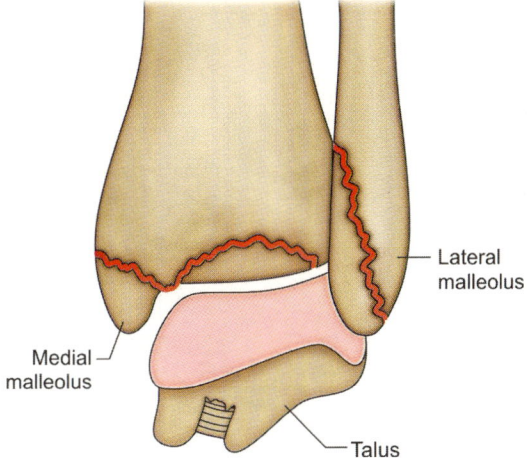

Fig. 15.10: Cotton's fracture due to external rotation injuries

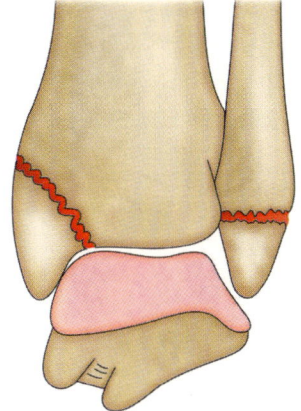

Fig. 15.11: Pott's fracture due to adduction injuries

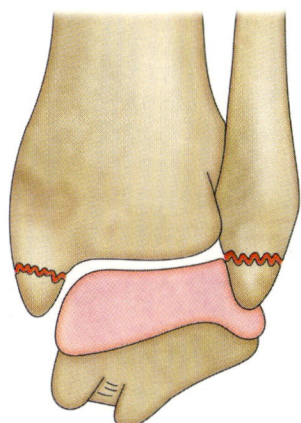

Fig. 15.12: Pott's fracture due to abduction injuries

ii. Rupture of deltoid ligament (C) and interosseous ligament of distal tibiofibular joint (D)
iii. Lateral subluxation of talus (E).

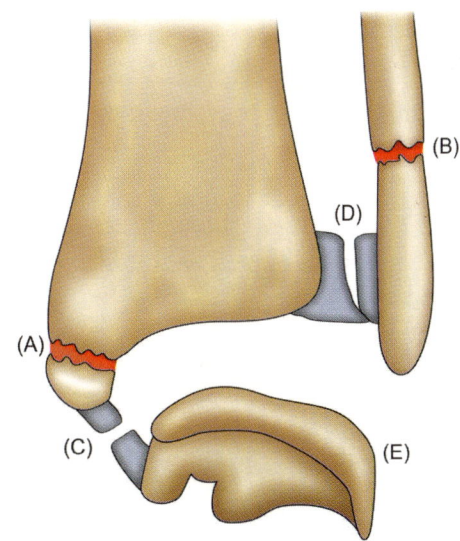

Fig. 15.13: Dupuytren's fracture. For explanation of letters (A to E) see literature

11. *Congenital absence of fibula* is more common than any other long bone of the body.

CHAPTER 16

The Tarsal Bones

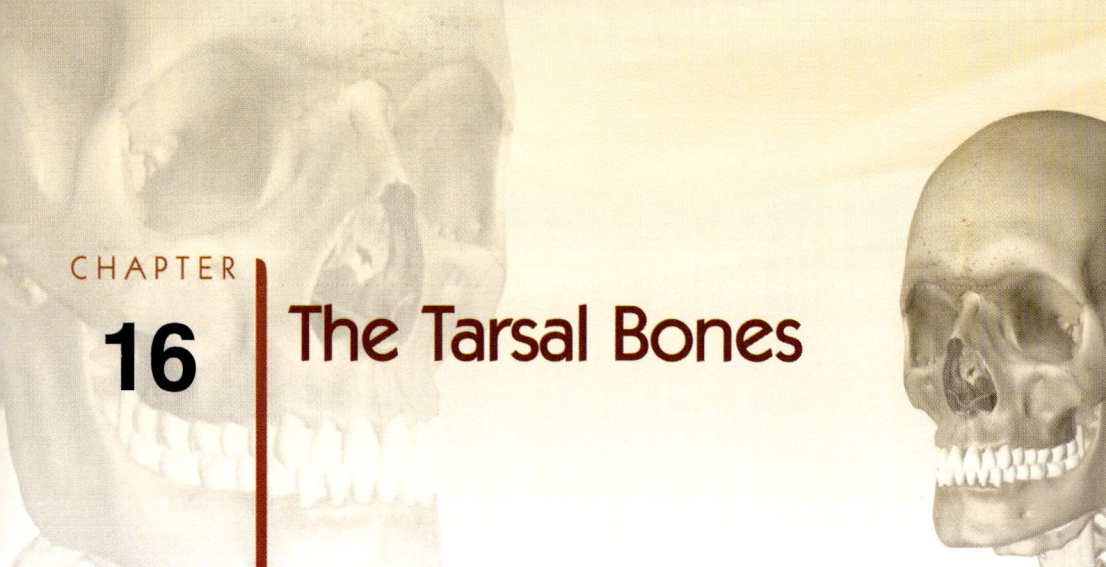

TARSUS

Seven tarsal bones together constitute the tarsus.

NAMES

7 tarsal bones are named as follows:
1. Talus.
2. Calcaneus.
3. Navicular bone
4. Cuboid bone
5. Medial cuneiform.
6. Intermediate cuneiform.
7. Lateral cuneiform.

Talus and calcaneus form *proximal tarsal row*. Cuboid bone and three cuneiforms constitute the *distal tarsal row*. Navicular bone lies between the two rows.

IDENTIFICATION OF TARSAL BONES IN FOOT SKELETON (Figs 16.1 and 16.2)

1. *Calcaneus* is the largest tarsal bone. It forms heel and is located below the talus.
2. *Talus* is the second largest tarsal bone. It rests over the superior aspect of calcaneus. It has a head which is directed forwards and medially.
3. *Navicular* bone is identified on the basis of deep concavity on the proximal surface which meets with the talar head.
4. *Cuboid* bone. is the next distal bone in the line of calcaneus.
5. *Cuneiforms* are the 3 small tarsal bones arranged from side to side along the distal surface of the navicular bone.

INDIVIDUAL TARSAL BONES

I. THE TALUS

Nomenclature

Talus is a Latin word meaning "ankle bone".

Peculiarities

1. It is the second largest tarsal bone.
2. There is no muscular attachment to this bone.
3. It participates in the formation of three joints, i.e. talocrural (ankle), talocalcaneal (subtalar) and talocalcaneonavicular.

Side determination

1. Keep the rounded head forwards.
2. Keep the trochlear articular surface (which is convex anteroposteriorly and concave from side to side) upwards.
3. Each side has got an articular surface. The one which is triangular, faces laterally while the comma shaped articular facet is directed medially.

The Tarsal Bones

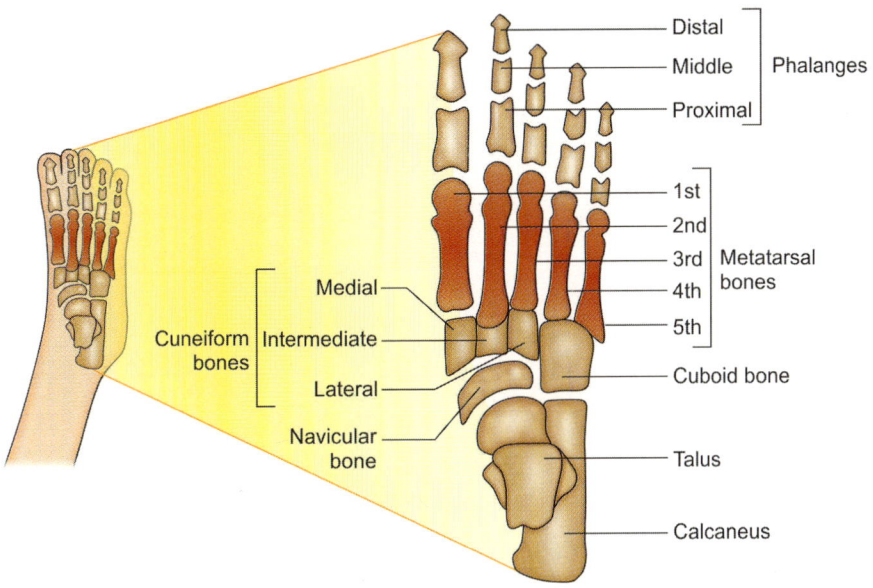

Fig. 16.1: Skeleton of the right foot : Dorsal aspect

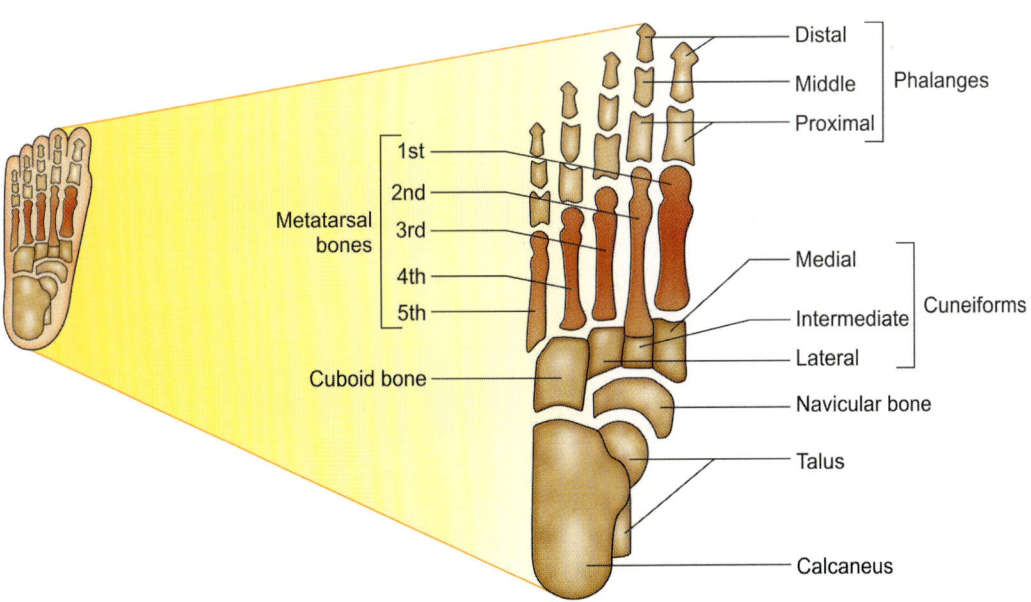

Fig. 16.2: Skeleton of right foot : Plantar aspect.

Features and attachments (Figs 16.3 to 16.6)

Talus has got a head, a neck and a body.

A. Head

1. It is directed forwards, downwards and medially.

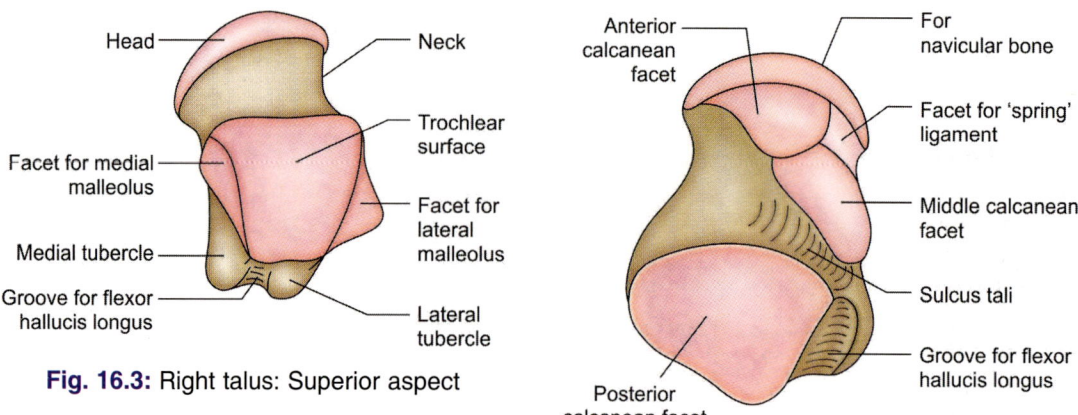

Fig. 16.3: Right talus: Superior aspect

Fig. 16.4: Right talus : Inferior aspect

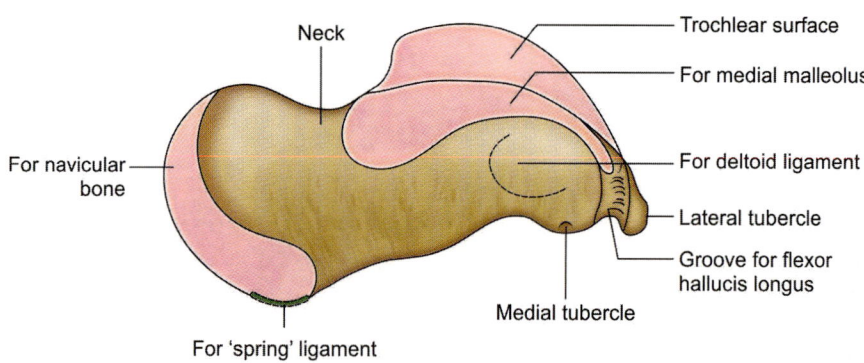

Fig. 16.5: Right talus : Medial aspect

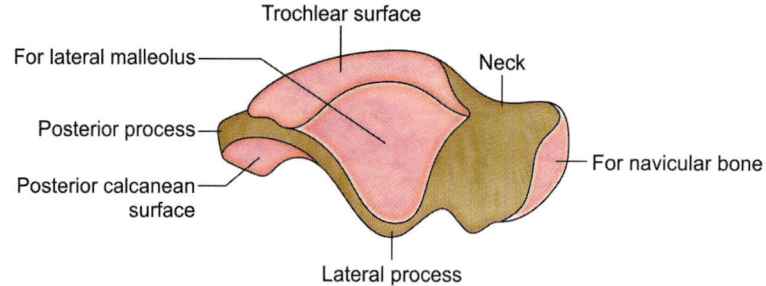

Fig. 16.6: Right talus: Lateral aspect

2. It has two surfaces, anterior and inferior.
3. Anterior surface is oval and convex to articulate with the concavity of navicular bone.
4. Inferior surface has 3 articular areas separated by ridges.

i. Posterior articular area is the largest and articulates with the middle facet of calcaneus.
ii. Medial facet articulates with the spring (*plantar calcaneonavicular*) ligament.

iii. Anterolateral facet articulates with the anterior facet of calcaneus.

B. Neck

1. It is the constriction between head and body.
2. Its long axis forms an angle of 150° with the long axis of body.
3. Distal part of its dorsal surface provides attachment to *dorsal talonavicular ligament* and *capsular ligament of ankle joint*.
4. Proximal part of dorsal surface is intracapsular.
5. Laterally, there is attachment of *anterior talofibular ligament*.
6. Plantar surface medially, is narrow and called as *sulcus tali*. It opposes the *sulcus calcanei* of calcaneus to form *sinus tarsi*.
7. Plantar surface of neck provides attachments to two ligaments, *interosseous talocalcanean* (medially) and *cervical* (laterally).

C. Body

It has five surfaces (superior, inferior, medial, lateral and posterior)

i. Superior surface

1. It bears *trochlear articular surface*.
2. Trochlear articular surface is convex from anterior to posterior and concave from side to side.
3. The articular surface is broader anteriorly and narrower posteriorly.
4. It participates in the formation of *ankle joint*.

ii. Inferior surface

1. It is entirely articular.
2. This articular surface is oval and concave.
3. It articulates with the posterior facet of calcaneus to form *subtalar joint*.

iii. Medial surface

1. It is articular above and nonarticular below.
2. Its articular area is comma shaped to articulate with the medial malleolus.
3. *Deep part of the deltoid ligament* is attached to the nonarticular part.

iv. Lateral surface

1. It shows a triangular articular area.
2. It articulates with lateral malleolus.
3. Its anterior border gives attachment to *anterior talofibular ligament*.
4. Its lower end forms the apex of triangle also called the *lateral process of talus*.

v. Posterior surface

1. It is also called as *posterior process of talus*.
2. *Tendon of flexor hallucis longus* grooves the posterior surface.
3. *Medial and lateral tubercles* bound the groove for flexor hallucis longus.
4. Deltoid ligament's superficial fibres (*posterior tibiotalar ligament*) are attached to the medial tubercle.
5. *Posterior talofibular ligament* is attached to the lateral tubercle.
6. *Os trigonum* is the name given to the lateral tubercle when it is a separate bone. Os trigonum is one of the examples of atavistic epiphysis.

Ossification

Talus ossifies from one centre which appears in its body during 6th month of intrauterine life.

Applied anatomy

1. *Fracture of talus* is rare. But forceful dorsiflexion of foot may result into fracture of neck of talus (Fig. 16.7).

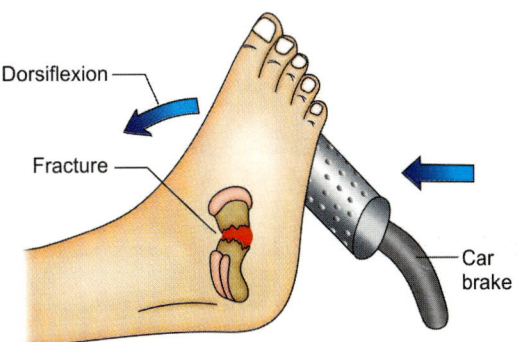

Fig. 16.7: Fracture of neck of talus

2. The fact which is important to be known in case of fracture, is the vascular pattern of talus. Arteries supplying the talus enter its neck and blood flow is mainly backwards. Hence a fracture across the neck of talus may be followed by the expected problems of nonunion and avascular necrosis (Fig. 16.8).

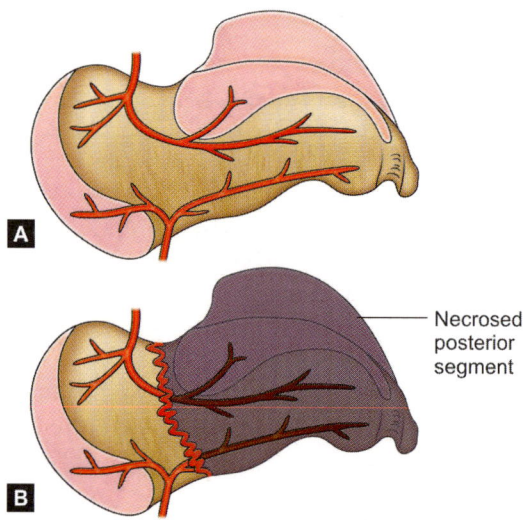

Fig. 16.8: Blood supply of talus (A) and its significance in fracture of neck of talus (B)

3. *Displaced fractures of talus* always require open reduction and internal fixation.
4. *Dislocation of talus* is rare, but if it occurs it is usually posterior.
5. Talus plays very active role in fractures of the ankle e.g. Pott's fracture. It is the talus which either hits or pulls off the lower ends of tibia and fibula to fracture them.
6. *Os trigonum*, if present, may be confused with talus fracture but the former can easily be identified by its position and by the fact that it is bilateral.
7. Most common benign tumour under 21 years of age is *osteoid talus*.

II. THE CALCANEUS

Terminology

It is a Latin word which means heel. Clinicians often name it as *os calis*.

Peculiarities

1. It is the largest bone of foot.
2. It is the strongest bone of foot.
3. It is the first tarsal bone to ossify.
4. It contributes to subtalar as well as midtarsal joints.

Side determination

1. Keep the long axis of bone anteroposteriorly.
2. Look for the anterior and posterior surfaces. Anterior surface is articular and concavoconvex. The posterior surface is larger and rough.
3. Keep the surface bearing large convex articular area dorsally.
4. Keep the concave surface medially. Medial surface is made concave by the shelf like projection called *sustentaculum tali*.

Features and attachments

It has six surfaces (anterior, posterior, superior, plantar, lateral and medial).

A. Anterior surface

1. It is the smallest of all.
2. It bears a concavoconvex articular facet.
3. It articulates with cuboid.

B. Posterior surface

1. It is divided into 3 areas.
2. Its upper part is smooth and is related to a bursa.
3. Its middle part receives insertion of *tendocalcaneus and plantaris*.
4. Its lowermost part is roughened. Dense fibrofatty tissue covers it. It is weight bearing during standing posture.

C. Superior surface (Fig. 16.9)

1. It is also called dorsal surface.
2. It is divided into 3 areas.
   i. Posterior 1/3rd is nonarticular.
   ii. Middle 1/3rd is articular.
   iii. Anterior 1/3rd is partly articular and partly nonarticular.

The Tarsal Bones | 129

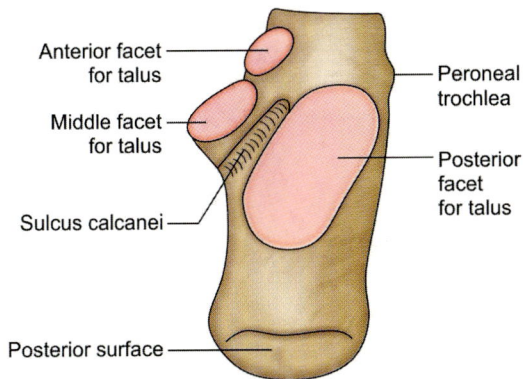

Fig. 16.9: Right calcaneus: Dorsal aspect

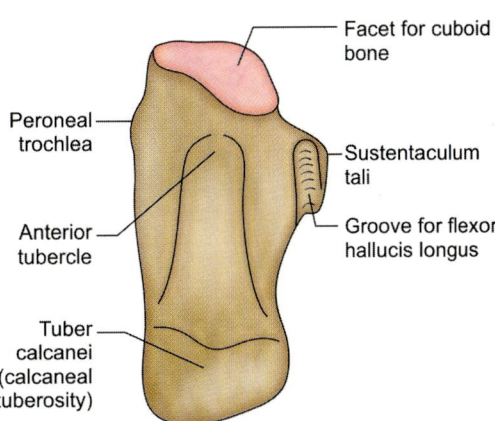

Fig. 16.10: Right calcaneus: Plantar aspect

3. Posterior 1/3rd is rough and is related to fibrofatty tissue between tendocalcaneus and ankle.
4. Middle 1/3rd forms the *posterior facet for talus*.
5. Anteromedial area of anterior 1/3rd possesses two articular facets called *middle and anterior facets for talus*. Middle facet is situated over sustentaculum tali.
6. Nonarticular part of anterior 1/3rd can be divided into medial narrow and lateral wide parts.
   a. Medial narrow part is grooved and known as *sulcus calcanei*. It receives attachments of:
      i. *Interosseous talocalcanean ligament* medially.
      ii. *Cervical ligament* laterally.
   b. Lateral part (area in front of the posterior facet for talus) provides attachments to:
      i. *Extensor digitorum brevis*.
      ii. *Stem of inferior extensor retinaculum*.
      iii. *Stem of bifurcated ligament*.

D. Plantar surface (Fig. 16.10)

1. It has a smaller tubercle at the anterior end called *anterior tubercle*.
2. The elevation at the posterior end is called *calcaneal teberosity*.
3. Calcaneal tubersity is further divided into *larger medial* and *smaller lateral processes*.
4. *Flexor retinaculum* and *abductor hallucis* are attached to the medial margin of medial process.
5. *Plantar aponeurosis* and *flexor digitorum brevis* are attached to the distal margin of medial process.
6. *Abductor digiti minimi* is attached to the distal margins of both the processes.
7. To the anterior tubercle is attached *short plantar ligament*.
8. Triangular area between the anterior tubercle and calcaneal tuberosity gives attachment to *long plantar ligament*.
9. Lateral margin of triangular area in front of lateral process provides attachment to *lateral head of flexor digitorum accessorius*.

E. Lateral surface (Figs 16.11 and 16.13)

1. It is almost flat.
2. Most of it is subcutaneous.
3. A small elevation in its anterior part is called *peroneal trochlea (tubercle)*.
4. Peroneal trochlea lies between the tendons of peroneus brevis above and peroneus longus below.
5. Inferior peroneal retinaculum is attached to the peroneal trochlea and margins of the grooves for peronei muscles.
6. *Calcaneofibular ligament* is attached to this surface about a cm behind the peroneal trochlea.

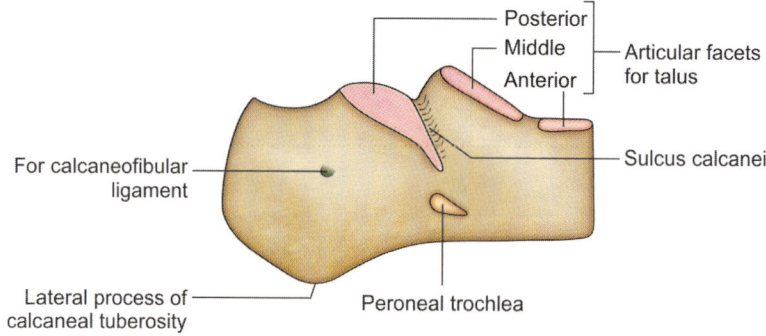

Fig. 16.11: Right calcaneus: Lateral aspect

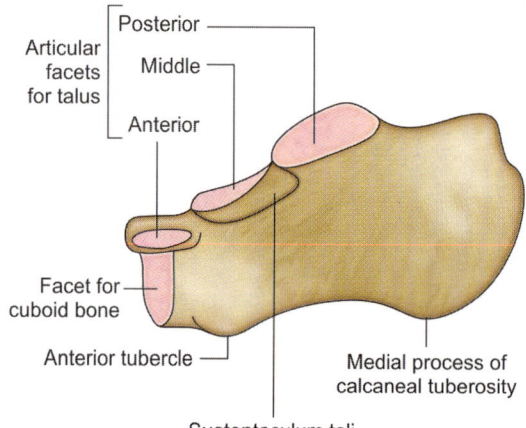

Fig. 16.12: Right calcaneus: Medial aspect

F. Medial surface (Figs 16.12 and 16.14)

1. It is concave from above downwards.
2. *Sustentaculum tali* is a shelf like projection from its upper anterior part.
3. Superior surface of sustentaculum tali has middle facet for talus which contributes to *talocalcaneonavicular joint*.
4. *Tendon of flexor hallucis longus* grooves the inferior surface of sustentaculum tali.
5. *Tendon of flexor digitorum longus* is related to medial surface of sustentaculum tali.
6. Medial surface of sustentaculum tali provides attachments to:
    i. *Spring ligament.*

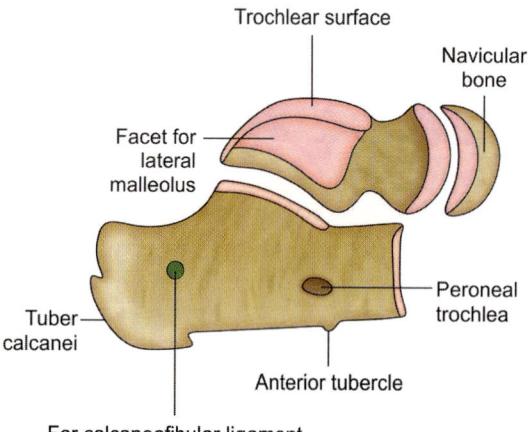

Fig. 16.13: Interrelationships between right talus, calcaneus and navicular bone: Lateral aspect

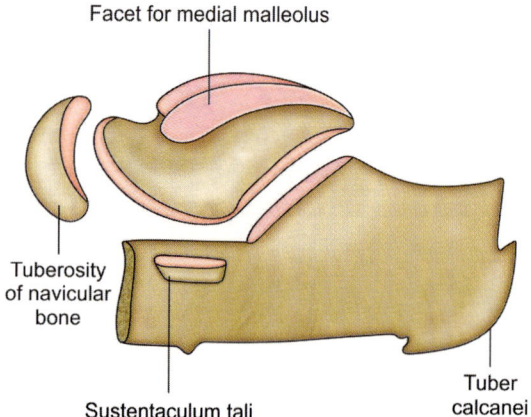

Fig. 16.14: Interrelationships between right talus, calcaneus and navicular bone: Medial aspect

ii. *Slip from tibialis posterior.*
iii. *Some fibres of superficial part of deltoid ligament.*
7. Medial head of *flexor digitorum accessorius* arises from the medial surface below the groove of flexor hallucis longus.

Ossification

Calcaneus ossifies from a centre which appears during 3rd month of intrauterine life.

Note: *Some times a secondary centre may appear for the posterior surface at the age of 6–8 years. If present, it fuses with the rest of bone at the age of 16 years.*

Applied anatomy

1. A *calcanean fracture* may result if a person falls on his heels from the height. Such fracture due to fall is commonly associated with fracture of vertebra (Fig. 16.15).
2. Calcanean fracture is usually comminuted, i.e. the bone breaks into many pieces.
3. Sometimes calcaneus makes a prominence posteriorly and laterally with a bump. This condition is usually associated with a tender bursa between the bump and skin.
4. *Osteochondritis of calcaneus (Sever's disease)* affects it during its developing stage. In this case the bone softens and forms fragments.

III. THE NAVICULAR BONE

Terminology

Navicular is a Latin word which means little ship.

Side determination

1. Deep concave surface faces posteriorly.
2. A prominent projection called *navicular tuberosity*, is directed medially.
3. A groove adjacent to tuberosity is the part of plantar surface and therefore faces inferiorly.

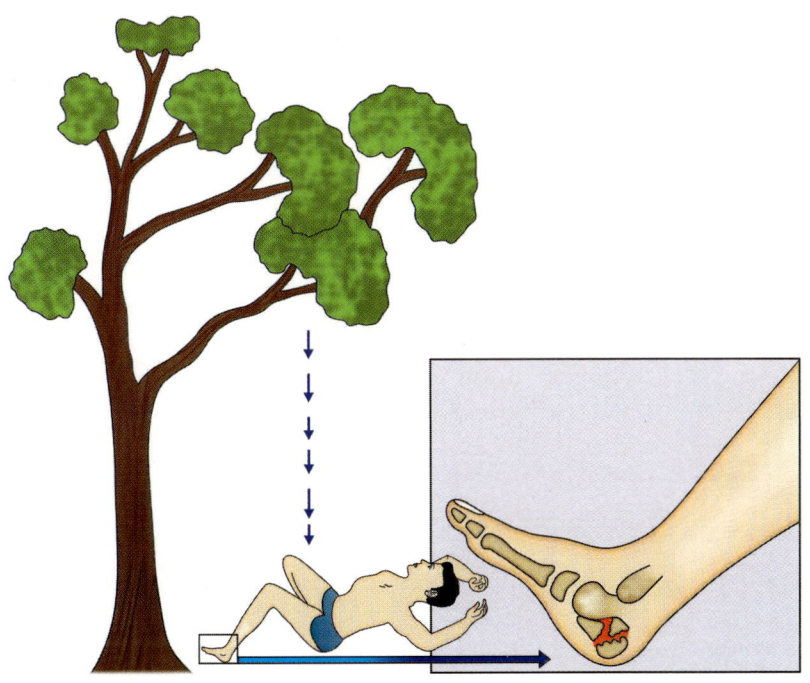

Fig. 16.15: Multiple fractures of calcaneus due to fall from height

Features and attachments (Figs 16.16 to 16.18)

Navicular has 6 surfaces:

A. Anterior surface

It has 3 facets for corresponding 3 cuneiforms.

B. Posterior surface

It is deeply concave for articulation with head of talus.

C. Dorsal surface

It receives attachments of:
1. Dorsal talonavicular ligament.
2. Dorsal cuneonavicular ligaments.
3. Dorsal cubonavicular ligament.

D. Plantar surface

1. Its medial part is marked by a groove through which passes *tendon of tibialis posterior*.
2. Its lateral part receives attachment of *plantar calcaneonavicular (spring) and plantar cuneonavicular ligaments*.

E. Medial surface

It presents the *navicular tuberosity* which receives the insertion of the main part of tendon of *tibialis posteriors*.

F. Lateral surface

It gives attachment to the *medial limb (calcaneonavicular part) of bifurcated ligament*.

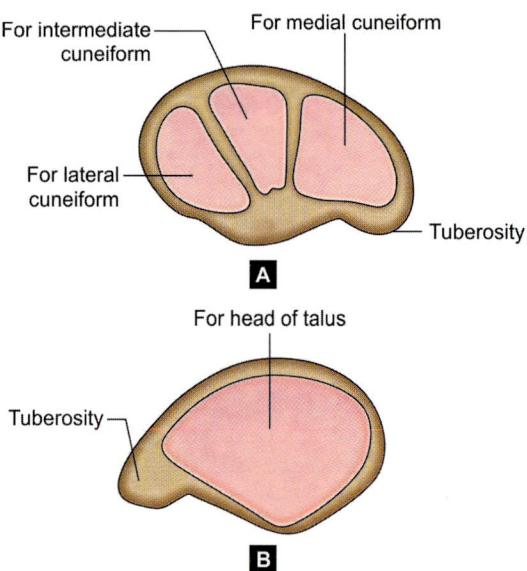

Fig. 16.16: The right navicular bone. (A) Distal aspect; (B) Proximal aspect

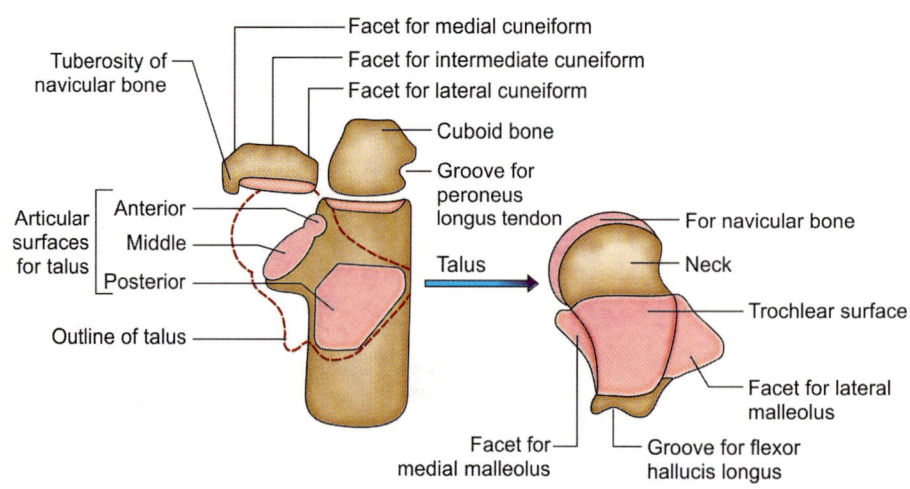

Fig. 16.17: Right talus, calcaneus and navicular and cuboid bones. Dorsal aspect

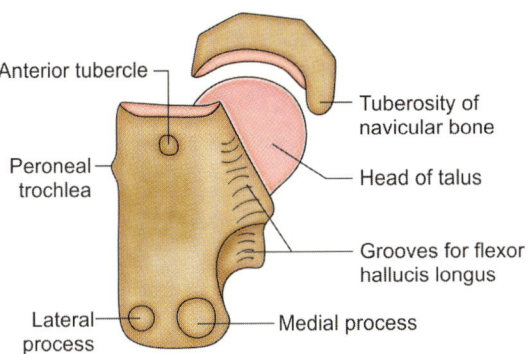

Fig. 16.18: Right talus, calcaneus and navicular bone: Plantar aspect

Ossification
Navicular bone ossifies from single centre which appears during 4th year.

Applied anatomy
1. Removal of navicular bone is an alternative technique in treatment of congenital flat foot. This will reduce the tension on the soft tissue medially.
2. *Navicular secundarium (accessory navicular bone, os tibiale)* is the most common accessory bone of foot. Pain and tenderness localized to this region indicate a strain of the syndesmosis or synchondrosis between this bone and navicular (Fig. 16.19).
3. *Stress fracture of navicular bone* if occurs, it is usually sagitally oriented and in the middle 1/3rd of bone.

IV. THE CUBOID BONE

Terminology
The name of bone is derived from its shape which is approximately cubical.

Side determination
1. Articular surfaces of the cuboid bone are anterior (distal) and posterior (proximal). The proximal surface is one and concavoconvex while distal surface is divided into two by a vertical ridge.

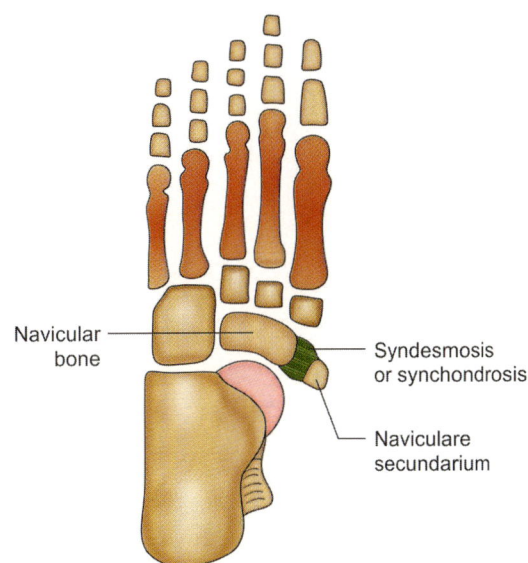

Fig. 16.19: Skeleton of right foot : Plantar view

2. Its inferior surface is marked by a groove.
3. Its lateral surface is less extensive and nonarticular while medial surface is more extensive and partly articular.

Features and attachments
Cuboid bone has got 6 surfaces:

A. Anterior surface
1. It is wholly articular.
2. It is divided by a vertical ridge into medial quadrangular and lateral triangular areas for the bases of 4th and 5th metatarsal bones respectively.

B. Posterior surface
It bears a concavoconvex surface for the anterior surface of calcaneus.

C. Plantar surface (Fig. 16.21)
1. A groove in this surface runs medially and forwards and is meant for *tendon of peroneus longus*.
2. There is a ridge behind the groove. This ridge and margins of groove provide attachments to *long plantar ligament*.

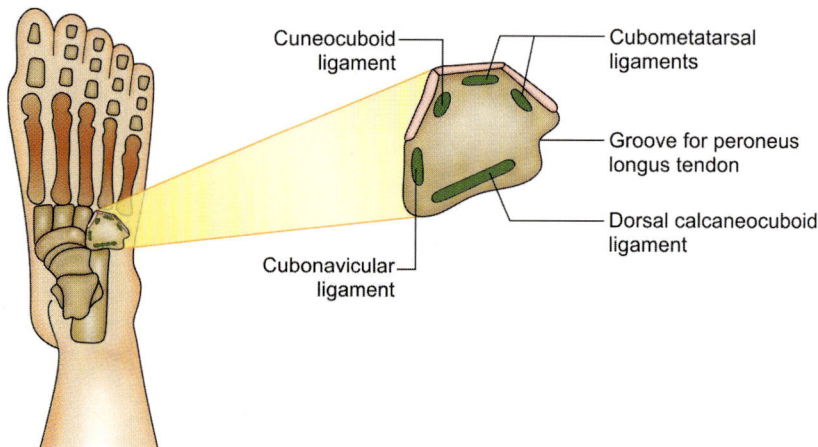

Fig. 16.20: Right cuboid bone : Dorsal view

3. Surface behind the ridge gives attachment to *short plantar ligament*.

D. Dorsal surface (Fig. 16.20)

It receives attachments of following ligaments:
1. *Dorsal calcaneocuboid.*
2. *Dorsal cubometatarsal.*
3. *Dsorsal cubonavicular.*
4. *Dorsal cuneocuboid.*

E. Medial surface

1. Its anterior part is articular for lateral cuneiform bone.
2. Its posterior part is nonarticular and gives attachments to:
   i. *Calcaneocuboid part of bifurcated ligament.*
   ii. *Interosseous cubonavicular ligament.*
   iii. *Interosseous cuneocuboid ligament*

F. Lateral surface

1. It is narrow and nonarticular.
2. The groove for peroneus longus begins here.

Ossification

Cuboid bone ossifies from one centre which appears just before birth, i.e. at 9th month of intrauterine life.

Applied anatomy

1. Decancellation of cuboid bone is the curetting of its interior through small

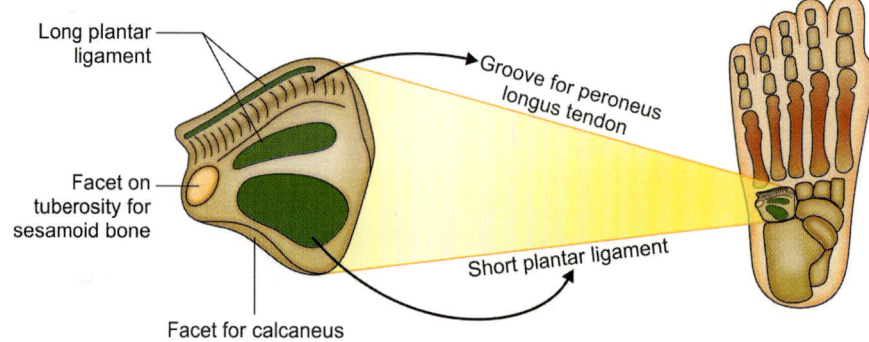

Fig. 16.21: Right cuboid bone : Plantar view

openings. The procedure is often adapted in the treatment of congenital club foot.

2. Most frequent mechanism of cuboid injury is lateral subluxation of the midtarsal joint which creates the nutcracker fracture.

3. Total dislocation of cuboid bone, although very rare but may accur.

V. THE CUNEIFORM BONES

Terminology

Cuneiform is a Latin word which means wedge shaped.

Names

There are three cuneiforms. These are named from medial to lateral as follows:

1. Medial or 1st cuneiform.
2. Intermediate or 2nd cuneiform.
3. Lateral or 3rd cuneiform.

Sizes

The medial cuneiform is largest while intermediate cuneiform is smallest.

Articulations (Fig. 16.22)

1. Proximal surfaces of cuneiforms articulate with navicular bone.
2. Distal surface of medial cuneiform articulates with the base of 1st metatarsal bone.
3. Distal surface of intermediate cuneiform articulates with the base of 2nd metatarsal bone.
4. Distal surface of lateral cuneiform articulates with the base of 3rd metatarsal bone.
5. Adjacent cuneiforms articulate with each other.
6. Medial and lateral cuneiform bones articulate with the corresponding sides of base of 2nd metatarsal.
7. Lateral surface of lateral cuneiform articulates with the base of 4th metatarsal and cuboid bones.

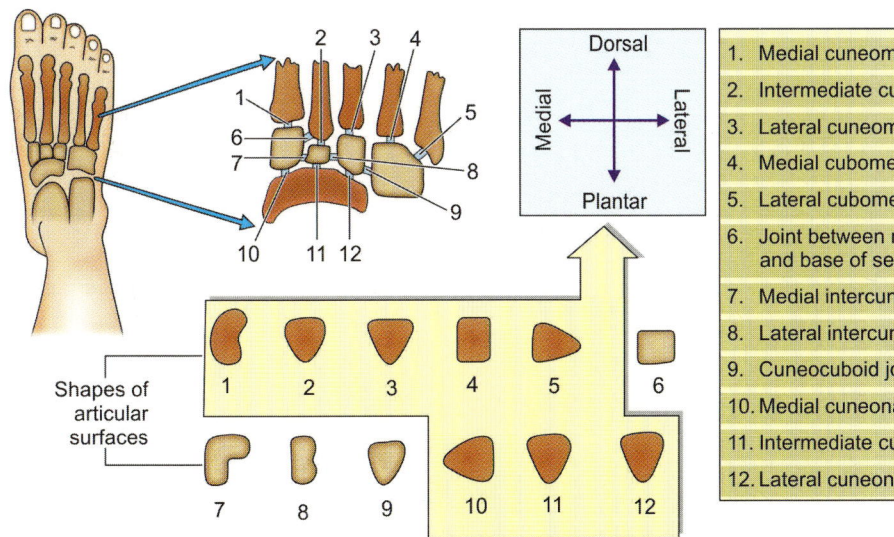

Fig. 16.22: Right cuneiform bones: Dorsal aspect

Attachments

1. Medial cuneiform receives attachments of *tibialis anterior* and *peroneus longus*.
2. Slips of *tibialis posterior* extend to plantar surfaces of all cuneiforms.
3. In general three cuneiforms receive attachments of interosseous, dorsal and plantar ligaments (Fig. 16.23).

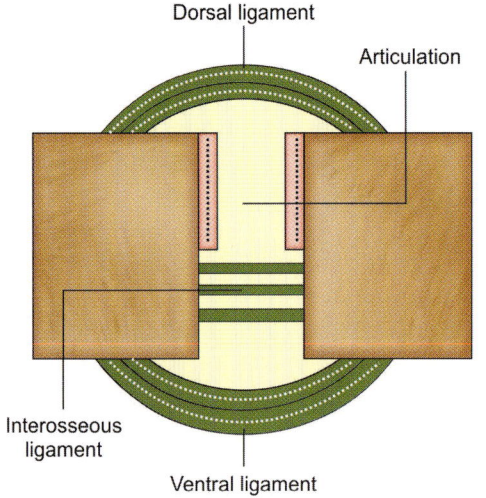

Fig. 16.23: Ligaments attached to cuneiform bones

Ossification

Each cuneiform ossifies from one centre, the time of appearance for which is as follows:

    Lateral cuneiform   : 1 year
    Medial cuneiform   : 2 years
    Intermediate cuneiform : 3 years

Applied anatomy

1. Isolated *fracture of the cuneiform bone* can occur from direct blow.
2. Isolated *dislocation of cuneiform bone* can occur although very rare. Dislocation of cuneiform bone is usually associated with involvement of adjacent bones.
3. *Lisfranc fracture* : It is fracture dislocation of tarsometatarsal joints (Fig. 16.24).

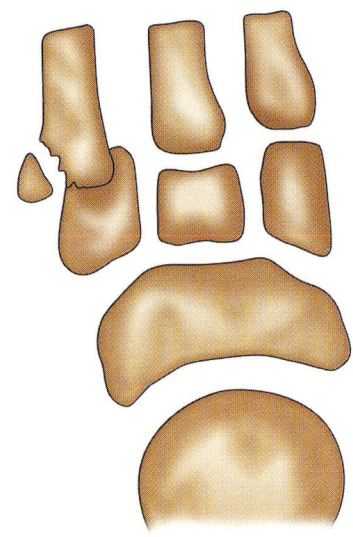

Fig. 16.24: Lisfranc fracture

CHAPTER 17
The Metatarsal Bones

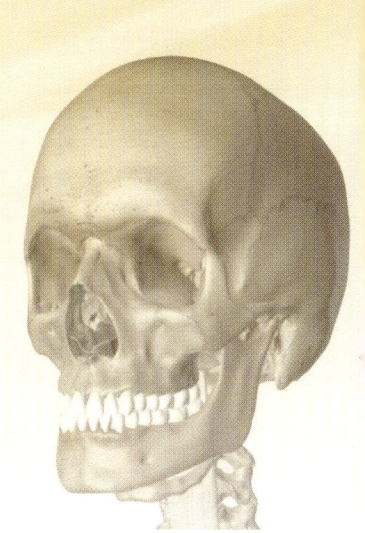

METATARSUS

Five metatarsal bones together constitute the metatarsus.

NAMING THE METATARSAL BONES (Fig. 17.1)

Metatarsal bones are named by numbering them. They are numbered from medial to lateral, i.e. the metatarsal bone along the great toe is called as 1st metatarsal bone and the metatarsal bone along the little toe is known as 5th metatarsal bone.

IDENTIFICATION OF METATARSAL BONES (Fig. 17.2)

1st metatarsal bone

1. It is shortest and thickest.
2. Proximal surface of its base possesses a kidney shaped articular surface.

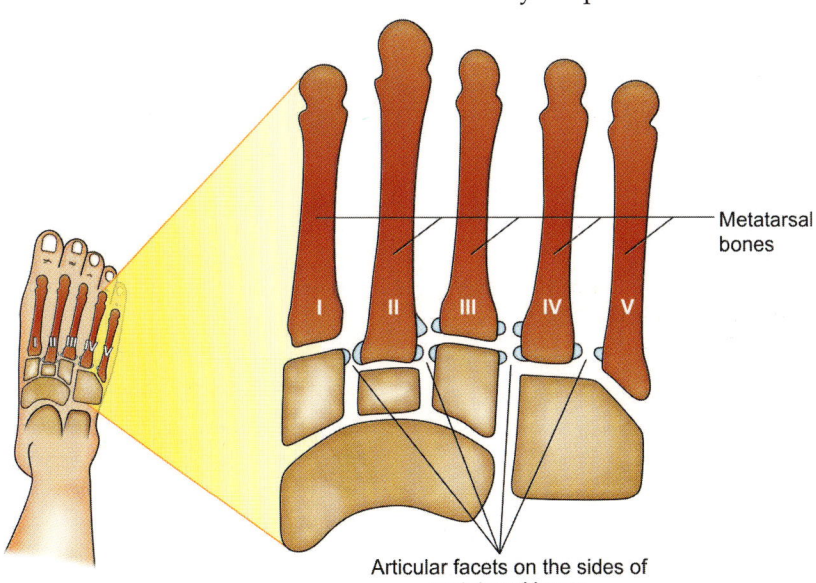

Fig. 17.1: Skeleton of right foot: Dorsal aspect

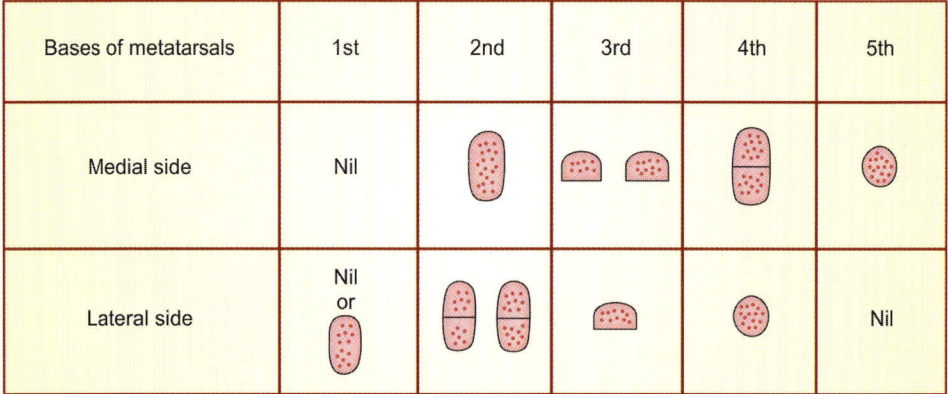

Fig. 17.2: Shapes of articular facets by the sides of bases of metatarsal bones

2nd metatarsal bone

1. Proximal surface of its base has triangular articular surface.
2. One side of the base has single facet while the other side possesses two facets divided into four.

3rd metatarsal bone

It has two facets on one side and one facet on the other side of the base.

4th metatarsal bone

It has a quadrilateral facet on the proximal surface of base and single facet on one side and one facet divided into two on the other side.

5th metatarsal bone

The lateral aspect of base projects proximally to form *styloid process*.

FEATURES AND ATTACHMENTS

Metatarsal bones are miniature long bones. Each metatarsal bone has got a distal end (head), a shaft or body and a proximal end (base).

I. HEAD

1. Its articular surface meets with the base of corresponding proximal phalanx.
2. Articular surface is more extensive on the plantar aspect.
3. Each side of the head shows a tubercle dorsally for callateral ligament of tarso-metatarsal joint.

II. SHAFT

1. It is concave on its plantar aspect.
2. Sides of the shaft provide attachments to interossei muscles.
3. Plantar aspect of 5th metatarsal bone gives origin to flexor digiti minimi.

III. BASE

1. Articulations of proximal surfaces and the shapes of articular surfaces are as follows:

Metatarsal bone	Proximal bone	Shape of the articular surface
1st	Medial cuneiform bone	Kidney shaped
2nd	Intermediate cuneiform bone	Triangular
3rd	Lateral cuneiform bone	Triangular
4th	Cuboid bone	Quadrangular
5th	Cuboid bone	Triangular

2. Both the sides of bases of middle 3 metatarsal bones and lateral side of 1st and medial side of 5th metatarsal bones possess articular facets the details of which are as follows:
3. Base of 1st metatarsal bone gives attachments to:
   i. Tibialis anterior.
   ii. Peroneus longus.

4. Plantar aspects of bases of middle 3 metatarsal bones provide attachments to:
    i. *Slips of tibialis posterior.*
    ii. *Oblique head of adductor hallucis.*
5. Base of 5th metatarsal bone receives insertions of:
    i. *Peroneus tertius.*
    ii. *Peroneus brevis.*

OSSIFICATION

A. Primary centres

One centre appears for the shaft of each metatarsal bone as follows:
1st metatarsal bone - 10th week of intrauterine life.
Rest of the metatarsal bone - 9th week of intrauterine life.

B. Secondary centres

Only one secondary centre appears for each metatarsal bone.

Location

1st metatarsal bone	: Base
Rest of the metatarsal bones	: Head
Appearance	: 3 years
Fusion	: 18 years

APPLIED ANATOMY

1. *Fracture of the base of 5th metatarsal bone* is common. It is usually due to inversion injury where peroneus brevis tendon pulls off the styloid process of 5th metatarsal bone. It is also called *Jones' fracture* after the name of Sir Robert Jones, an orthopaedic surgeon who himself sustained this injury while dancing (Fig. 17.3).
2. Metatarsal bones are the sites for *march fracture* due to prolonged repeated minor trauma as in military recruits. Typically the shaft or neck of 2nd or 3rd metatarsal bone is affected. Neck of the 2nd metatarsal bone is said to be the commonest site.
3. *Metatarsalgia* (pain in the forefoot) may be due to excessive pressure exerted usually by the 2nd or 3rd metatarsal heads.

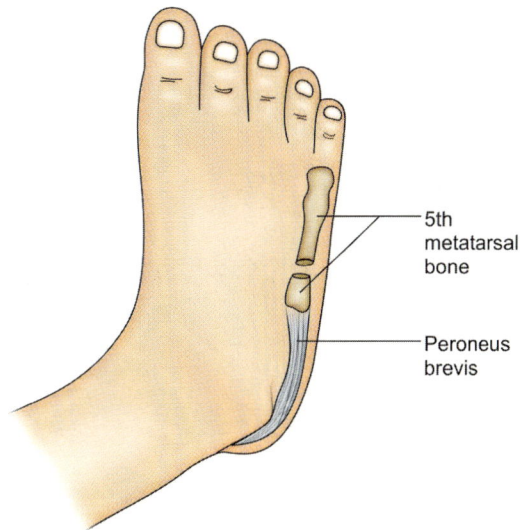

Fig. 17.3: Fracture of 5th metatarsal base

4. *Hallux valgus* (lateral displacement of great toe) exposes the first metatarsal head creating in *medial bump* or *bunion* (Fig. 17.4).

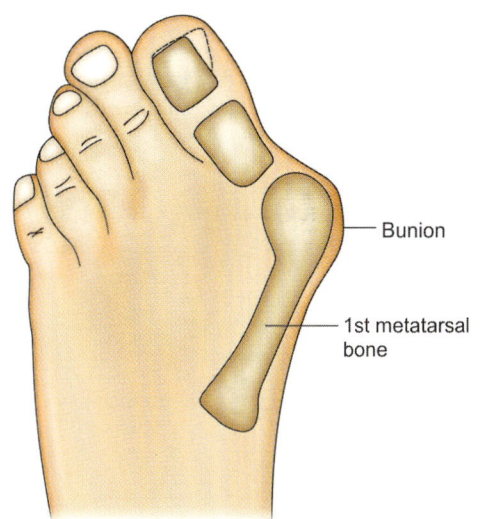

Fig. 17.4: Hallux valgus

5. *Gout* is one condition which shows affinity for 1st metatarsophalangeal joint. In chronic cases there is destruction of head of metatarsal bone and base of proximal phalanx, easily observed in radiographs.
6. *Freiberg's disease* is the infarction of the distal epiphysis of the 2nd metatarsal bone.

CHAPTER 18

The Phalanges of the Foot

The total number of phalanges in each foot is 14. Great toe has got only two phalanges, i.e. proximal and distal. Rest of the toes have got three phalanges each, i.e. proximal, middle and distal (Fig. 18.1).

CHARACTERISTICS

1. Phalanges of the foot are very much similar to those of hand as far as features are concerned but in foot they are relatively smaller.
2. Each phalanx has *base* (proximal end), *shaft* and *head* (distal end).
3. Articular surfaces show similarities with those of phalanges of hand.
4. The distal phalanx of each toe bears a roughened tuberosity on the plantar aspect of its distal end. This gives attachment to the pulp of the tip of the toe and provides a wider area to take pressure.

OSSIFICATION

A. Primary centre

One centre appears for the shaft as follows:
    Proximal phalanx   : 12th week of IUL.

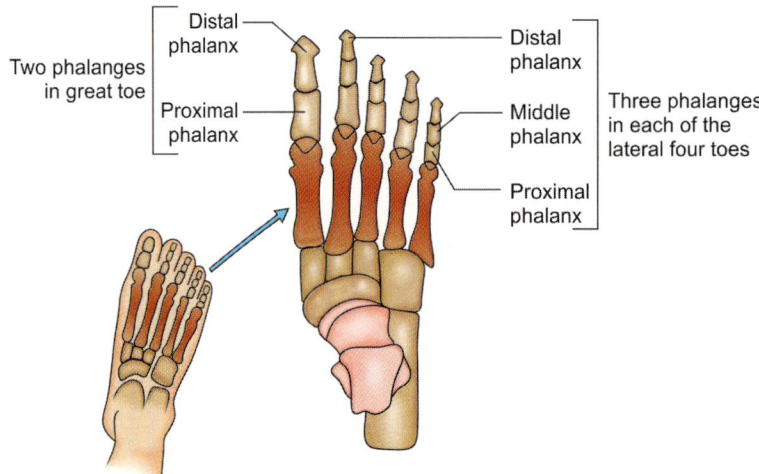

Fig. 18.1: Skeleton of right foot. Dorsal aspect

Middle phalanx : 15th week of intrauterine life
Distal phalanx : 9th week of intrauterine life

B. Secondary centre
One centre appears for the base of each phalanx.

Appearance
Proximal phalanx : 2 years
Middle phalanx : 4 years
Distal phalanx : 6 years
Fusion : 18 years

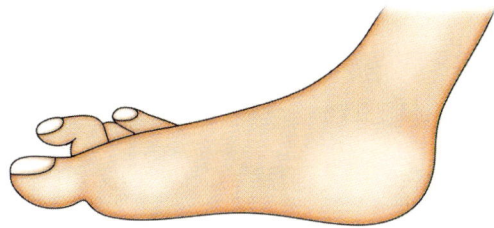

Fig. 18.2: Hammer toe

APPLIED ANATOMY

1. *A hammer toe* usually involves 2nd toe where it is fixed in dorsiflexion at metatarsophalangeal joint and plantar flexion at distal joints (Fig. 18.2).
2. In *claw toe* both interphalangeal joints are flexed but the metatarsophalangeal joints are hyperextended.
3. *Ainhum* (constriction band around the base of toe) usually involves 5th toe. There is always rarefying osteitis of phalanges distal to constriction. It leads to *auto-amputation*.
4. Phalanges are indispensable in walking. Amputation of *great toe* poses difficulty in take off. The amputation of 2nd toe produces *hallux valgus*. Amputation of 5th toe results into least disturbance.
5. *Congenital overlapping usually involves little toe* which is dorsiflexed, adducted over the 4th toe and rotated in such a way that dorsal surface faces laterally. The condition is usually bilateral.
6. *Phalangeal fracture*: Proximal phalanges of foot are more commonly injured than all other phalanges. The commonest mechanism of injury is direct blow due to fall of heavy weight on foot.

CHAPTER 19

The Vertebrae

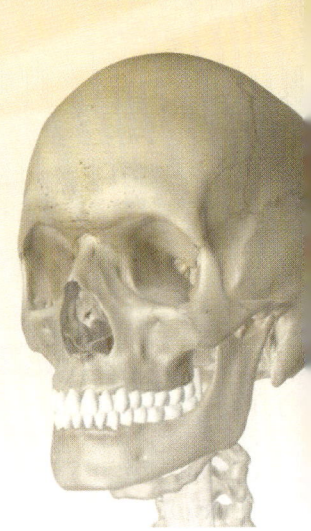

GENERAL CONSIDERATIONS

1. Vertebral column is made up of a number of irregular bones called vertebrae.
2. Vertebral column forms the central axis of the body.
3. There are 33 vertebrae.
4. Vertebrae are named according to regions they belong.
5. Following is the classification of vertebrae:

   Cervical vertebrae   7
   Thoracic vertebrae   12
   Lumbar vertebrae   5
   Sacral vertebrae   5 (These fuse to form single *sacrum*)
   Coccygeal vertebrae   4 (These fuse to form single *coccyx*)

6. Vertebrae are mobile or fixed.
7. Mobile vertebrae are called *true vertebrae* while fixed vertebrae are called *false vertebrae*.

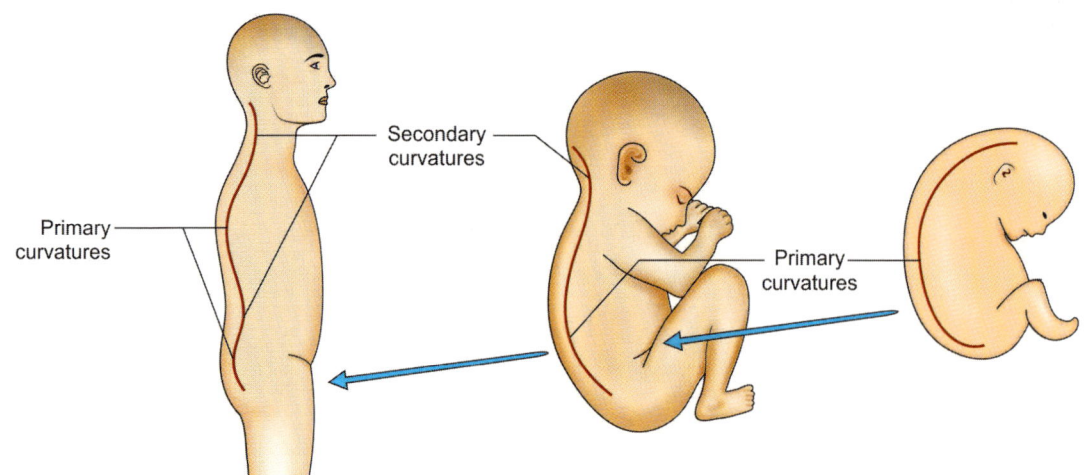

Fig. 19.1: Curvatures of vertebral column

8. Movable vertebrae are cervical, thoracic and lumbar.
9. Sacral and coccygeal vertebrae are immobile.

CURVATURES OF VERTEBRAL COLUMN (Fig. 19.1)

a. Primary curvatures

1. During intrauterine life the whole vertebral column is concave ventrally and convex dorsally. This is *primary curvature*.
2. In adult primary curvatures are retained only in thoracic and sacral regions.
3. They are mainly due to the shape of vertebrae.

b. Secondary curvatures

1. Secondary curvatures are convex forwards.
2. They develop after birth.
3. They develop due to posture.
4. They are mainly due to the shape of intervertebral discs.
5. Secondary curvatures are observed in cervical and lumbar regions.
6. Cervical curvature appears around 6–9 months when the child starts holding his head by himself.
7. Lumbar curvature appears at about 12–18 months when the child starts walking.

MOVEMENTS OF VERTEBRAL COLUMN

Vertebral column shows following movements:
1. *Flexion* – Forward bending.
2. *Extension* – Backward bending.
3. *Lateral flexion* – Side bending.
4. *Rotation* – Twisting of trunk.
5. *Circumduction* – Combination of all the above movements.

FEATURES OF A TYPICAL VERTEBRA (Fig. 19.2)

A typical vertebra is made up of 2 parts, body and vertebral arch.

a. Body

1. It is ventral part of a vertebra.
2. It is cylindrical in shape.
3. It has 4 surfaces, anterior, posterior, superior and inferior.
4. Anterior surface is convex from side to side and concave from above downwards.
5. Posterior surface is slightly concave from side to side but flat from above downwards. It has number of foramina for exit of *basivertebral veins*. It forms anterior boundary of vertebral foramen.
6. Upper and lower surfaces are rough for the intervertebral discs.

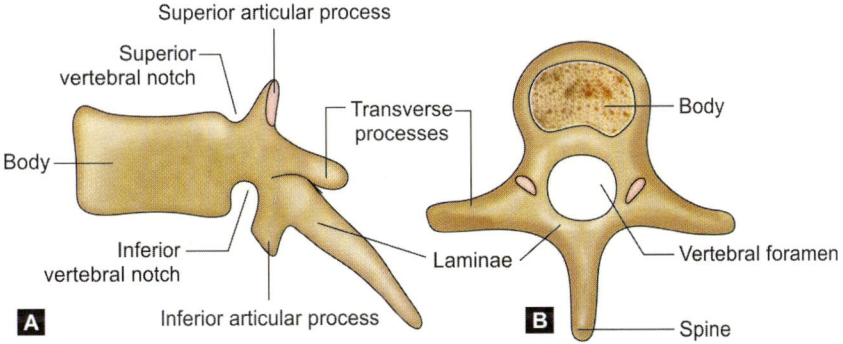

Fig. 19.2: A typical vertebra. (A) Left lateral view; (B) Superior view

b. Vertebral arch

It consists of a pair of pedicles, a pair of laminae and seven processes (one spinous, four articular and two transverse).

i. Pedicles

1. These are pair of short thick processes which project backwards from the body.
2. Between the adjacent pedicles are *intervertebral foramina*.

ii. Laminae

1. These are bony plates extending backwards and medially from posterior end of the pedicles.
2. Posteriorly they fuse to form spine in the midline.
3. Body, pedicles and laminae together enclose the foramen of vertebra called *vertebral foramen*.

iii. Transverse process

It projects laterally on each side from the junction of pedicle and lamina.

iv. Articular processes

1. They are two on each side and four in total.
2. They are *superior and inferior articular processes* projecting upwards and downwards respectively from the junction of pedicle and lamina.

v. Spinous process (spine)

It projects backwards in the midline from the meeting point of laminae.

DISTINGUISHING FEATURES (Fig. 19.3)

1. *Cervical vertebra* is characterized by the presence of a foramen in each transverse process. This foramen is named as *foramen transversarium*.
2. *Thoracic vertebra* is recognized by the presence of *costal facets* on the sides of body.
3. *Lumbar vertebra* is larger in size and lacks both *foramen transversarium* as well as *costal facets*.
4. There is no isolated sacral vertebra. Five *sacral vertebrae* fuse to form single piece of triangular and curved **sacrum**.
5. Similarly there is no isolated coccygeal vertebra. Four *coccygeal vertebrae* fuse to form single piece of **coccyx**. Coccyx is relatively very small in size than sacrum.

REGIONAL VERTEBRAE

I. CERVICAL VERTEBRAE

These are classified as *typical* and *atypical*. 3rd to 6th cervical vertebrae are typical. 1st, 2nd and 7th cervical vertebrae are atypical.

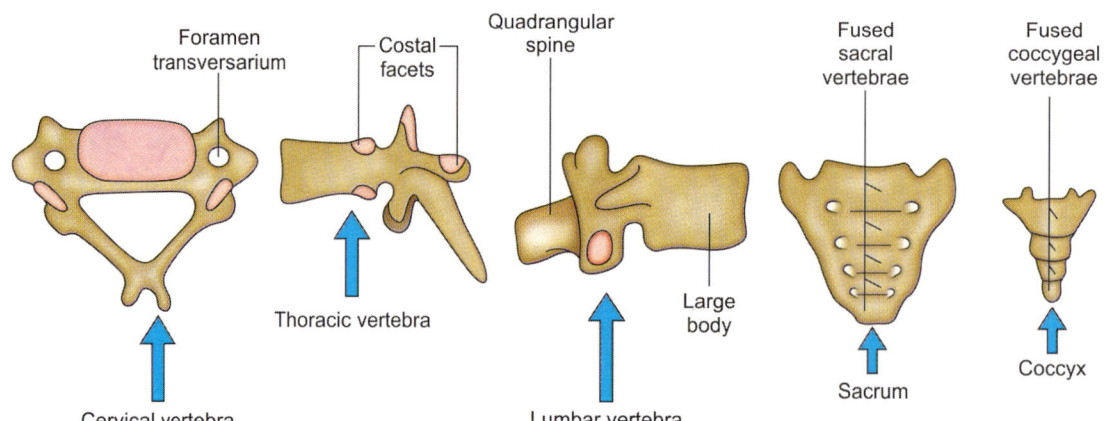

Fig. 19.3: Distinguishing features of vertebrae

A. Typical cervical vertebra (Fig. 19.4)

It has a *body* and a *vertebral arch*. These enclose a *vertebral foramen*.

a. Body

1. It is smallest among all vertebrae.
2. It is narrower anteroposteriorly.
3. It has 4 surfaces; *superior, inferior, anterior* and *posterior*.
4. Its superior surface is concave from side to side with an upward projecting lip on either side. This surface is mainly related to *intervertebral disc*.
5. The inferior surface is convex from side to side. The anterior border of inferior surface projects downwards to hide the intervertebral disc. Inferior surface, like superior surface is also related to *intervertebral disc*.
6. Anterior surface provides attachments to *anterior longitudinal ligament* in the middle and *longus colli muscle* on either side of it.
7. Posterior surface has number of foramina for *basivertebral veins*. Its superior and inferior margins provide attachments to *posterior longitudinal ligament*.

b. Vertebral foramen

1. It is triangular in shape.
2. It is bigger than the body.

c. Vertebral arch

It is comprised of *pedicles, laminae*, the *superior* and *inferior articular processes*, the *transverse processes* and *spine*.

i. Pedicles (Fig. 19.5)

1. They are directed backwards and laterally. It is this direction which is

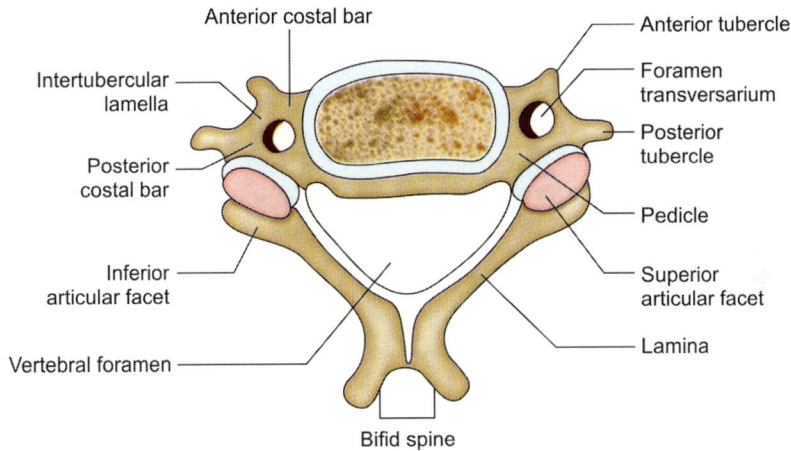

Fig. 19.4: Typical cervical vertebra : Superior aspect

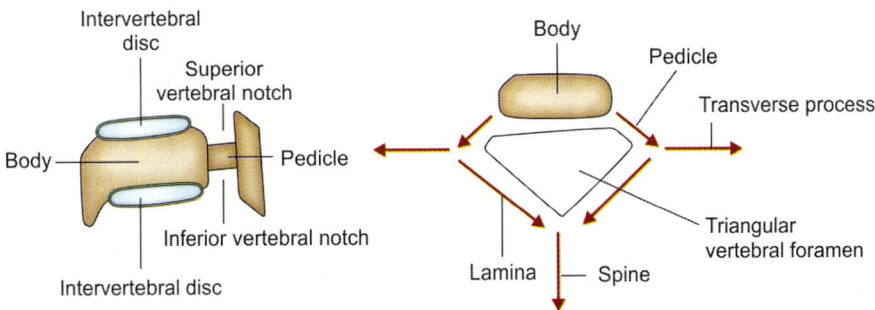

Fig. 19.5: The pedicle of cervical vertebra

responsible for triangular shape of vertebral foramen.
2. Above and below the pedicles are *superior* and *inferior vertebral notches* respectively. These notches are equal in size.

ii. Laminae (Fig. 19.6)

1. They are long and narrow.
2. The superior border is thinner than the inferior border.
3. *Ligamentum flavum* is attached to its superior border and lower part of its anterior surface.

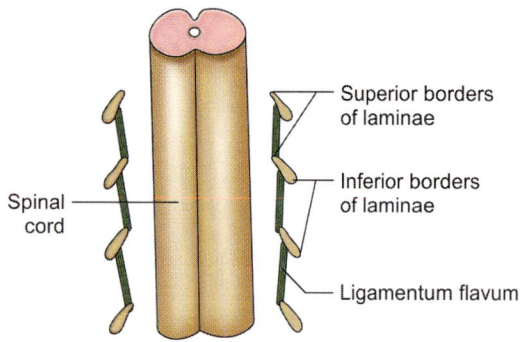

Fig. 19.6: The laminae of cervical vertebrae: Cross sectional view

iii. Articular processes

1. *Superior* and *inferior articular processes* are located on each side, above and below the junction of pedicle and lamina.
2. *Superior articular process* faces upwards and backwards.
3. *Inferior articular process* is directed downwards and forwards.
4. Superior articular process of a vertebra articulates with inferior articular process of the vertebra above.
5. Articular processes lie in one line forming an *articular pillar*.

iv. Transverse process

1. It has got a foramen called *foramen transversarium*, which forms a characteristic feature of *cervical vertebra*.
2. *Vertebral artery, vertebral vein* and *sympathetic nerves* pass through foramen transversarium (vertebral artery passes through upper 6 foramina only).
3. The foramen transversarium is bounded anteriorly and posteriorly by *anterior and posterior roots* respectively.
4. The lateral ends of the anterior and posterior roots are connected by *costotransverse bar* or *intertubercular lamella* (Fig. 19.7).

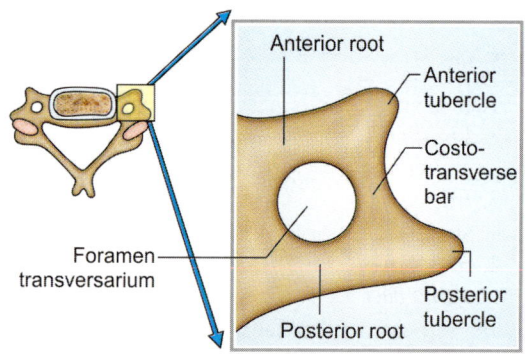

Fig. 19.7: Foramen transversarium

5. Junctions of anterior and posterior roots with costotransverse bar are marked by *anterior and posterior tubercles* respectively.
6. The enlarged anterior tubercle of the sixth cervical vertebra is called *carotid tubercle*. This is related to *common carotid artery*.
7. Anterior tubercles give origins to *scalenus anterior, longus capitis* and *longus colli muscles*.
8. Posterior tubercles provide attachments to *levator scapulae, scalenus medius, scalenus posterior* and some *deep muscles of the back*
9. The anterior root, anterior tubercle, costotransverse bar, posterior tubercle and adjoining (lateral part of) posterior root represent the *costal element* while the medial part of posterior root represents the *transverse element* of the developing vertebra (Fig. 19.8).

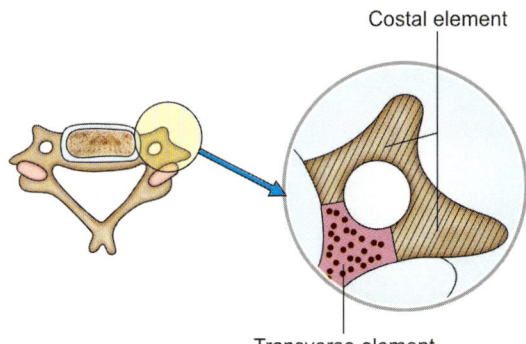

Fig. 19.8: Costal and transverse elements of transverse process

v. Spine
1. It is small and bifid.
2. *Ligamentum nuchae* is attached to the *spinous notch*.
3. *Interspinous ligaments* are attached to its superior and inferior borders.
4. Sides provide attachments to *deep muscles of the back* (Fig. 19.9).

B. Atypical cervical vertebrae
First cervical vertebra
Terminology
It is also named as *atlas* because it supports the skull. According to Greek mythology, Atlas is the God who supported the earth on his shoulders.

Distinguishing features
1. It is ring shaped with narrow anterior and posterior arches.
2. It has no body.
3. It has no spine.
4. It has a large *lateral mass* on either side.
5. The two *transverse processes* are widest apart relative to other cervical vertebrae.

Normal anatomical position
1. Two arches lie in same horizontal plane.
2. *Anterior arch* is smaller than the *posterior arch*.
3. *Superior articular facets* on lateral masses are elongated.

Features and attachments
(Figs 19.10 and 19.11)

Atlas has got an *anterior arch*, a *posterior arch* and two *lateral masses*.

a. Anterior arch
1. It is smaller than the posterior arch.
2. It connects the two lateral masses.

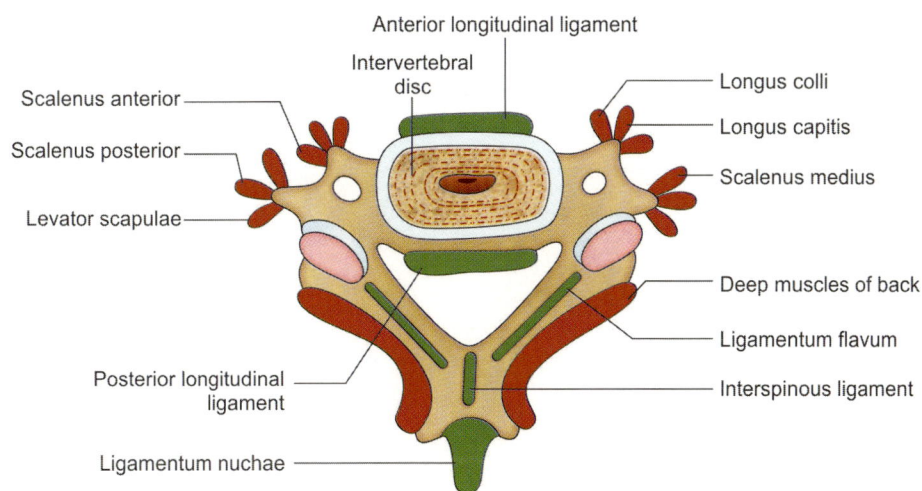

Fig. 19.9: Main attachments and relations of typical cervical vertebra

148 | Human Osteology

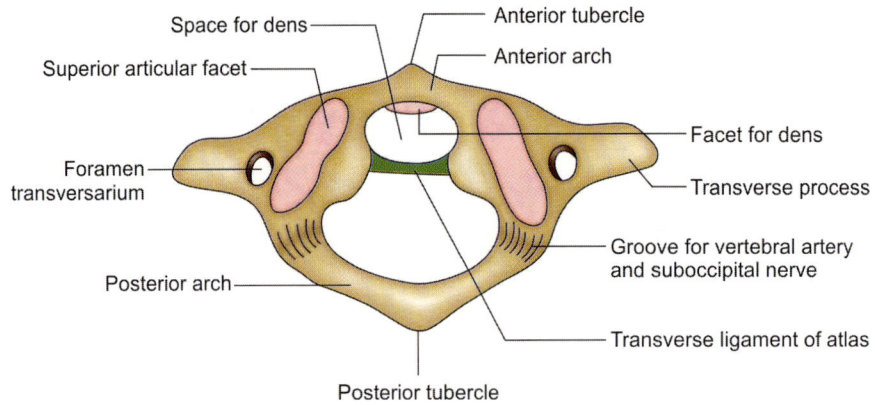

Fig. 19.10: Atlas: Superior aspect

3. *Anterior tubercle* is present on its anterior aspect in the midline. Midline part of upper end of *anterior longitudinal ligament* is attached to it.
4. Its anterior surface on each side of anterior tubercle provides attachment to *longus colli muscle*.
5. An *oval facet* is present on its posterior surface in the midline for articulation with dens of 2nd cervical vertebra to form the *atlantoaxial joint*.
6. *Anterior atlanto-occipital membrane* is attached to the upper border of anterior arch.
7. Lateral part of upper end of *anterior longitudinal ligament* is attached to the lower border of anterior arch.

b. Posterior arch

1. It is longer than the anterior arch.
2. Midline *posterior tubercle* on its posterior surface represents the spine.
3. *Ligamentum nuchae* is attached to the posterior tubercle.
4. On each side of posterior tubercle is attached the *rectus capitis posterior minor*.
5. *Vertebral artery (3rd part)* and *first cervical nerve* lie in the shallow groove on the

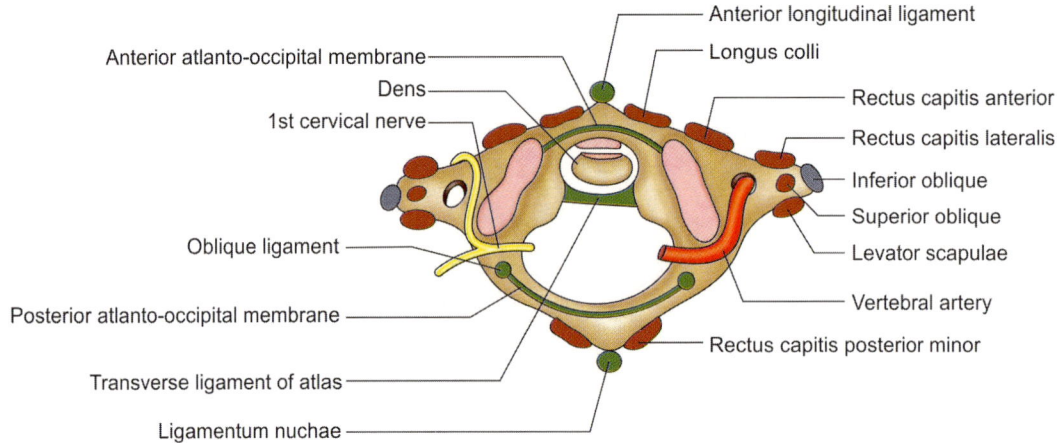

Fig. 19.11: Attachments and relations of atlas: Superior view

superior surface of posterior arch just behind the lateral mass.
6. *Posterior atlanto-occipital membrane* is attached to the superior border behind the grooves.
7. *Ligamentum flavum* is attached to its lower border on each side of midline.

c. **Lateral masses**

Each lateral mass has got two articular facets (superior and inferior), two surfaces (anterior and medial) and a transverse process.
1. *Superior articular facet* is concave and elongated. It articulates with occipital condyle to from *atlanto-occipital joint*.

Note: *Remember, we say 'No' at atlanto-axial joint, i.e. move the head from side to side while we say 'Yes' at atlanto-occipital joint, i.e. perform nodding movement of the head.*

2. *Inferior articular facet* is flat and circular. It articulates with axis.

3. *Medial surface* has got a *tubercle for transverse ligament of atlas*.
4. *Anterior surface* gives origin to *rectus capitis anterior*.
5. *Transverse process* is long and strong. It has *foramen transversarium* which transmits *vertebral artery, vertebral vein* and *sympathetic nerve*. Rectus capitis lateralis, levator scapulae and superior oblique muscles are attached to its superior aspect around the foramen transversarium. Inferior oblique muscle is attached to its inferior surface. Anterior aspect of transverse process is related to *ventral ramus of 1st cervical nerve* and *accessory nerve*.

Second cervical vertebra (Figs 19.12 and 19.13)

Terminology

It is also called *axis* because atlas carrying the skull rotates on it.

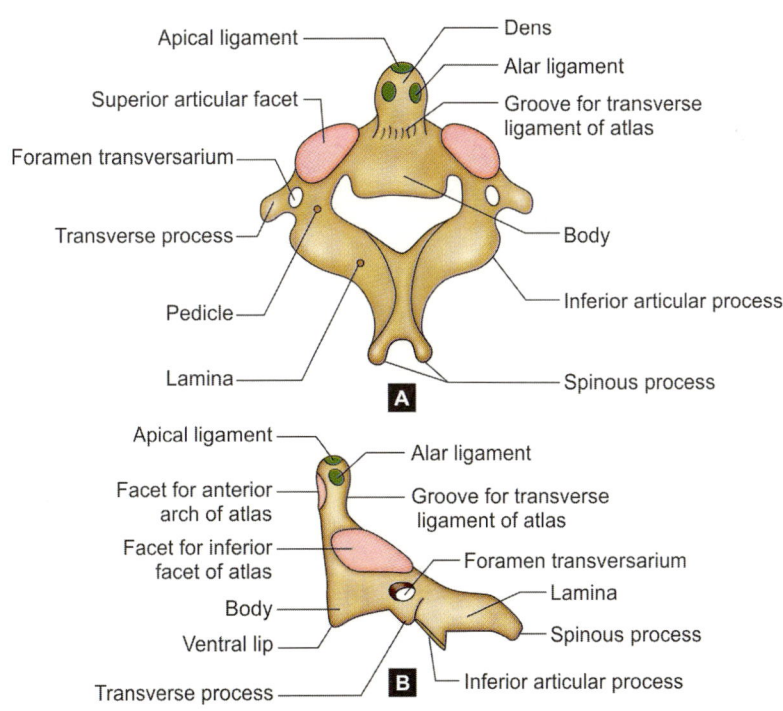

Fig. 19.12: Axis: (A) Posterosuperior aspect; (B) Lateral aspect

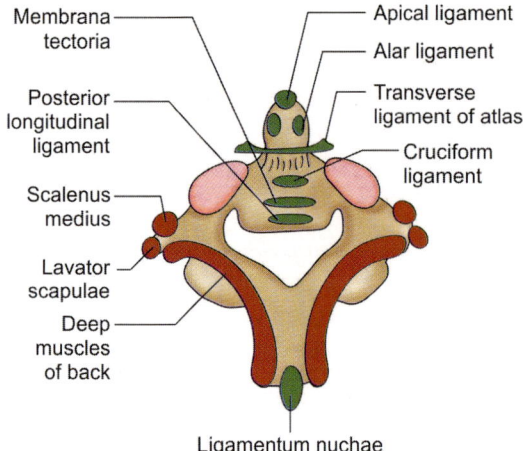

Fig. 19.13: Attachments and relations of axis: Postero-superior view

Peculiarities

1. It is strongest of the cervical vertebrae.
2. It is easily identified by the presence of an *odontoid process* (*dens*) which is a strong tooth like projection from the superior surface of body.

Features and attachments

a. Body and odontoid process

1. Apex of odontoid process gives attachment to *apical ligament*.
2. On each side of the apex, the sloping gives attachment to *alar ligament*.
3. Anterior surface of odontoid process possesses an oval facet for articulation with anterior arch of atlas.
4. Posterior surface of odontoid process is grooved to lodge *transverse ligament of atlas*.
5. Inferior surface of body is related to *intervertebral disc*.
6. The anterior surface of body gives attachments to *anterior longitudinal ligament* in the midline and *longus colli muscle* on each side.
7. The posterior surface of the body provides attachments to following 3 structures from above downwards:
    i. *Lower vertical limb of cruciform ligament.*
    ii. *Membrana tectoria.*
    iii. *Posterior longitudinal ligament.*
8. *Superior articular facet* (for articulation with the inferior facet of atlas) is situated lateral to odontoid process, partly over the body and partly on the pedicle.

b. Vertebral arch

1. The pedicle passes backwards from the upper part of body.
2. *Superior articular facet* is large, flat and circular. It is directed upwards and laterally.
3. *Inferior articular facet* is situated posterior to transverse process and is directed downwards and forwards.
4. *Spine* is short, thick and strong. Its tip is bifid and receives attachment of *ligamentum nuchae*.
5. *Ligamentum flavum* is attached to superior border and lower part of anterior surface of *lamina on each side*.
6. Side of spine provides attachment to *rectus capitis posterior major*.
7. External surface of lamina is meant for the attachment of *inferior oblique* in its upper part and *deep muscles of back* in its lower part.
8. *Transverse processes* are very small. They represent the true posterior tubercles only.
9. The tip of transverse process receives attachments of following 3 muscles from anterior to posterior:
    i. *Scalenus medius*
    ii. *Levator scapulae*
    iii. *Deep muscles of back*

Seventh cervical vertebra

Terminology

It is also called *vertebra prominens* because it has a very long spine which may be palpated under the skin of lower part of the back of neck.

Peculiarities (Fig. 19.14)
1. *Spine* is long, horizontal and nonbifid.
2. *Transverse process* is large with prominent posterior tubercle.
3. *Foramen transversarium* is smaller and some times may be absent.

Important attachments and relations
1. *Spine* provides attachments to *ligamentum nuchae, trapezius, rhomhoideus minor* and *deep muscles of back*.
2. *Posterior tubercle* of transverse process receives attachments of *suprapleural membrane* and *scalenus minimus*.
3. *Foramen transversarium* transmits *accessory vertebral vein*.

Note: *Vertebral artery occupies the foramina transversaria of the upper 6 cervical vertebrae only*

II. THORACIC VERTEBRAE

There are 12 thoracic vertebrae. They can be classified as *typical* and *atypical*. 2nd to 8th thoracic vertebrae are typical while 1st and 9th to 12th thoracic vertebrae are atypical.

A. Typical thoracic vertebra
Peculiarities
1. *Articular facets* are present by the side of body and on front of transverse processes.
2. *Body* is heart shaped.
3. *Vertebral foramen* is circular.
4. *Spinous process* is long, pointed and directed downwards.
5. *Pedicle* is attached to the upper part of the body making the *inferior vertebral notch* deeper.

Features and attachments (Figs 19.15 to 19.17)

Typical thoracic vertebra has got a *body* and a *vertebral arch*. These enclose a relatively smaller and circular vertebral foramen.

a. Body
1. It is heart shaped.
2. Its anteroposterior and transverse dimensions are almost equal.
3. On each side, the body is characterized by the presence of 2 *costal facets, superior* and *inferior*.

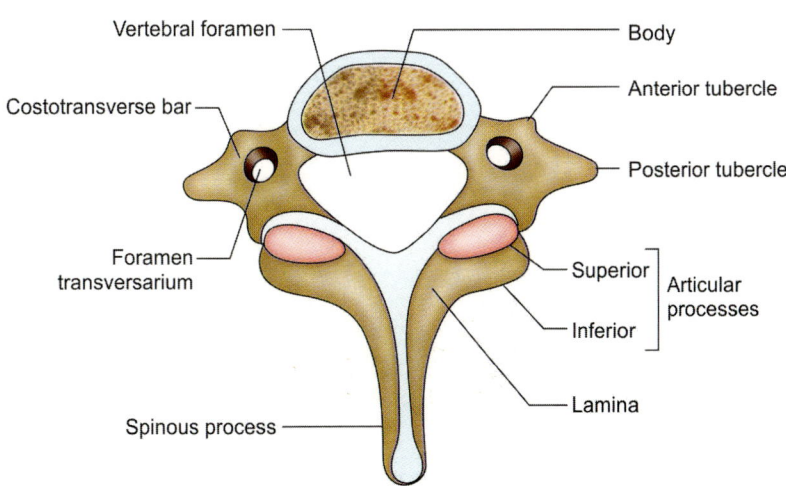

Fig. 19.14: Vertebra prominens : Superior aspect

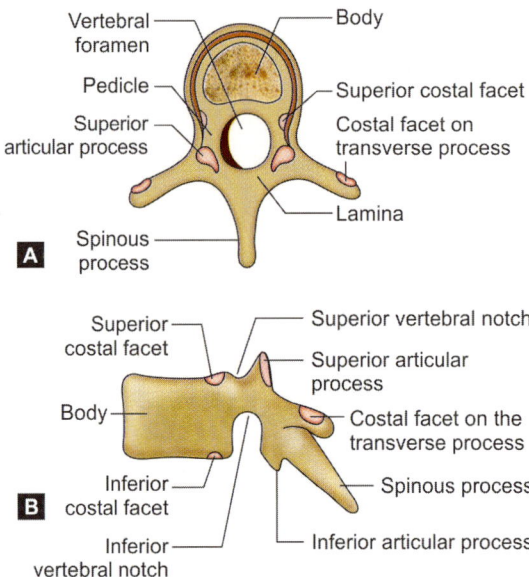

Fig. 19.15: Typical thoracic vertebra. (A) Superior aspect; (B) Left lateral aspect

4. *Superior costal facet* is larger and situated on the upper border of body near the pedicle.
5. *Inferior costal facet* is smaller and placed near the lower border just in front of inferior vertebral notch.
6. Anterior surface of body provides attachment to anterior *longitudinal ligament*.
7. Posterior surface is marked by *vascular foramina for basivertebral veins* which are covered by *posterior longitudinal ligament*. The latter is attached to the upper and lower borders of the posterior surface of body.

b. **Vertebral arch**

Vertebral arch consists of a pair of *pedicles, laminae,* the *superior* and *inferior articular processes*, the *transverse processes* and a *spine*.

i. **Pedicles**

1. These are directed backwards, i.e. do not diverge and therefore making the vertebral foramen circular.

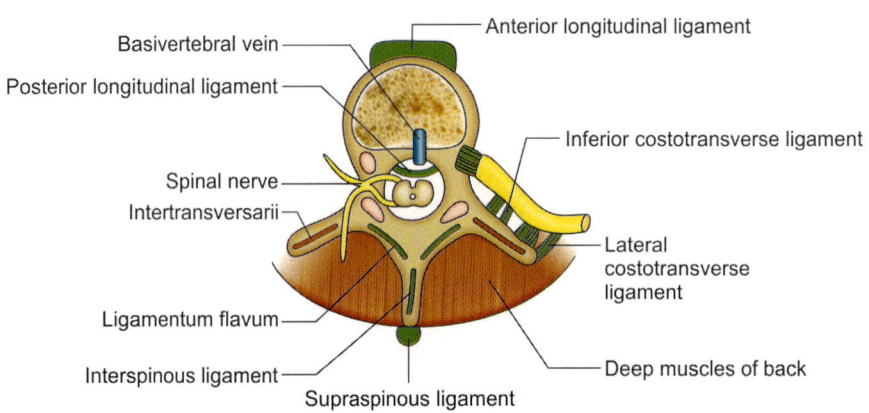

Fig. 19.16: Attachments and relations of thoracic vertebra : Superior view

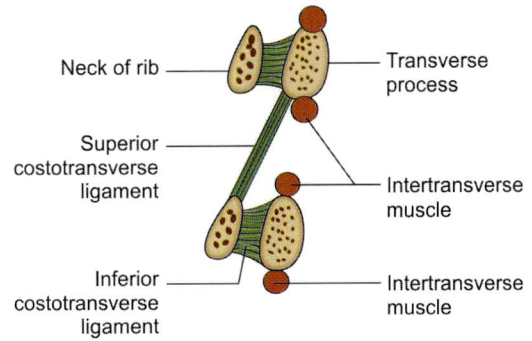

Fig. 19.17: Attachments of transverse process of a thoracic vertebra

    2. Pedicles are attached nearer the superior border of body and thus the *superior vertebral notch* is shallow where as the *inferior vertebral notch* is deep.
- ii. **Laminae**
  1. They overlap each other from above downwards.
  2. *Ligamenta flava* are attached to their upper borders and lower parts of anterior surfaces.
  3. *Deep muscles of back* are attached to the posterior surfaces of laminae.
- iii. **Superior articular processes**
  1. These are flat surfaces located on the superior aspects of junctions of pedicles and laminae.
  2. These facets are directed *backwards* and slightly laterally.
- iv. **Inferior articular processes**
  1. They are fused with the lateral ends of laminae.
  2. Each articular facet is flat and faces forwards and little downwards and medially.
- v. **Transverse processes**
  1. They project backwards and laterally from the junction of pedicles and laminae between the superior and inferior articular processes.
  2. A *facet* is observed on its anterior surface near the tip for articulation with the tubercle of numerically corresponding rib.

3. Tip provides attachment to *lateral costotransverse ligament*.
4. Its anterior surface medial to facet receives attachment of *(inferior) costotransverse ligament*.
5. *Superior costotransverse ligament* is attached to lower border of transverse process.

Note: *Superior costotransverse ligament is superior in relation to the neck of rib below.*

6. *Intertransverse mucles* are attached to superior and inferior borders of transverse processes.
7. Posterior surfaces of transverse processes near their lateral ends provide attachments to *levatores costarum*.

- vi. **Spine**

It is long, pointed and in general directed downwards.

Note: *In the middle four vertebrae the spinous processes are almost vertical.*

Thoracic spines provide attachments to the following structures:
1. *Trapezius* (all the thoracic spines) and *latissimus dorsi* (lower six thoracic spines) muscles.
2. *Interspinous and supraspinous ligaments*.
3. *Rhomboideus major* (2nd to 5th thoracic spines) and rhomboideus minor (1st thoracic spine) muscles.
4. *Serratus posterior superior* (upper three thoracic spines) and *serratus posterior inferior* (lower two thoracic spines) muscles.
5. *Deep muscles of the back*.

B. Atypical thoracic vertebrae (Fig. 19.18)

First thoracic vertebra

1. Its *body* is more like a cervical vertebra with the upper surface of body showing lateral lipping and is bevelled anteriorly.
2. *Superior costal facet* on the lateral aspect of body is complete for articulation with the head of 1st rib.

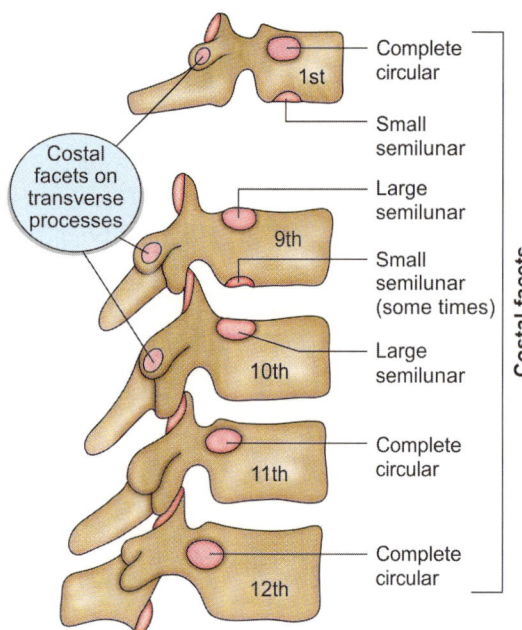

Fig. 19.18: Atypical thoracic vertebrae: Right lateral aspect

3. *Inferior costal facet* is half (demifacet) for 2nd rib.
4. *Spine* is nearly horizontal.
5. *Superior vertebral notches* are well marked.

Ninth thoracic vertebra

1. *Body* has got only *superior costal facets* (demifacets).
2. Inferior costal facets are absent.

Tenth thoracic vertebra

1. *Body* has single complete *costal facet* on each side superiorly.
2. *Costal facets* extend on the roots of pedicles.

Eleventh thoracic vertebra

1. *Body* has single *costal facet* on each side.
2. *Costal facet* extends on the upper part of pedicle.
3. *Transverse process* has no articular facet.

Twelfth thoracic vertebra

1. Shape is similar to lumbar vertebra.

2. Single *costal facet* is seen on each side of vertebra.
3. *Costal facet* is more on lower part of pedicle than on the body.
4. Transverse process has no articular facet but has *superior, inferior* and *lateral tubercles*.
5. The *superior articular facets* are thoracic in type whereas the *inferior articular facets* are lumbar in type.

III. LUMBAR VERTEBRAE

Peculiarities (Fig. 19.19)

1. A lumbar vertebra has *massive body*.
2. *Vertebral foramen* is triangular.
3. *Spine* is quadrangular.
4. *Superior articular facet* is concave.
5. *Inferior articular facet* is convex.
6. Posteroinferior part of root of transverse process has a rough elevation called *accessory process*.

Classification

There are 5 lumbar vertebrae. They are classified as *typical* and *atypical*. First to fourth lumbar vertebrae are typical. Last (5th) lumbar vertebra is atypical.

A. Typical lumbar vertebra (Figs 19.20 and 19.21)

a. Body

1. It is large.
2. Its transverse diameter is more than the anteroposterior diameter.
3. Its upper and lower surfaces are covered by *hyaline cartilages* which in turn are related to *intervertebral discs*.
4. Anterior surface in the midline provides attachment to the *anterior longitudinal ligament*.
5. *Crura of diaphragm* are attached to anterior surface on either side of anterior longitudinal ligament. Right crus is attached to upper three while left crus to upper two lumbar vertebrae.

The Vertebrae 155

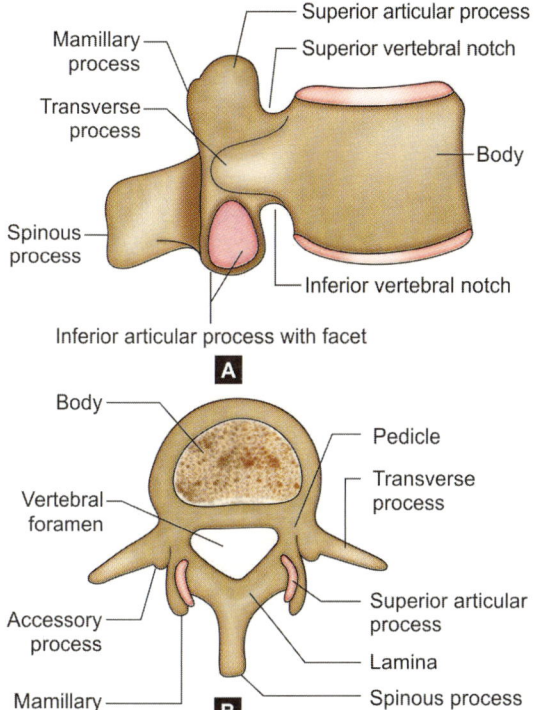

Fig. 19.19: Typical lumbar vertebrae. (A) Right lateral aspect; (B) Superior aspect

6. *Psoas major and its tendinous arches* are attached to upper and lower margins of sides of body.
7. *Posterior longitudinal ligament* is attached to margins of its posterior surface.

Note: *Remember, when lumbar vertebral body is seen from the side, attachments of following structures are appreciated from anterior to posterior; (i) anterior longitudinal ligament, (ii) crus of diaphragm, (iii) psoas major and (iv) posterior longitudinal ligament.*

b. Vertebral foramen

1. It is triangular in cross section.
2. Outer two spinal meninges, i.e. *dura mater* and *arachnoid mater*, are found in the vertebral foramina of all the lumbar vertebrae.
3. *Conus medullaris with pia mater* occupies the vertebral foramen of 1st lumbar vertebra.
4. *Cauda equina* is contained in the foramina of lower four lumbar vertebrae.

c. Vertebral arch

i. Pedicles
1. They are short and strong.
2. *Inferior vertebral notches* are deeper than the superior vertebral notches.
3. Vertebral notches of adjacent vertebrae complete the formation of *intervertebral foramen*.
4. Intervertebral foramina are traversed by *spinal nerves* and *radicular vessels*.

ii. Laminae
1. These are short and thick.
2. They are directed posteromedially.

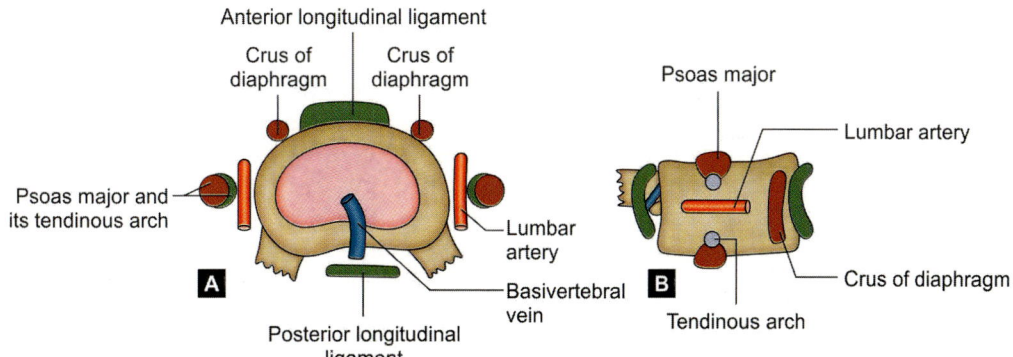

Fig. 19.20: Attachments and relations of body of lumbar vertebra. (A) Superior view; (B) Right lateral view

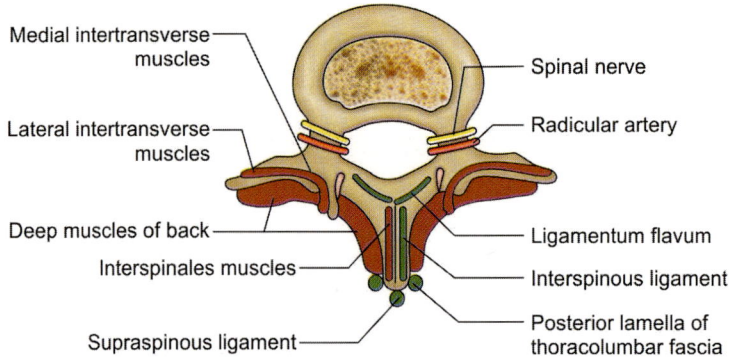

Fig. 19.21: Relations and attachments of vertebral arch of lumbar vertebra

3. *Ligamentum flavum* is attached to its upper border and lower half of its anterior surface.
4. Posterior surface of lamina gives attachments to *deep muscles of back*.

iii. **Spine**
   1. It is quadrilateral in shape.
   2. Its posterior border provides attachments to *supraspinous ligament* in the midline and *posterior lamella of thoracolumbar fascia* on each side.
   3. Its superior and inferior borders receive attachments of *interspinous ligaments* in the midline and *interspinales muscles* on each side.
   4. Sides of spine give attachments to *deep muscles of back*.

iv. **Transverse processes**
   1. They are tapering and thin.
   2. They are homologous with the ribs in the thoracic region.
   3. *Medial and lateral arcuate ligaments* are attached to the tip of transverse process of 1st lumbar vertebra.
   4. *Iliolumbar ligament* is attached to the tip of 5th lumbar vertebra.
   5. *Middle lamella of thoracolumbar fascia* is attached to the tips of transverse processes of all vertebrae.
   6. The anterior surface is marked by a faint ridge to which is attached the *anterior lamella of thoracolumbar fascia*.
   7. Its anterior surface medial to ridge gives attachment to *psoas major* while the area lateral to ridge receives attachment of *quadratus lumborum muscle*.
   8. Posterior surfaces of transverse processes are meant for attachments of *deep muscles of back*.
   9. The upper and lower borders of transverse processes give attachments to *intertransversarii muscles*.
   10. *Accessory process* gives attachment to medial intertransverse (medial part of intertransversarii) muscle.

v. **Articular processes**
   1. *Superior articular facet* is concave and faces mainly medially while *inferior articular facet* is convex and faces mainly laterally.
   2. The distance between the superior articular processes is relatively more than that between inferior articular processes in upper three lumbar vertebrae. This relation is reversed in case of 5th lumbar vertebra. In 4th lumbar vertebra both superior and inferior articular processes are at equal distances (Fig. 19.22).
   3. Posterior border of superior articular process is marked by a roughened elevation called *mamillary process*.

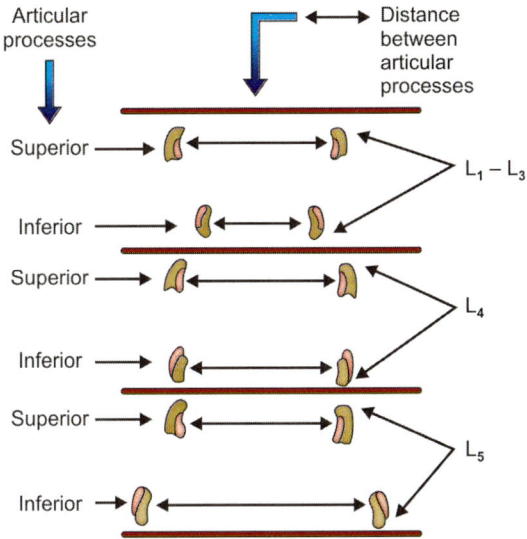

Fig. 19.22: Interrelationships of distances between lumbar articular processes

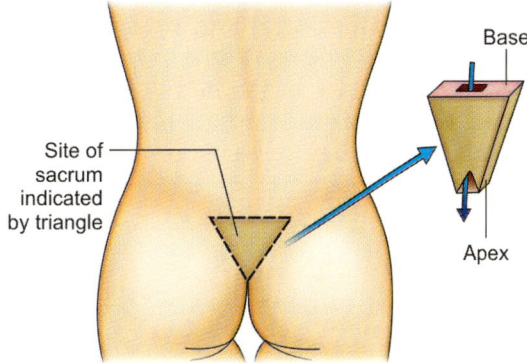

Fig. 19.23: Wedge shaped sacrum (arrow is passing through the sacral canal)

4. Mamillary process provides attachments to *medial intertransverse muscles* and *deep muscles of back*.

B. Atypical (5th) lumbar vertebra

1. Thick and short *transverse processes* are connected to whole of the pedicles and part of body.
2. The distance between *inferior articular processes* is more than that between *superior articular processes*.
3. The *body* is very much deeper anteriorly than posteriorly.

IV. SACRUM

Terminology

The word sacrum is derived from the Latin word 'sacred'. It is considered to be a 'sacred bone' because it occupies the lowest part of the back which is invariably covered as mark of respect.

General form (Fig. 19.23)

Sacrum is a wedge shaped triangular bone. The base of wedge is superior and forms the base of sacrum. Edge of the wedge forms the inferior apex. It has 4 surfaces, *pelvic (anterior), dorsal (posterior)* and 2 *lateral*. The canal of sacrum is called *sacral canal*.

Anatomical position (Fig. 19.24)

1. Sacrum is a midline bone placed between hip bones (on each side), 5th lumbar

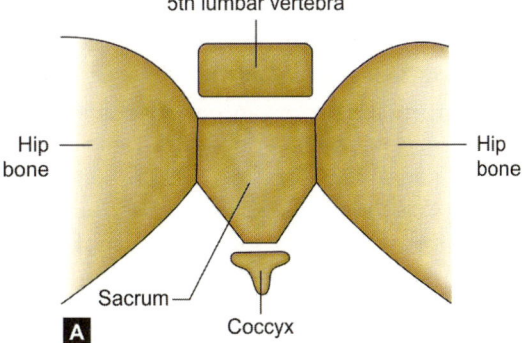

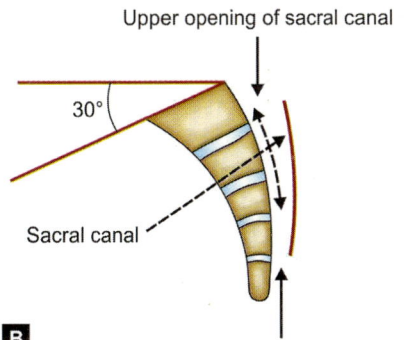

Fig. 19.24: Position of sacrum. (A) Posterior view; (B) Side view

vertebra (superiorly) and coccyx (inferiorly).
2. Superior surface of the body of 1st sacral vertebra slopes forward at an angle of 30°.
3. Anterior surface of sacrum faces downwards and forwards.
4. The upper end of sacral canal is directed upwards.

Features and attachments

A. Base

For the sake of description it can be divided into a central portion and 2 lateral parts (*ala*).

a. Central portion

It shows features of a typical vertebra.

i. Body

1. Its transverse diameter is greater than the anteroposterior diameter, i.e. it is lumbar in type.
2. Its anterior border projects forwards as *sacral promontory*.
3. It articulates with 5th lumbar vertebra to form *lumbosacral joint*.
4. The angle between anterior surface of 5th lumbar vertebra and ventral surface of 1st sacral vertebra (*lumbosacral angle*) is approximately 210° (Fig. 19.25).
5. Anterior and posterior surfaces of body of 1st sacral vertebra provide attachments to lowest fibres of *anterior and posterior longitudinal ligaments* respectively.

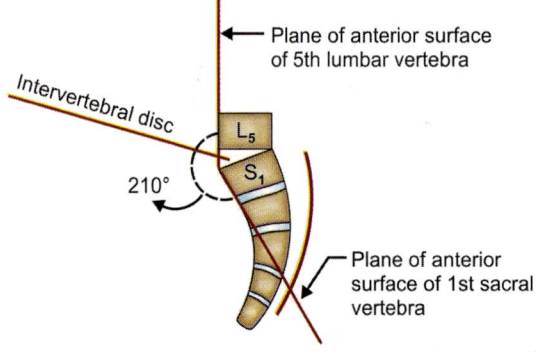

Fig. 19.25: Lumbosacral angle

ii. Vertebral foramen

1. It is triangular.
2. It faces upwards, i.e. it lies in horizontal plane during erect position of body.
3. It leads into sacral canal.

iii. Vertebral arch

1. *Pedicle* is short and directed backwards and laterally.
2. *Laminae* are directed backwards, medially and downwards. Lowest pair of *ligamenta flava* are attached to them.
3. Spine forms 1st *spinous tubercle*.
4. *Superior articular processes* project upward and bear concave surfaces for inferior articular processes of 5th lumbar vertebra.

b. Ala

1. It is on either side of body.
2. It is formed by the fusion of transverse process and costal element of primitive vertebra.
3. It has smooth medial and rough lateral parts.
4. Both the parts are covered by *psoas major* muscle.
5. The smooth part is related to (from lateral to medial):
    i. Obturator nerve.
    iii. Lumbosacral trunk.
    ii. Iliolumbar artery.
    iv. Sympathetic chain.

Note: *One can remember the formula of OILS to realize the relations of ALA in which O = Obturator nerve, I = Iliolumbar artery, L = Lumbosacral trunk and S = Sympathetic chain.*

6. Lateral rough part gives attachments to *iliacus* anteriorly and *ventral sacroiliac ligament* posteriorly.

B. Apex

1. It is formed by the inferior surface of 5th sacral vertebra.
2. It articulates with coccyx.

C. Surfaces

a. Pelvic surface (Fig. 19.26)
1. It is smooth and concave.
2. This surface faces downwards and forwards.
3. *Four transverse ridges* and *four pairs of pelvic sacral foramina* at the lateral ends of these ridges, represent the junctions of 5 fused sacral vertebrae.
4. Pelvic sacral foramina transmit:
   i. *Ventral rami of upper 4 sacral nerves.*
   ii. *Lateral sacral arteries.*
5. Pelvic sacral foramina communicate with the *sacral canal* through *intervertebral foramina*.
6. Median area between pelvic sacral foramina of two sides represent the bodies of 5 sacral vertebrae. This area is related to (Fig. 19.27):
   i. *Median sacral vessels* in the midline.
   ii. *Sympathetic trunks* along the medial margins of ventral sacral foramina.
   iii. *Peritoneum and pelvic mesocolon* to bodies of upper 2½ pieces.
   iv. *Rectum* to lower 2½ pieces.
   v. *Superior rectal artery.*

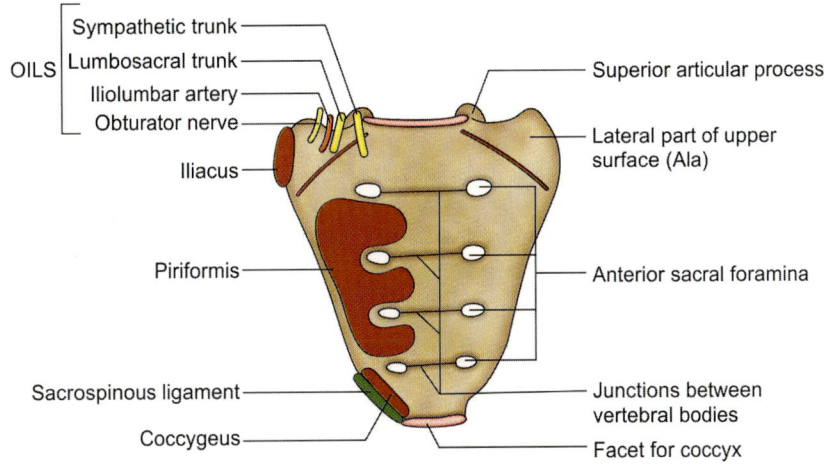

Fig. 19.26: Sacrum: Pelvic surface

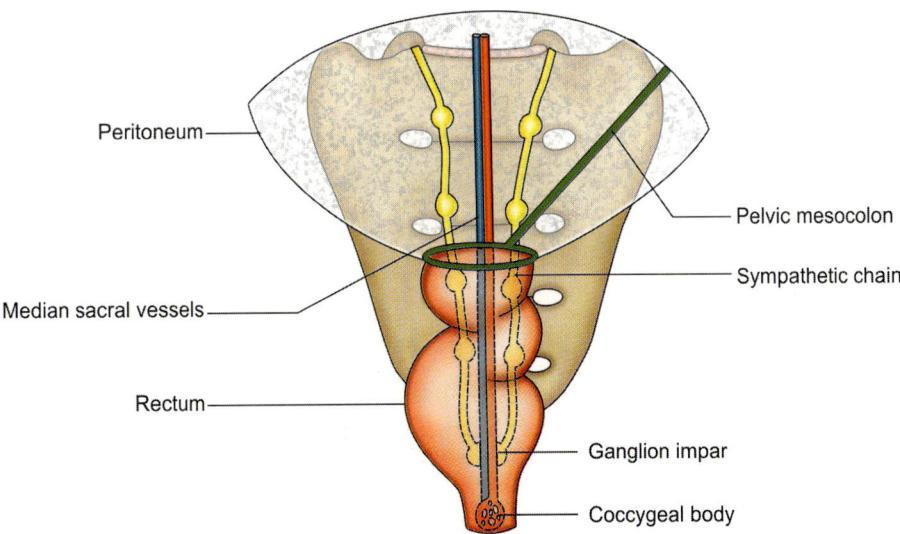

Fig. 19.27: Median relations of pelvic surface of sacrum

7. The *lateral mass* (bony mass lateral to pelvic sacral foramina) is formed by the fusion of costal elements with each other and with the transverse processes of sacral vertebrae.
8. *Piriformis* orginates from the middle 3 pieces of sacral vertebrae.

b. Dorsal surface (Fig. 19.28)

1. This surface is relatively rough.
2. It is convex and faces backwards and upwards.
3. Five vertical uneven ridges are the most prominent features on the dorsal surface.
4. A median ridge called *median sacral crest* is formed by the fusion of sacral spines. Elevations along this crest are therefore known as *spinous tubercles*.
5. On either side of median sacral crest is *intermediate sacral crest*. Tubercles along the crest are called *articular tubercles* because this crest is formed by the fusion of articular processes of sacral vertebrae.
6. The lower end of the intermediate sacral crest projects as *sacral cornu*. This represents the inferior articular process of 5th sacral vertebra.
7. Most lateral crest, on each side, is called *lateral sacral crest*. Its tubercles are called *transverse tubercles* because this crest is formed by the fusion of transverse processes of sacral vertebrae.
8. There are four pairs of *dorsal sacral foramina*. These are located just lateral to intermediate sacral crest (Fig. 19.29).
9. Dorsal sacral foramina communicate with the sacral canal through intervertebral foramina.

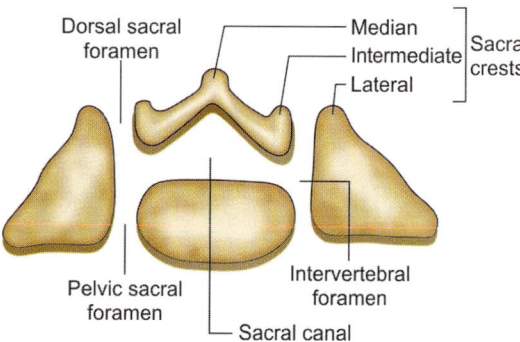

Fig. 19.29: Sacral canal and its communications

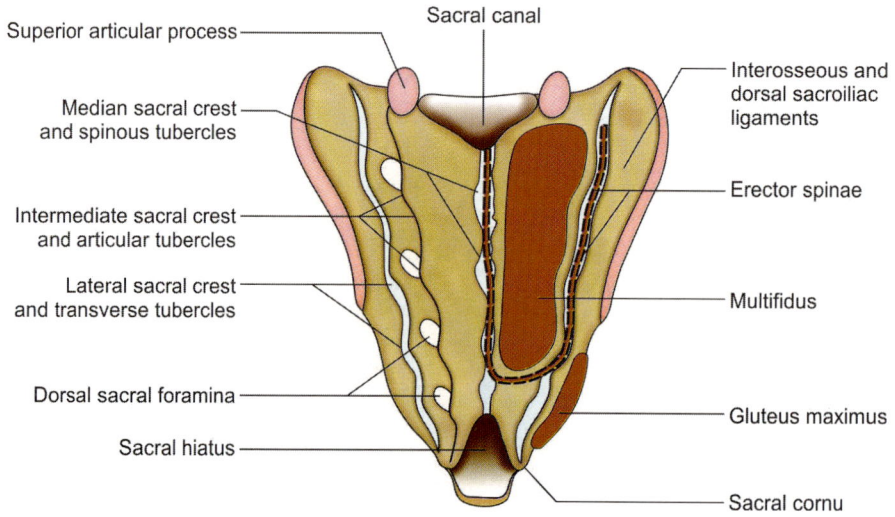

Fig. 19.28: Sacrum : Dorsal surface

10. The *erctor spinae* muscle takes origin in a 'U' shaped manner from lateral and median sacral crests on each side.
11. The area enclosed by 'U' gives origin to *multifidus muscles*.

c. Lateral surface (Fig. 19.30)

It is tapering, being wider above and narrower below.

i. Upper wider part

1. Anteriorly it has an 'L' shaped articular surface called *auricular surface*. Angle between the two limbs of 'L' faces backwards.

Note: *It is named as auricular surface because it is shaped like the auricle or pinna. Remember that 'auricular' is 'articular'.*

2. Auricular surface articulates with ilium to form *sacroiliac joint*.
3. Anterior and inferior margins of auricular surface provide attachment to *ventral sacroiliac ligament*.
4. *Interosseous sacroiliac ligament* is attached to the area just behind the auricular surface.
5. More posteriorly is attached the *dorsal sacroiliac ligament*.

ii. Lower narrower part

It gives attachments to following structures from anterior to posterior:
   i. *Coccygeus muscle*.
   ii. *Sacrospinous ligament*.
   iii. *Sacrotuberous ligament*.
   iv. *Gluteus maximus muscle*.

Note: *Remember on the lower narrow part of the lateral area there are 2 muscles and 2 ligaments. We can also say that 2 ligaments are sandwiched between two muscles.*

D. Sacral canal

1. It is formed by sacral vertebral foramina.
2. It is triangular in cross section.
3. The laminae of 5th sacral vertebra do not fuse giving rise to *sacral hiatus* which marks the lower end of sacral canal.
4. Sacral canal communicates with the pelvic and dorsal sacral foramina through four *intervertebral foramina* present in its lateral wall on each side.
5. The contents of sacral canal are as follows:
   i. Lower part of *cauda equina* (sacral and coccygeal nerve roots).
   ii. *Filum terminale*.

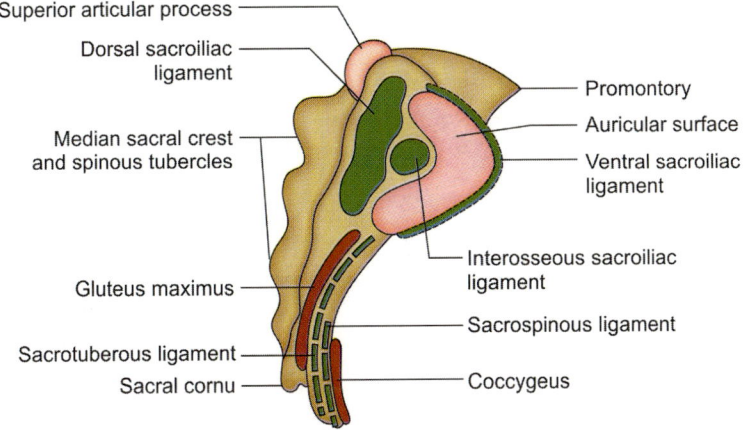

Fig. 19.30: Sacrum : Right lateral aspect

iii. *Spinal meninges.*
iv. *Lateral sacral vessels.*
6. Following structures emerge through sacral hiatus:
    i. *5th Sacral nerves.*
    ii. *Coccygeal nerves.*
    iii. *Filum terminale.*

Note: *Remember that the 2nd sacral vertebra marks the lower limit of dura mater, arachnoid mater and subarachnoid space.*

7. Lower part of sacral hiatus is bounded on each side by *sacral cornu* which represents the inferior articular process of 5th sacral vertebra. Sacral cornu gives attachment to *intercornual ligament.*

Sex differences (Table 19.1)

Table 19.1: Sexual dimorphism in sacrum

Features	Male sacrum	Female sacrum
1. Length	More	Less
2. Ratio between the transverse width of body of 1st sacral vertebra and the entire width of sacral base.	More than 1/3rd	Less than 1/3rd
3. Auricular surface	Relatively longer, encroaches on the 3rd segment also in addition to upper two segments.	Smaller, occupies only upper two segments of sacrum
4. Anterior surface of sacrum	Shallower	Deeper
5. Sacral index $\left(\dfrac{\text{Breath of the base}}{\text{Lenght}} \times 100\right)$	Lesser	Greater
6. Width	Relatively narrower	Wider
7. Curvature	Uniformly curved	Flattened in the upper part but sharply curved in the lower part

V. COCCYX

Terminology

The word coccyx is derived from Greek word 'cuckoo', the name of a bird. This is due to the fact that the bone resembles the beak of a bird. Another name of coccyx is 'tail bone' because it is highly developed in animal with tail.

Normal anatomical position

Coccyx is directed downwards and forwards.

Features and attachments (Fig. 19.31)

Coccyx is formed by the fusion of four coccygeal vertebrae. It is triangular in shape with the base upwards and apex downwards. It has two surfaces (pelvic and dorsal) and two lateral borders (right and left).

A. Base

1. It is formed by the superior surface of the body of 1st coccygeal vertebra.
2. It articulates with the apex of sacrum.
3. *Coccygeal cornua* project from the posterolateral part of the base.
4. Coccygeal and sacral cornua are connected by *intercornual ligaments.*
5. *Transverse process* projects laterally from the base.

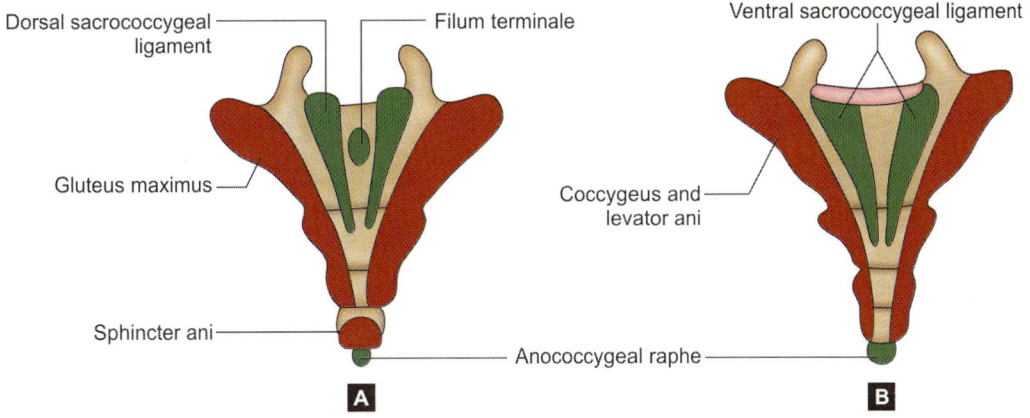

Fig. 19.31: Coccyx. (A) Dorsal aspect; (B) Ventral aspect

B. Apex
It is formed by the last coccygeal segment. It provides attachment to *anococcygeal raphe*.

C. Surfaces
a. Pelvic surface
1. *Ganglion impar* is related to it.
2. It provides attachment to *ventral sacrococcygeal ligament*.
3. *Coccygeus* and *levator ani* are attached to either side of it.

b. Dorsal surface
It provides attachments to following structures:
   i. Gluteus maximus.
   ii. Sphincter ani externus.
   iii. Dorsal sacrococcygeal ligament.
   iv. Filum terminale.

Note: *Remember filum terminale is a fibrous cord which connects the tip of spinal cord with the dorsum of coccyx.*

D. Lateral borders
Following ligaments are attached to either side (lateral border) of coccyx:
   i. Sacrotuberous ligament.
   ii. Sacrospinous ligament.

OSSIFICATION OF VERTEBRAE

1. GENERAL MODE OF OSSIFICATION
A. Primary centres: 3 in all, one for body (centrum) and one for each half of the vertebral (neural) arch.

  Appearance : 9–16 weeks of intrauterine life
  Fusion : Each half of the neural arch with each other : 1 year
        : Neural arch with centrum : 3–6 years.

Note: *Before fusion, neural arch is united with centrum by synchondrosis called neurocentral joint.*

B. Secondary centres: 5 in total, one each for circumferential parts (*annular epiphyseal ring*) of upper and lower surfaces of the body, one each for tips of transverse processes and one for the tip of spine.

  Appearance : Puberty
  Fusion : 25 years.

II. EXCEPTIONS TO GENERAL MODE OF OSSIFICATION
a. Atlas : 3 centres in all.
1 each for lateral mass and half of posterior arch.

1 for anterior arch.

Appearance : For lateral mass – 7 weeks of intrauterine life.
For anterior arch – 1 year

Fusion : Two halves of posterior arch (derived from lateral mass) fuse with each other : 4 years
Anterior arch with each lateral mass : 7 years.

b. Axis: 5 Primary and 2 secondary centres appear for axis.

Appearance

Primary centres:

1 for centrum : 2 months of intrauterine life.

2 for vertebral arch : 4 months of intrauterine life

2 for dens : 6 months of intrauterine life

These two centres for dens fuse to form one centre just before birth

Secondary centres

1 for tip of dens : 2 years
1 for lower surface of body : Puberty

Fusion

Two halves of the neural arches,
with each other : 3 years
Body with neural arch and dens : 4 years
Apex of dens with rest of
the dens : 12 years
Body with the inferior
epiphyseal plate : 25 years

c. 7th cervical vertebra

A separate centre appears for each costal element of transverse process at 6 months of intrauterine life. This fuses with the body and transverse element of transverse process at 6 years. Sometimes this part of the vertebra remains independent and then forms cervical rib.

d. Lumbar vertebrae

Two additional centres appear, one each for mamillary process.

e. Sacrum

Sacrum ossifies from 21 primary and 14 secondary centres. Primary centres appear in the bodies (5), arches (10) and costal elements (6). Secondary centres appear in the epiphyses of bodies (10), auricular surfaces (2) and margins below auricular surfaces (2).

i. Primary centres

Appearance : 2–8 Months of intrauterine life

Fusion : 2–8 years

ii. Secondary centres

Appearance : Puberty

Fusion : 25 years

f. Coccyx

Coccyx ossifies from 4 primary centres, one each for individual coccygeal vertebra.

Appearance : 1–10 years
Fusion : 20–30 years

APPLIED ANATOMY

Note: *Clinicians usually use the word 'spine' instead of vertebral column.*

1. **Congenital anomalies of vertebral column**

   Minor anomalies may remain unnoticed. Many times anomalies are detected on routine examination for some other diseases. Some of the interesting congenital anomalies are as follows:

   i. *Cervical rib* (Fig. 19.32)

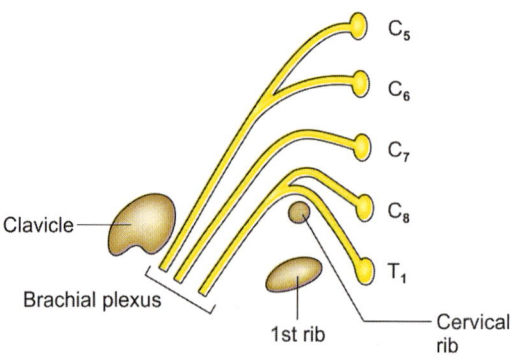

Fig. 19.32: Cervical rib

In 1 per cent individuals costal element of the 7th cervical vertebra remains as separate entity. This is called cervical rib. The contribution of 1st thoracic nerve to the brachial plexus passes above the cervical rib leading to neurological pressure symptoms.

ii. Sacrum may consist of six vertebrae.

iii. *Sacralization of 5th lumbar vertebra*

5th Lumbar vertebra fuses with the base of sacrum either partially or completely.

iv. *Lumbarization of sacrum* (Fig. 19.33)

1st Sacral vertebra remains partially or completely free from the rest of the sacrum.

v. *Agenesis of segments of vertebral column* is rare and usually occurs in its terminal portions (Fig. 19.34). Extreme degree of involvement is incompatible with life.

vi. First lumbar vertebra has a pair of ribs (*lumbar ribs*) in 7 per cent of skeletons.

vii. Defective closure of the two halves of the neural arch leads to bony gap (Fig. 19.35). Following are some of the important conditions:

   a. *Spina bifida.*
   b. *Gap in the upper sacrum.*
   c. *Larger or smaller sacral hiatus.*

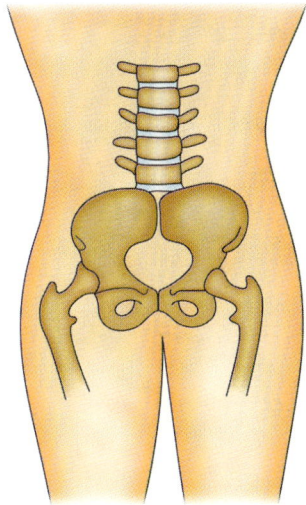

Fig. 19.34: Congenital absence of sacrum and coccyx

viii. The body of vertebra may ossify from two primary centres. If one fails to develop, a wedge shaped vertebra develops. This is one of the causes of *scoliosis* (lateral curvature of spine) (Fig. 19.36).

Note: *Remember both spina bifida and scoliosis usually occur in the lumbar region of vertebral column.*

ix. *Klippel-Feil Syndrome* is a condition of congenitally fused and deformed cervical vertebrae (Fig. 19.37).

x. Congenital fusion of the ring of atlas to the base of occiput (*atlas occipi-*

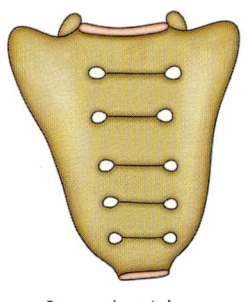
6 sacral vertebrae

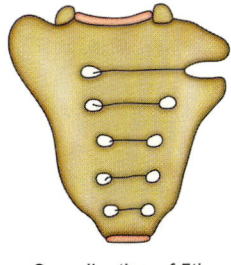
Sacralization of 5th lumbar vertebra

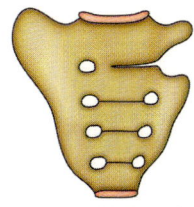
Lumbarization of sacrum

Fig. 19.33: Numerical anomalies of sacrum

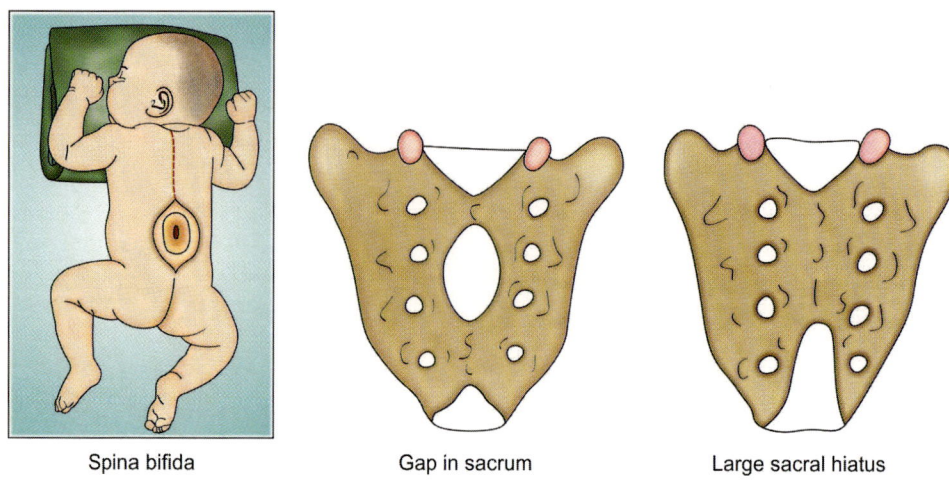

Fig. 19.35: Defective closure of neural arch

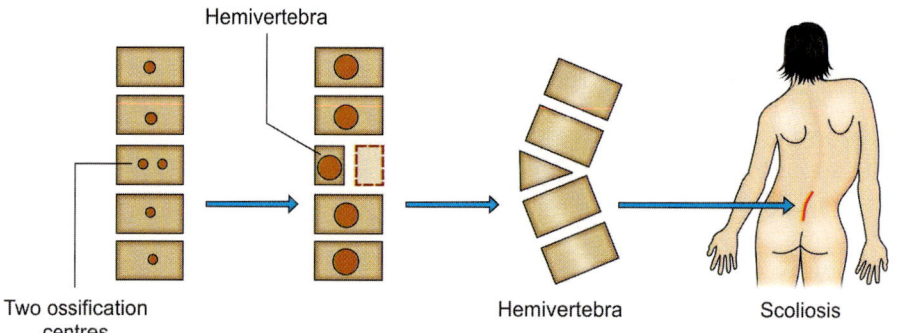

Fig. 19.36: Scoliosis due to hemivertebra

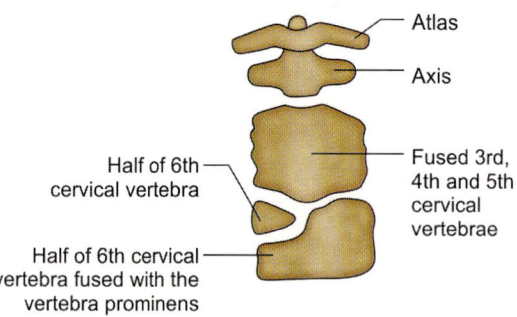

Fig. 19.37: Klippel-Feil Syndrome

talization) is one of the most common abnormalities of upper cervical vertebrae.

xi. Anomalies of odontoid process of axis are rare, but if present, result in atlanto-axial instability leading to pain and neurological symptoms. Some anomalies are as follows:

   a. *Os Odontoideum*

      This is also called hypoplasia of odontoid process.

   b. *Os Terminale*

      Nonfusion of tip of odontoid process with the rest of it.

xii. *Diastematomyelia*

   It is a congenital longitudinal fissure in the spinal cord. It is due to a midline osseous septum. Dura mater usually splits making the lesion extradural (Fig. 19.38).

xiii. Vertebral anomalies lead to vertebral column deformities which are of following types:
   a. Kyphosis.
   b. Lordosis.
   c. Scoliosis.
   d. Combination of these.

Basic reasons for the above deformities are usually two folds:

a. *Failure of segmentation* (Fig. 19.39)
   Deformity depends upon the location of failure.

Anterior failure : *Kyphosis.*
Posterior failure : *Lordosis.*
Lateral failure : *Scoliosis.*

b. *Defect of formation* (Fig. 19.40)
   If the anterior part of vertebra has not fully developed then the vertebral column shows angular kyphosis. Defective formation of the lateral part of the vertebra leads to *scoliosis*.

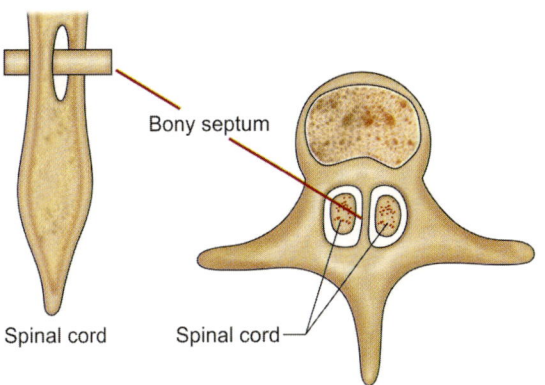

Fig. 19.38: Diastematomyelia

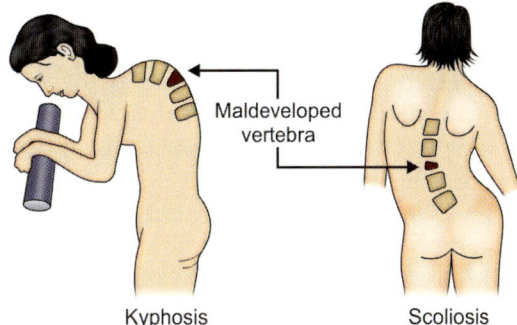

Fig. 19.40: Defective formation of vertebra

2. The vertebral bodies and intervertebral discs can very well bear the compression forces but the column is not very strong in terms of shearing forces, i.e. transverse and rotational forces. To bear the latter

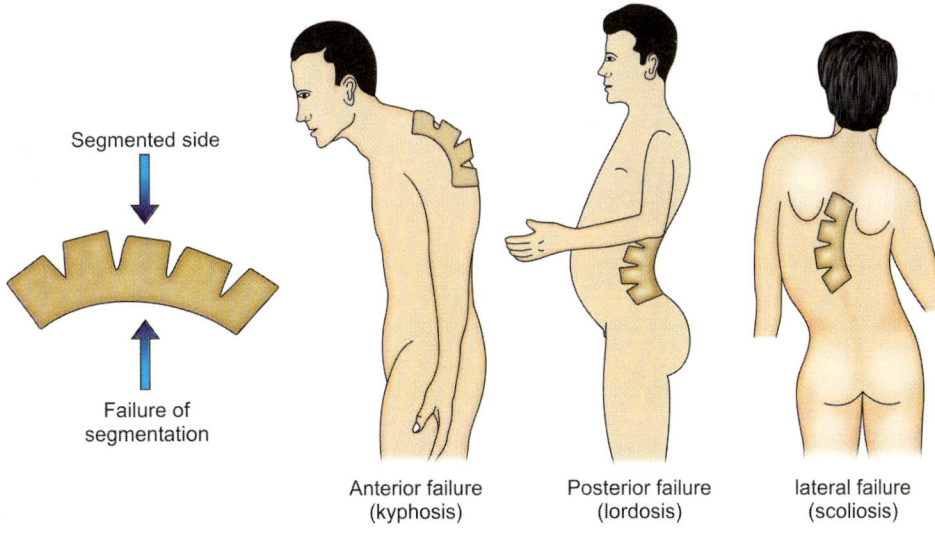

Fig. 19.39: Vertebral column deformities

there are additional ligaments to stabilize the vertebral column. These include anterior and posterior longitudinal ligaments, ligamenta flava and intertransverse, interspinous and supraspinous ligaments. All these ligaments together constitute *"the posterior ligament complex"* (Fig. 19.41).

3. *Conus medullaris* (lower end of spinal cord) is located at the level of 1st lumbar vertebra. Spinal cord injury is commonly noted at 12th thoracic and 1st lumbar vertebral levels. This frequently involves the bladder as the sacral nerves supplying the bladder appear from conus.

4. All the spinal cord segments are accommodated between 1st cervical to 1st lumbar vertebrae. Therefore one should know about the numerical relations of spinal cord segments with vertebral levels to localize the lesion in spinal cord when it is compressed by the vertebrae.

5. For proper management of *vertebral injuries*, one should always determine whether spinal cord has been involved or not. If the spinal cord is spared then the management is totally different.

6. Some of the interesting facts regarding the thoracic vertebrae are as follows:
   i. Out of all the thoracic vertebrae, 12th vertebra is most commonly fractured.
   ii. *Pott's spine* (tuberculosis of vertebral column) is commonest at dorsolumbar junction.
   iii. Bodies of T_{4-8} vertebrae are directly related to descending thoracic aorta. If there is aneurysm (localized dilatation) of aorta in this region then the vertebrae may be partly eroded by aortic pressure.
   iv. As the vertebral canal is small and circular in the thoracic region, the chances of compression of the spinal cord is more as compared to other regions.

7. *Intervertebral foramen* is very important clinically due to its contents (spinal nerve in its upper part and redicular vessels in its lower part) which are vulnerable to disc prolapse and zygapophyseal lesions (Fig. 19.42).

Table 19.1: Interrelationship between spinal cord segments and vertebral levels. '+1', '+2' and '+3' are the numbers to be added to vertebral levels to determine spinal segments.

Vertebral segments	Spinal cord segments
Cervical (C_{1-7})	+1
Upper thoracic (T_{1-6})	+2
T_{7-9}	+3
T_{10}	$L_{1,2}$
T_{11}	$L_{3,4}$
T_{12}	L_5, S_1
L_1	$S_2–Co_1$

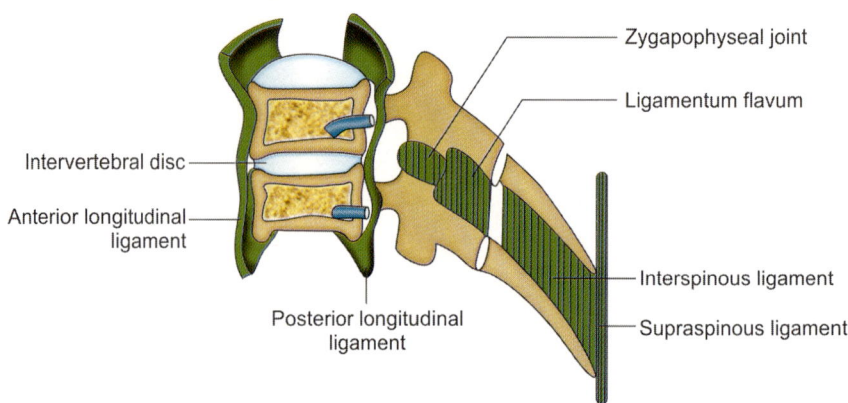

Fig. 19.41: Right halves of bodies and vertebral arches of two adjacent vertebrae; Medial view

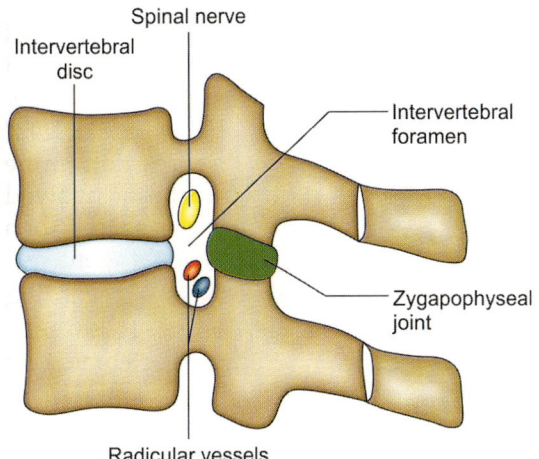

Fig. 19.42: Intervertebral foramen

8. *Disc degeneration* causes disc narrowing. This mechanical alteration predisposes the posterior intervertebral joints to osteoathrosis.
9. During old age, due to *degeneration of intervertebral discs*, some reduction in height usually occurs.
10. *Locking of the cervical vertebrae* may occur owing to dislocation of vertebral arches.
11. Thoracic vertebrae are considered to be relatively more protected because of ribs. The junction between protected and unprotected spines (thoracolumbar and cervicothoracic) are considered to be vulnerable to rotational shearing forces.
12. *Spinal tuberculosis (Pott's spine)* typically arises in a disc space but may also arise in the vertebral body itself. Some of the complications of such lesion are as follows:
    i. *Angular kyphosis*
    ii. *Paravertebral abscess*
    iii. *Cold abscess*, some distance away from the site of infection (e.g. psoas abscess) (Fig. 19.43).
13. Some of the interesting facts regarding the infection of the vertebral column are as follows:
    i. It begins usually in disc space which later erodes the adjacent bone.
    ii. It usually takes a chronic course.
    iii. Majority of infections are caused by blood-borne organisms.
14. *Spondylolisthesis* is usually due to defect in the pars interarticularis of 4th or 5th lumbar vertebra. In this case the upper vertebra begins to shift forwards on lower one (Fig. 19.44).

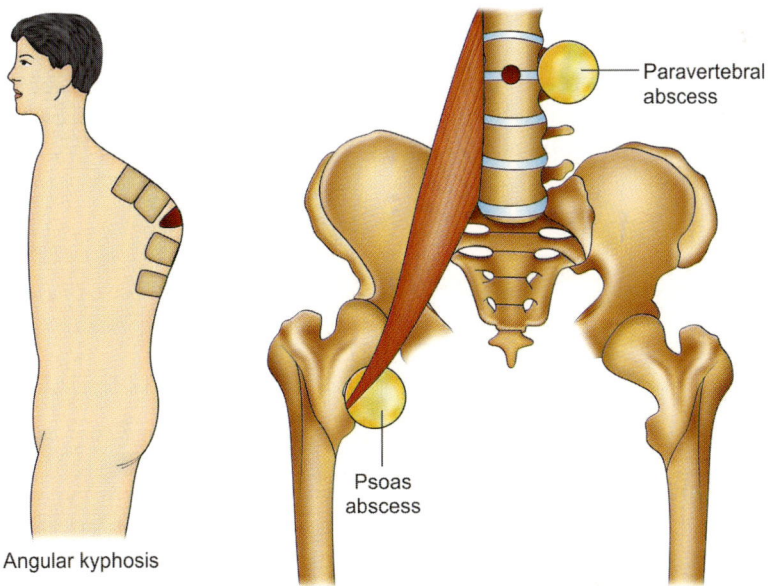

Fig. 19.43: Complications of Pott's spine

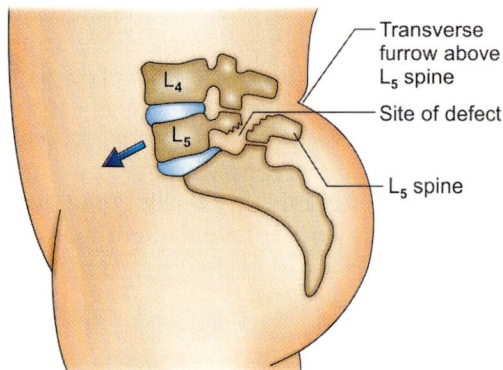

Fig. 19.44: Spondylolisthesis

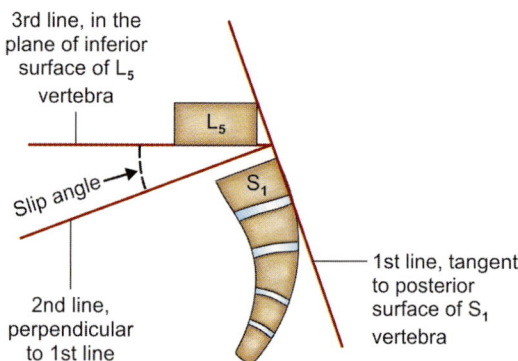

Fig. 19.46: Measuring slip angle in spondylolisthesis

Radiologically in a side view the spondylolisthesis can be graded as follows (Fig. 19.45):
a. First degree: Less than 25% of forward slip.
b. Second degree: 25% to 50% of slipping.
c. Third degree : More than 50% but less than 75% of slipping.
d. Fourth degree: More than 75% slip.

A transverse furrow on the back just above the 5th lumbar spine is often observed. *Slip angle* in case of spondylolisthesis determines the degree of instability and potential for progression. This angle is measured as shown in fig. 19.46.

15. Back pain persistently present and not relieved by rest is most likely due to tumour encroaching on painful structures.

16. Sacral cornua form important landmarks for locating the sacral hiatus between them. *Epidural (caudal) anaesthesia* is given through sacral hiatus.

17. Both the surfaces of coccyx are palpable. Its posterior surface can be palpated in the natal cleft while anterior surface can be felt by per rectal examination.

18. Coccyx moves backwards at sacrococcygeal joint to facilitate child birth.

19. *Coccydynia* refers to any condition causing pain in the region of coccyx. Majority of cases are due to trauma and therefore usually there is history of fall in sitting position.

20. The mode of injury determines the type of vertebral lesions. Some examples are as follows (Fig. 19.47):

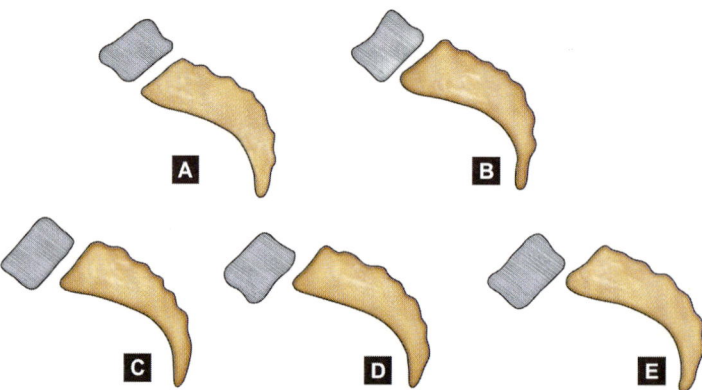

Fig. 19.45: Radiological classification of spondylolisthesis. (A) Normal; (B) First degree; (C) Second degree (D) Third degree; (E) Fourth degree

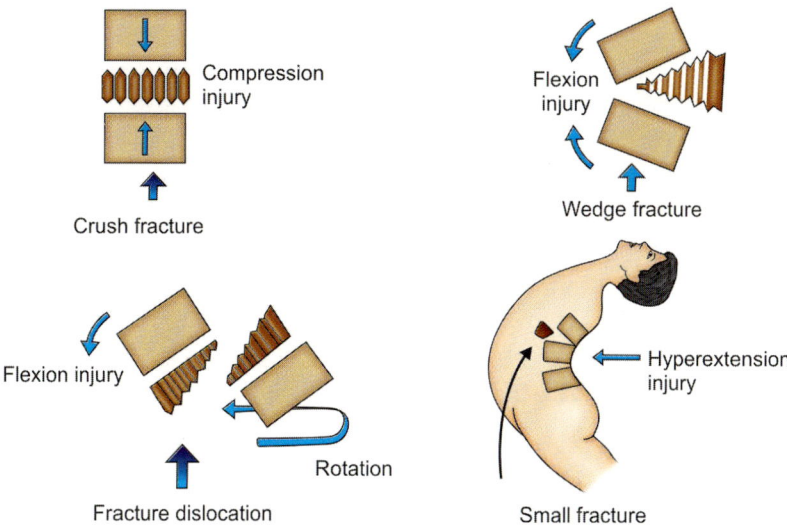

Fig. 19.47: Different types of vertebral fractures

i. Compression injury leads to *crush fracture*.
ii. Flexion injury results into *wedge fracture*.
iii. Flexion injury associated with rotation causes *fracture dislocation*.
iv. Hyperextension injury usually results into *small fracture*.

21. If the back pain appears on forward bending, the pathology is in disc (discogenic). On the other hand, pain on extension tends to originate in joint pathology (arthrogenic) (Fig. 19.48).

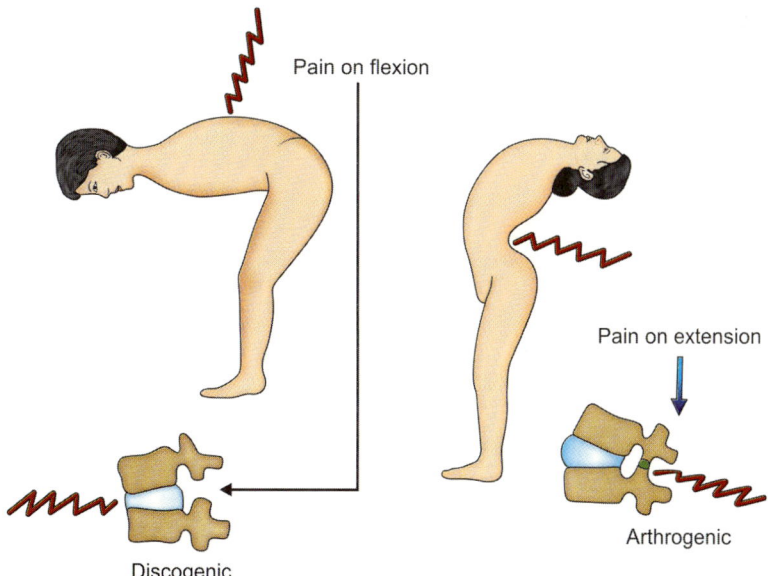

Fig. 19.48: Correlation between low backache and vertebral column (spinal) lesions

22. The normal spine (vertebral column) has a gradual thoracic kyphosis and lumbar lordosis. Normal thoracic kyphosis is defined as 20° to 40° and normal lumbar lordosis as 40° to 60°. Following is the method to measure these angles (Fig. 19.49):

23. *Scheuermann's disease*

    It is osteochondritis of vertebral column. It leads to gradual kyphosis which is due to wedging of vertebrae.

24. An *angular kyphosis* indicates bone collapse anteriorly.

25. *Idiopathic scoliosis*

    To distinguish progressive from nonprogressive curve of scoliosis, following criteria are taken into consideration in radiographs:

    i. *Relation of head of rib with vertebra*. If the head of the rib is distinct from vertebra, it is classified as phase 1. If the head of rib overlaps with vertebra, it is classified as phase 2 (Fig. 19.50).

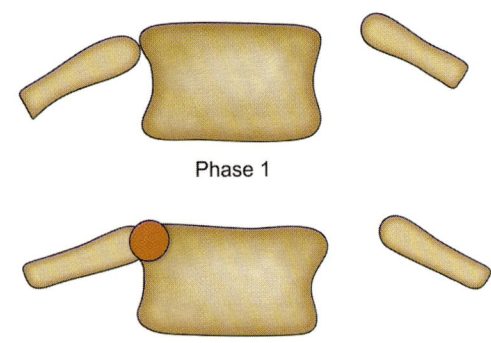

Fig. 19.50: Two types of scoliosis in radiographs

ii. *Mehta's method*

In this case *rib-vertebral angle difference* (RVAD) is measured as shown below (Fig. 19.51):

Phase 2 relationship and RVAD of more than 20° are associated with high likelihood of progression.

26. *Grading of vertebral rotation by Nash and Moe method* (Fig. 19.52)

In the radiograph, draw a vertical line in the middle of vertebral body considered

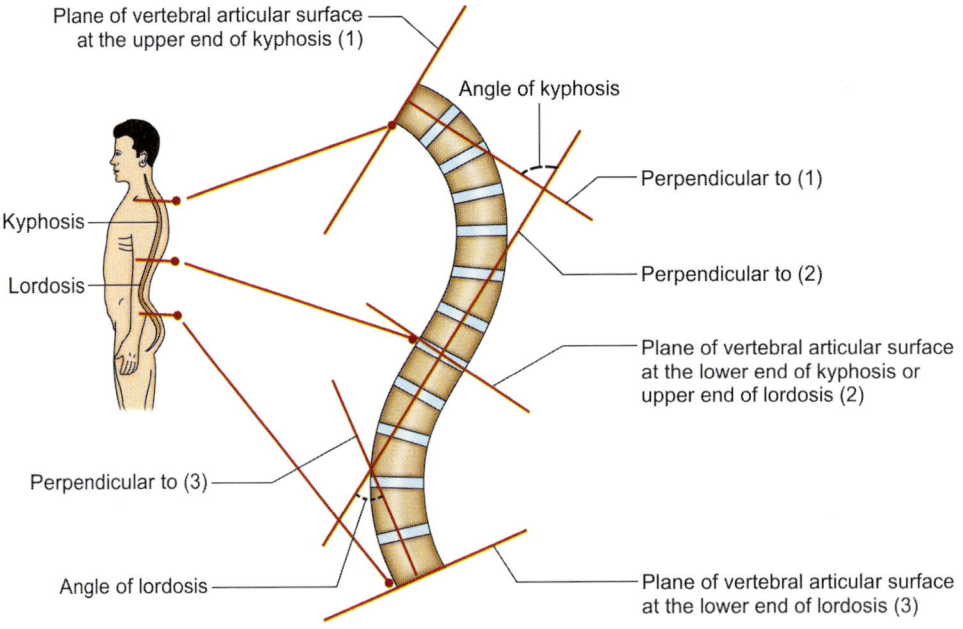

Fig. 19.49: Method of measuring angles of kyphosis and lordosis

The Vertebrae

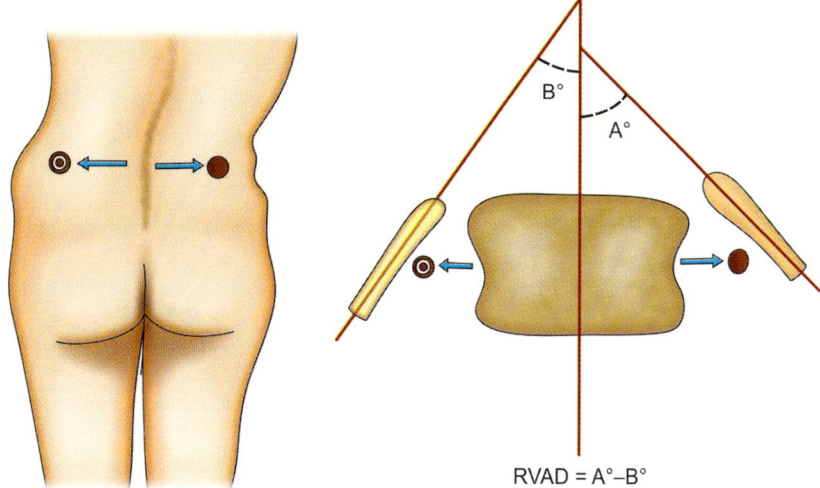

Fig. 19.51: Measuring RVAD

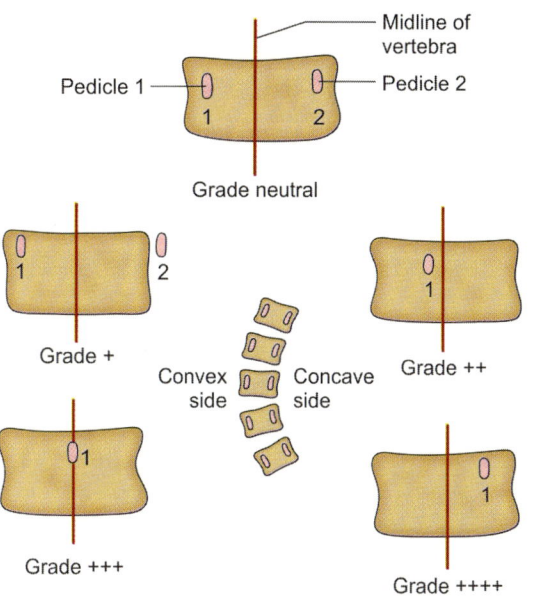

Fig. 19.52: Grading vertebral rotation

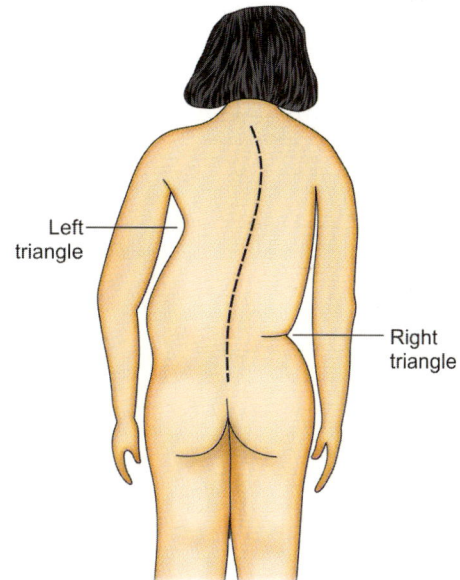

Fig. 19.53: Asymmetry of triangles between arms and trunk in scoliosis

and see its relations with the images of pedicles as shown below:

27. In case of spinal deformity especially in scoliosis, the triangles formed between the arms and patient's trunk are asymmetrical (Fig. 19.53).
28. Spinal curve types in cerebral palsy (Fig. 19.54)

Two basic curve patterns are observed in cerebral palsy.
  i. *Type 1 curve:* It is a balanced curve pattern, i.e. without pelvic obliquity.
  ii. *Type 2 curve:* Here the curve is associated with significant pelvic obliquity.

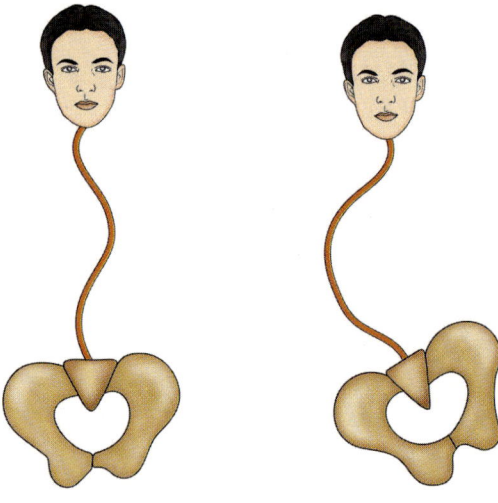

Fig. 19.54: Spinal curve types in cerebral palsy

29. Diagnosing scoliosis on clinical examination (Fig. 19.55)

    Observe the body from behind in erect position. The patient is said to be balanced when the base of neck is over sacrum. A visible tilt on one side is called 'scoliosis' (Fig. 19.55).

30. To detect the rotational deformity of spine, ask the patient to bend forwards and observe the back from behind. A hump on one side indicates a rotational deformity (Fig. 19.56).

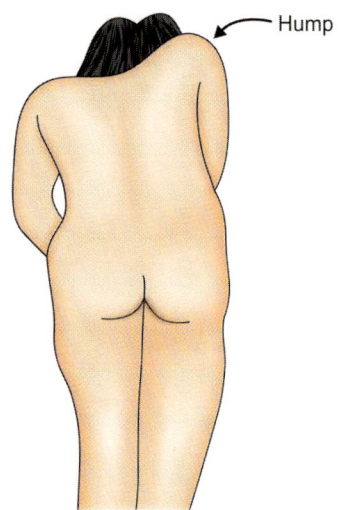

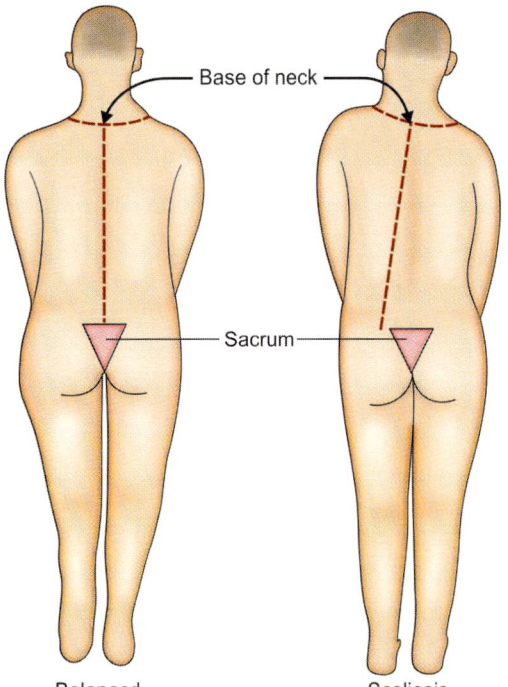

Fig. 19.55: Diagnosis of *scoliosis* on clinical observation

Fig. 19.56: Rotational deformity of spine

31. *Schmorl's node* is a radiological finding showing protruded nucleus pulposus into the vertebral body.
32. Minimal intradiscal pressure in vertebral column is seen when a person is lying flat.
33. Vertebra is the most common site of fracture in senile osteoporosis.
34. *Clay Shoveler's fracture*: It is avulsion fracture of a spinous process, most often the C_7 vertebra.
35. *Hangman's fracture*: It is bilateral avulsion fracture through the pedicles of axis.
36. *Fracture of coccyx* is commonly due to direct fall on the buttock.
37. *The three column concept* is the latest description of the spine stability (Fig. 19.57):

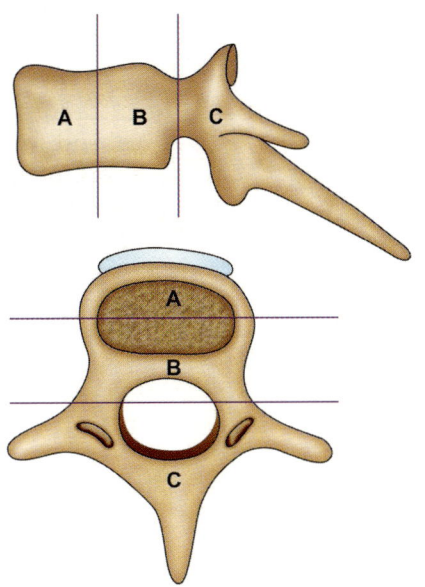

Fig. 19.57: Three column concept of spine stability. (A) Anterior column; (B) Middle column; (C) Posterior column

i. *Anterior column* consists of anterior half of vertebral body, anterior part of disc and anterior longitudinal ligament.

ii. *The middle column* consists of posterior half of the body and disc and the posterior longitudinal ligament.

iii. *Posterior column* consists of vertebral arch.

One column injury is stable. Two column injury is often unstable. Three column injury is invariably unstable. Spinal cord is at risk, in cases of an unstable spine.

38. *Odontoid process fracture* (Anderson and Dolondo's classification) (Fig. 19.58):

    Type I : Fracture of upper part of the odontoid process.

    Type II : Fracture at the junction of odontoid process and body

    Type III : Fracture through the upper part of the body of axis.

39. Patients with osteoporosis exhibit progressive loss of height due to kyphosis and vertebral compression.

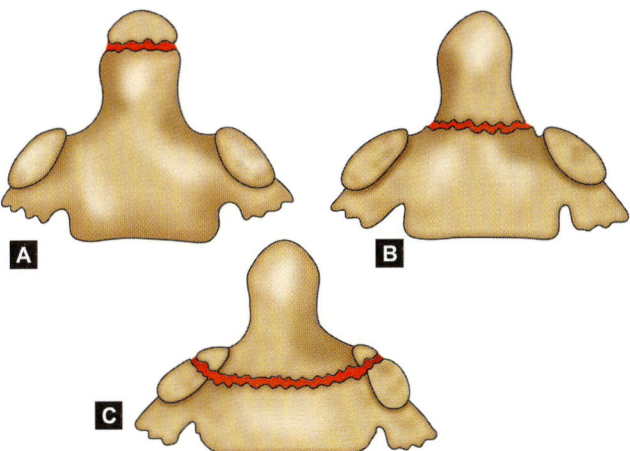

Fig. 19.58: Anderson and Dolondo's classification of fracture of odontoid process. (A) Type I; (B) Type II; (C) Type III

CHAPTER 20

The Sternum

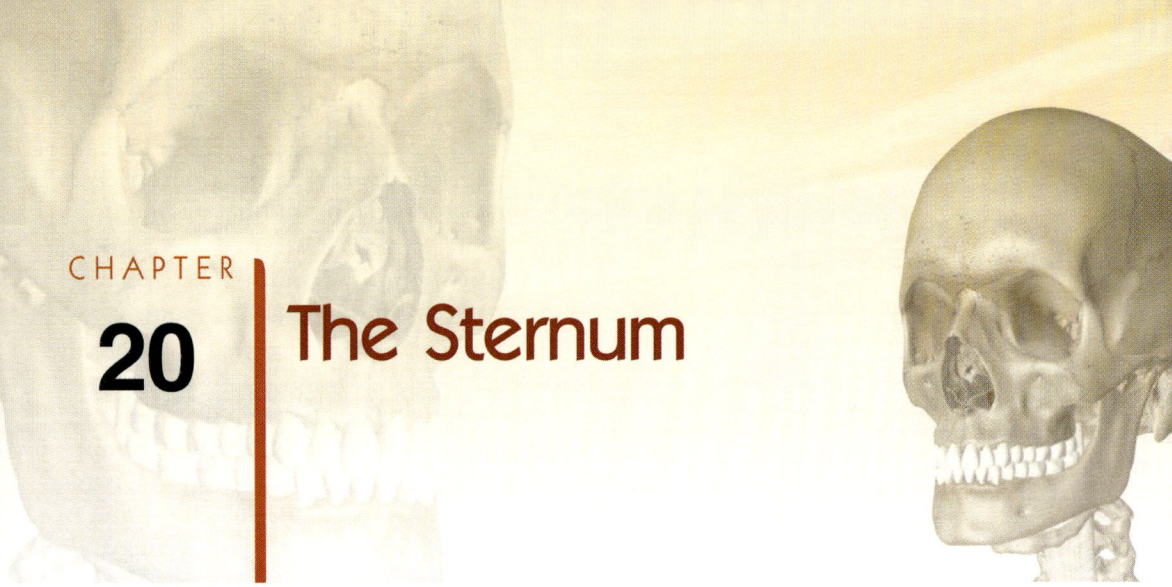

TERMINOLOGY

'Sternum' is derived from Greek word 'sternon' which means chest. Sternum is also called 'breast bone'. It has three parts, *manubrium*, *body* and *xiphoid process*. Manubrium is a Latin word which means 'handle'. Term 'xiphoid' is borrowed from greek word 'xiphos' which means 'sword'.

LOCATION (Fig. 20.1)

It is a flat bone whose long axis is vertical. It lies in the median part of anterior thoracic wall. Its surfaces are anterior and posterior. Its anterior surface also faces a little upwards.

LENGTH

It is about 7 inches (17 cm) long.

STRUCTURE

It is made up of mainly spongy bone and thus it is rich in red bone marrow.

FEATURES AND ATTACHMENTS

Sternum is made up of three pieces from above downwards:
   I. Manubrium.
  II. Body.
 III. Xiphoid process.

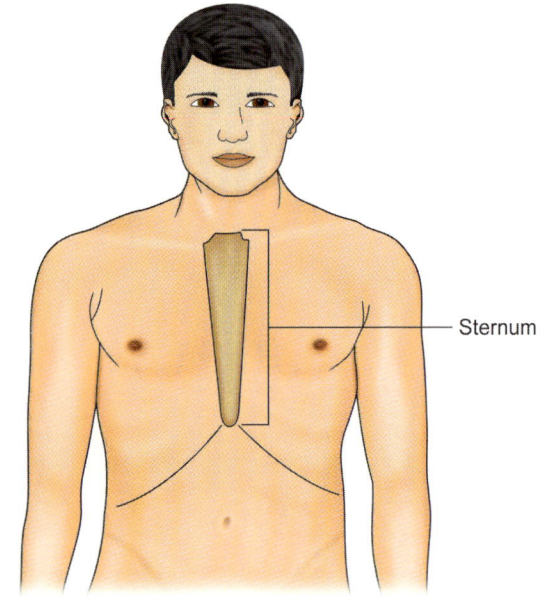

Fig. 20.1: Location of sternum

I. MANUBRIUM (PRESTERNUM OR EPISTERNUM)

It is somewhat triangular in shape and is wider above than below. It has two surfaces (anterior and posterior) and four borders (superior, inferior and 2 lateral).

A. Surfaces

a. Anterior surface (Fig. 20.2)

1. *Pectoralis major* originates from this surface on each side.
2. *Sternal head of sternocleidomastoid* takes origin from each side of its upper part.

b. Posterior surface (Figs 20.4 and 20.5)

1. It forms anterior boundary of the superior mediastinum (Fig. 20.3).
2. Two muscles originate from this surface:
   i. *Sternohyoid* at the level of the clavicular notch.
   ii. *Sternothyroid* at the level of facet for 1st costal cartilage.
3. Each half is related to corresponding parietal pleura.
4. Following vessels are related to this surface:
   i. *Arch of aorta* in its lower half.

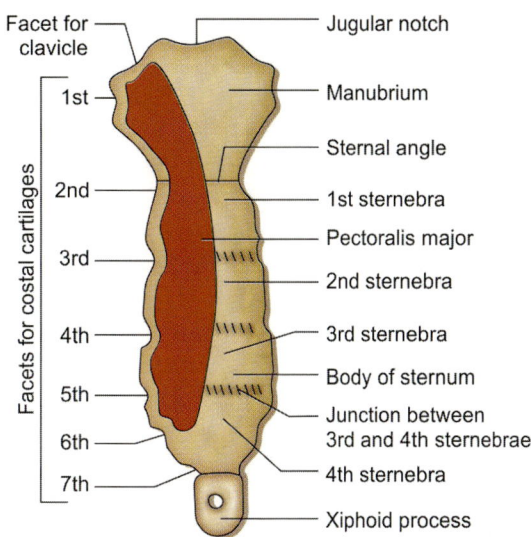

Fig. 20.2: Sternum: Anterior aspect

ii. *Left brachiocephalic vein, brachiocephalic artery, left common carotid artery* and *left subclavian artery* in its upper half.

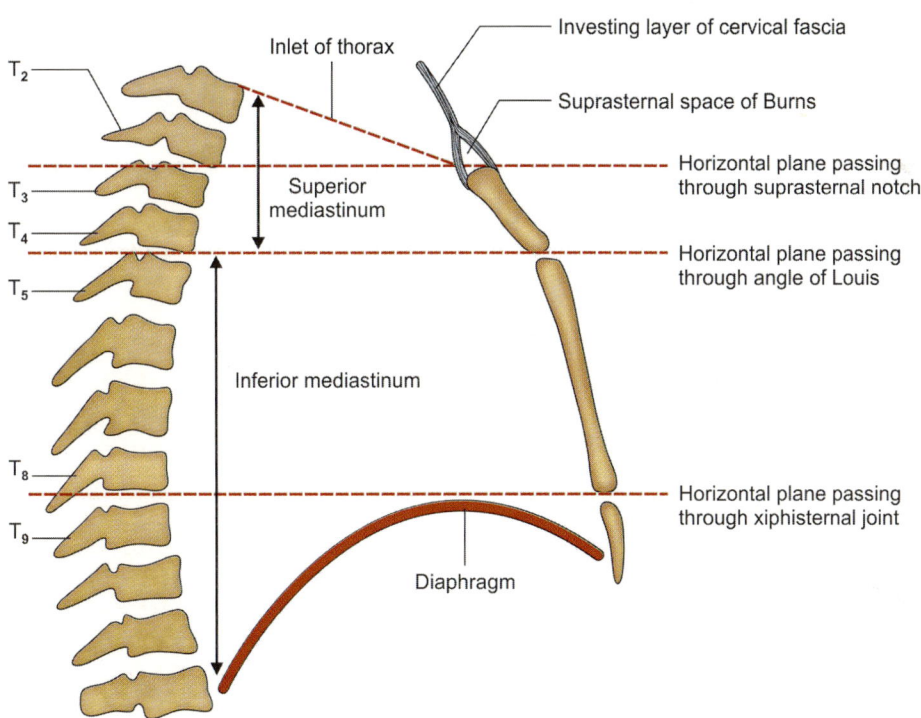

Fig. 20.3: Side views of sternum and thoracic vertebrae

B. Borders

a. Superior border
1. It is thick and rounded.
2. Its concavity in the middle is called suprasternal notch (*jugular notch*).
3. *Deep cervical fascia (investing layer)* and *interclavicular ligament* are attached to suprasternal notch.
4. *Clavicular notch* on either side of suprasternal notch forms *sternoclavicular joint* with the medial end of clavicle.

b. Inferior border
1. It articulates with the upper end of body of sternum to form *manubriosternal joint* which is a secondary cartilaginous joint.
2. Manubrium forms little angulation at its junction with body. This is called *angle of Louis* or *sternal angle*.
3. Sternal angle articulates on either side with the 2nd costal cartilage, thus forms an important landmark for counting the ribs.

c. Lateral borders (Fig. 20.6)
1. There are two lateral borders, right and left.
2. Its upper part forms primary cartilaginous joint with the first costal cartilage.
3. A demifacet is seen on the lower part of the lateral border which along with similar one on the upper angle of the body, forms two synovial joints with the 2nd costal cartilage.

II. THE BODY (MESOSTERNUM OR GLADIOLUS)

It has two surfaces (anterior and posterior), two borders (right lateral and left lateral) and two ends (upper and lower).

A. Surfaces

a. Anterior surface (Fig. 20.2)
1. Body of the sternum is formed by the fusion of 4 small segments called *sternebrae*.
2. The sites of fusion of sternebrae are represented on the anterior surface of body in the form of 3 ill defined horizontal ridges.
3. *Pectoralis major* originates from its corresponding half.

b. Posterior surface (Figs 20.4 and 20.5)
1. The transverse lines are less prominent than those on anterior surface.
2. *Transversus thoracis* originates from both the lower halves.

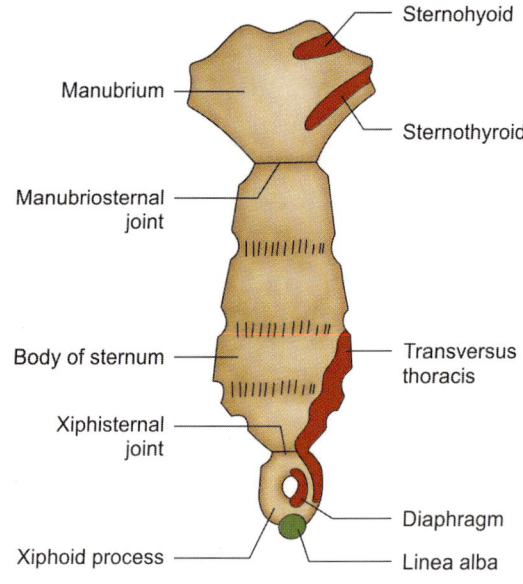

Fig. 20.4: Sternum: Posterior aspect

3. *Right lung and pleura* are related to the posterior surface on the right side of median plane.
4. *Left lung and pleura* are related to the upper two pieces on the left of midline.
5. *Pericardium* is related to lower two pieces on the left of the median plane.

B. Lateral borders (Fig. 20.6)
1. At their upper and lower ends, they articulate on either side with the lower part of 2nd and upper part of 7th costal cartilages by demifacets respectively.
2. It has 4 complete facets for 3rd to 6th costal cartilages.
3. Facets for the 3rd, 4th and 5th costal cartilages lie at the junction of sternebrae

The Sternum

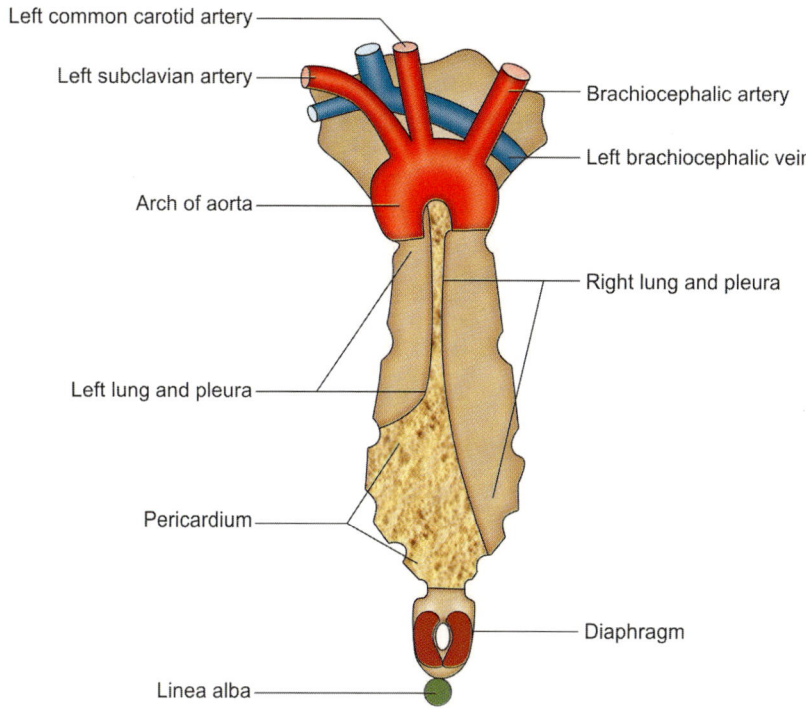

Fig. 20.5: Sternum. Posterior aspect

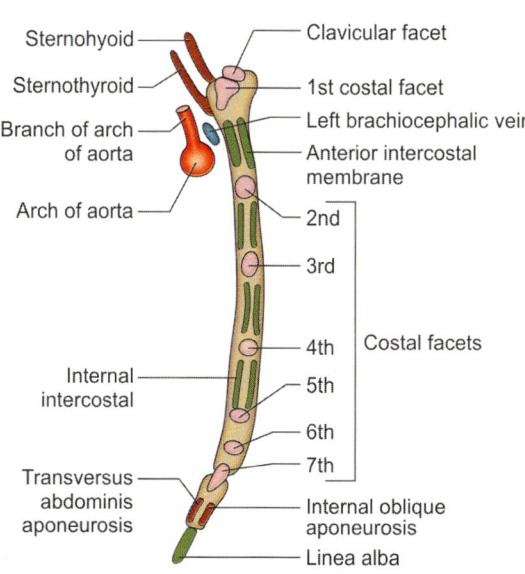

Fig. 20.6: Right lateral view of sternum

while that for 6th one lies at the side of 4th sternebra.

4. To the margins between the facets, following structures are attached:
   i. *Internal intercostal muscles.*
   ii. *External intercostal membranes.* Attachment of (ii) is anterior to (i).

C. Ends

a. Upper end

1. It is oval in shape.
2. It articulates with the lower end of the manubrium sterni to form *manubriosternal joint* which is secondary cartilaginous joint.

b. Lower end

1. It is quite narrow.
2. It articulates with xiphoid process to form *xiphisternal joint* which is a secondary cartilaginous joint.

3. Xiphisteral joint usually becomes a synostosis by 40th year.

III. XIPHOID PROCESS (XIPHISTERNUM OR METASTERNUM OR ENSIFORM CARTILAGE)

It is lowest and smallest part of sternum and is of variable shapes. It has two surfaces (anterior and posterior), two borders (right lateral and left lateral) and two ends (upper and lower).

A. Surfaces

a. Anterior surface

It gives insertions to following:
  i. *Rectus abdominis muscle.*
  ii. *Aponeuroses of external and internal oblique muscles* (anterior lamina of rectus sheath).

b. Posterior surface

1. It gives origin to following:
    i. *Diaphragm.*
    ii. *Transversus thoracis*
2. It is related to *liver*.

B. Lateral borders

1. Each gives attachments to *aponeuroses of internal oblique and transversus abdominis muscles* (posterior lamina of rectus sheath).
2. The superior angle possesses a demifacet for 7th costal cartilage.

C. Ends

a. Upper end

It articulates with lower end of body to form *xiphisternal joint.*

b. Lower end

It gives attachment to *linea alba.*

SEX DIFFERENCES

Body of sternum in males is more than twice the length of manubrium. In females, the body is shorter and less than twice the length of manubrium.

OSSIFICATION

Sternum ossifies from 6 centres, one for manubrium, 4 for sternebrae (one for each sternebra) and one for xiphoid process.

A. *Appearance*

Centres appear as follows:

Manubrium : 5th month
1st sternebra : 6th month
2nd sternebra : 7th month } Intrauterine life
3rd sternebra : 8th month
4th sternebra : 9th month

Xiphisternum : 3rd year

B. *Fusion:*

Between manubrium and 1st sternebra	: Ununited
Upper 3 sternebrae	: Between puberty and 25years
Between 3rd and 4th sternebrae	: Puberty
Between 4th sternebra and xiphoid process	: 40 years

APPLIED ANATOMY

1. Sternal angle is an important landmark for counting the ribs. The 2nd costal cartilage can be easily felt at the side of the angle and the ribs are then counted down.
2. Some times sternebrae ossify by double centres which fail to fuse in the midline. The defect ranges from *'sternal foramen'* to *'cleft sternum'*. The latter may be associated with 'ectopic cordis' (Fig. 20.7).
3. *Sternal puncture* is a useful procedure for haematological examination. In this procedure a thick needle is introduced into red bone marrow of sternum to get the sample.
4. *Sternal fracture* is common in automobile accidents. A backward displacement of

The Sternum | 181

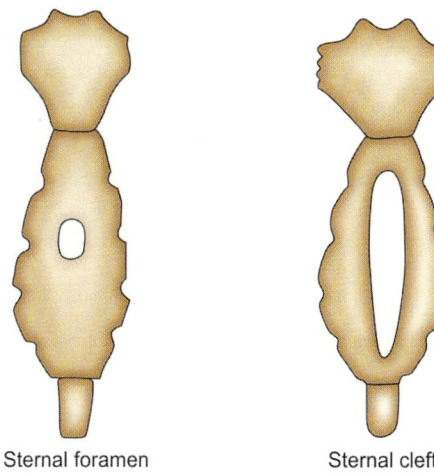

Fig. 20.7: Nonfusion of bilateral sternebrae

sternal fragments may lead to aortic, cardiac or liver damage, resulting into severe bleeding. This may be fatal.

5. *Midsternotomy* (dividing the sternum in median plane) is an important step for access to the heart and great vessels for surgery.

6. There are two abnormal shapes of thorax which are associated with anomalies of sternum (Fig. 20.8).

  i. *Funnel chest:* In this case the chest is compressed anteroposteriorly and sternum is pushed backwards compressing the heart.

  ii. *Pigeon chest:* In this case chest is compressed from side to side and sternum is projected forwards.

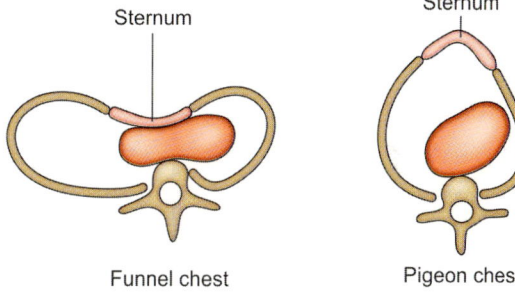

Fig. 20.8: Two abnormal shapes of thorax

CHAPTER
21 | The Ribs

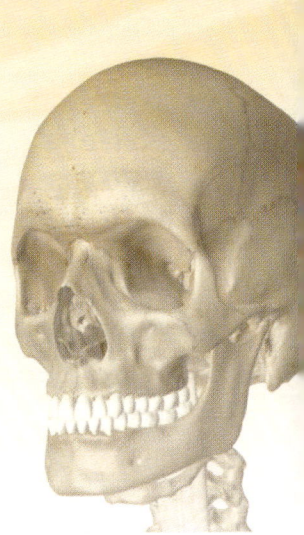

GENERAL CONSIDERATIONS (Fig. 21.1)

1. Ribs are bilateral bony arches forming greater part of the thoracic wall.
2. Normally there are 12 pairs of ribs which are numbered from above downwards.
3. The length of the ribs increases from 1st to 7th rib and then decreases from 7th to 12th rib. Therefore the 7th rib is the longest rib.
4. The ribs are arranged obliquely, i.e. the anterior end is at a lower level than the posterior end. The obliquity is maximum in the 9th rib.
5. The 8th rib is the most laterally projected rib.
6. Width of the rib gradually reduces from above downwards.
7. Intercostal spaces (gaps between adjacent ribs) are deeper in front than behind and deeper in the upper part than the lower part.

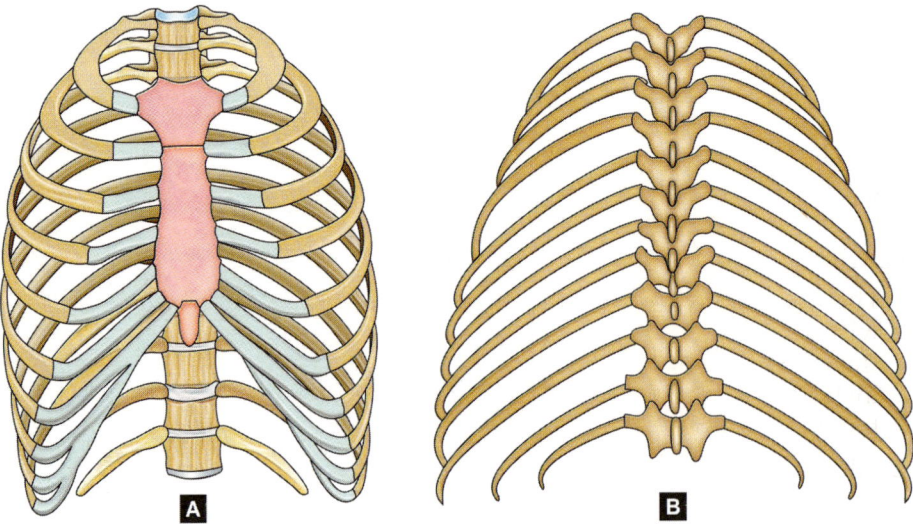

Fig. 21.1: The thoracic cage. (A) Anterior view; (B) Posterior view

CLASSIFICATION OF RIBS

The ribs can be classified differently.
- **A. According to the similarities and dissimilarities of features**
  - **a. Typical ribs**
    1. These are the ribs which are having same features.
    2. 3rd to 9th ribs are typical ribs.
  - **b. Atypical ribs**
    1. They have some special features and therefore can be differentiated from rest of the ribs.
    2. 1st, 2nd, 10th, 11th and 12th ribs are the examples of atypical ribs.
- **B. According to the relations of ribs with the sternum**
  - **a. True ribs**
    1. These are the ribs which articulate with sternum anteriorly.
    2. Upper seven ribs are true ribs.
  - **b. False ribs**
    1. These are not connected to sternum anteriorly.
    2. 8th to 12th ribs are false ribs.
- **C. According to articulation of ribs**
  - **a. Vertebrosternal ribs**
    1. Ribs which are connected posteriorly with vertebrae and anteriorly (directely or indirectly through its cartilage) with sternum, are called vertebrosternal ribs.
    2. Upper seven ribs are examples of vertebrosternal ribs.
  - **b. Vertebrochondral ribs**
    1. These ribs are connected posteriorly with the vertebrae but anteriorly they don't reach the sternum, instead their cartilages are joined together.
    2. 8th, 9th and 10th ribs are examples of vertebrochondral ribs.
  - **c. Vertebral ribs**
    1. Posteriorly they are attached to vertebrae but anteriorly they are free.
    2. Last two ribs (11th and 12th) are vertebral ribs.
- **D. According to state of anterior end**
  - **a. Floating ribs**
    1. If the anterior end is free and does not articulate with sternum or adjacent cartilage then the rib is said to be floating rib.
    2. 11th and 12th ribs are floating ribs.
  - **b. Nonfloating ribs**
    1. If anterior end of bone is fixed due to its attachment to sternum or the adjacent cartilage then it is called as nonfloating rib.
    2. All the ribs are nonfloating except last two.

Note: *Remember 'nonfloating rib' is usually not considered as terminology but has been used to differentiate it from 'floating rib'. Some of the terms used in classification reflect similar meaning, e.g. True ribs = Vertebrosternal ribs and Floating ribs = Vertebral ribs. The 10th rib is also floating in Japanese.*

DESCRIPTION OF RIBS

I. TYPICAL RIB (Figs 21.2, to 21.4)

Side determination
The side of a typical rib can be determined by considering the following points:
1. The end of the rib having head, neck and tubercle is directed posteriorly.
2. Concavity of the rib faces medially.
3. The sharp border of the rib is inferior.

Normal anatomical position
Keep the bone on the corresponding side in such a way that the posterior end is higher and nearer the median plane than the anterior end.

Human Osteology

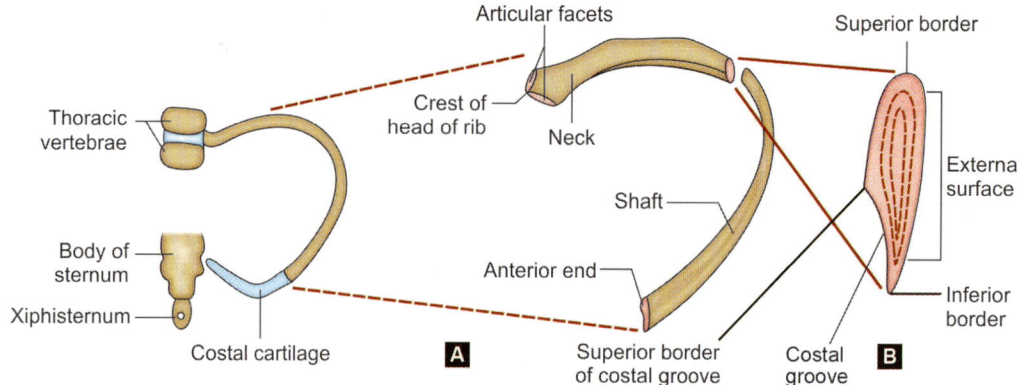

Fig. 21.2: Left typical rib. (A) Anterior aspect; (B) Cross section

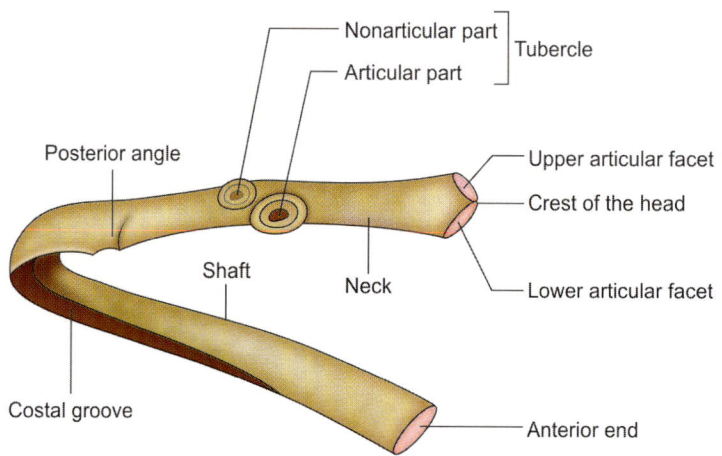

Fig. 21.3: Left typical rib: Posterior aspect

Features and attachments

Each rib has an anterior end, a posterior end and a shaft.

A. Anterior end

1. It is oval in shape.
2. It has a cup shaped depression.
3. Anterior end forms *costochondral joint* (a primary cartilaginous joint) with the lateral end of corresponding costal cartilage.

B. Posterior end

It consists of head, neck and tubercle.

a. Head

1. The head lies at the junction of two vertebrae and therefore comprises of two *articular facets* (Fig. 21.5).
2. The lower articular facet is larger and meets with the corresponding vertebra.

Note: *Remember 'L' for 'Lower' and 'L' for Larger*

3. The upper smaller facet articulates with vertebra above.

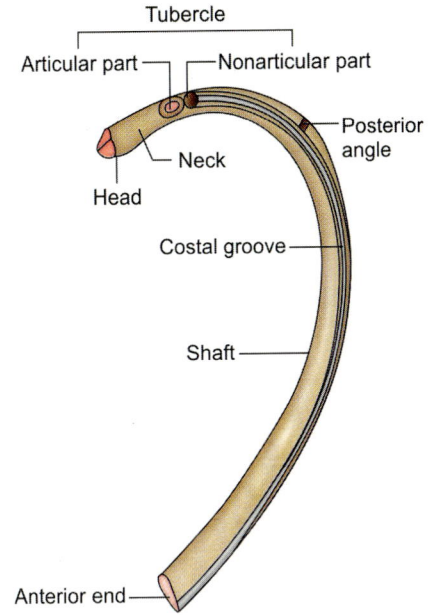

Fig. 21.4: Right typical rib: Inferior aspect

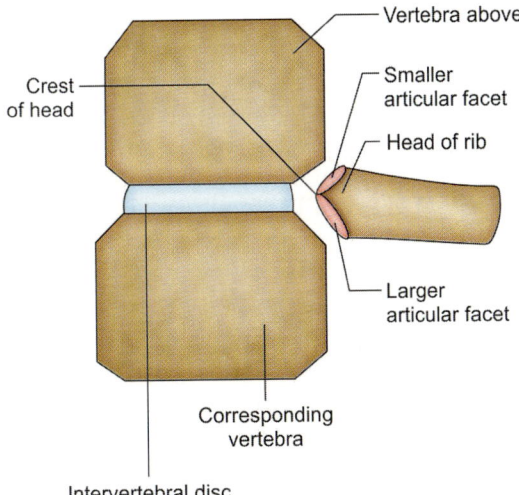

Fig. 21.5: Relations between the head of a typical rib and vertebrae

Note: *Remember 'S' for 'Superior' and 'S' for 'Smaller'*

4. The articular facets are separated from each other by a transverse ridge called as the *crest of head* which lies opposite the intervertebral disc.

5. *Capsular ligament* is attached to margins of articular facets while *intra-articular ligament* is attached to the crest of head.
6. *Radiate ligament* is attached to the front of head (Fig. 21.6).
7. Anterior aspect of head is also related to costal pleura and sympathetic chain.

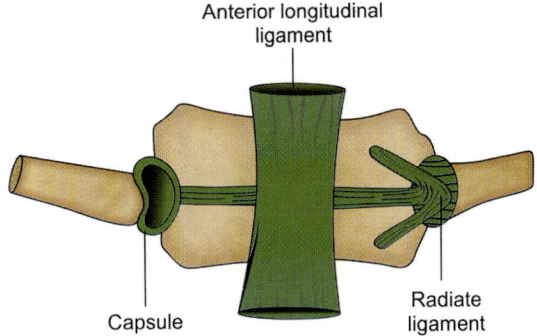

Fig. 21.6: Attachments on the head of 1st rib: Anterior view

b. Neck (Fig. 21.7)
1. It lies in front of the transverse process of corresponding vertebra.
2. It is flat part of rib adjacent to head.
3. It is 1 cm in length.
4. It has 2 borders (superior and inferior) and 2 surfaces (anterior and posterior).
    i. *Superior border*
        1. It is also called *crest of neck*.
        2. It is thin and sharp.
        3. *Superior costotransverse ligament* is attached to it.

Note: *Remember there are two crests at the posterior end of rib. Crest of head is between two articular facets while crest of neck is its sharp superior border.*

   ii. *Inferior border*
        1. It is smooth and round.
        2. It receives attachment of *internal (posterior) intercostal membrane*.
  iii. *Anterior surface*
        1. It is divided by an *oblique ridge* into an upper medial area and a lower lateral area.

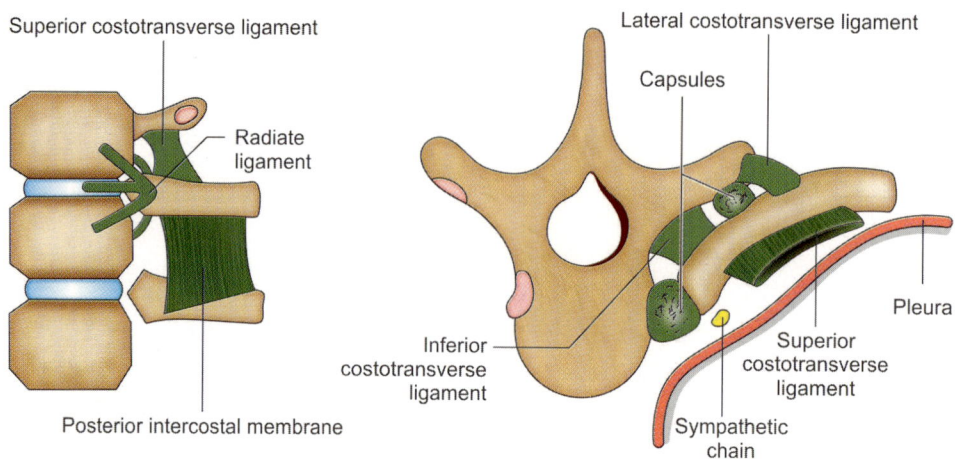

Fig. 21.7: Attachments on the posterior end of a typical rib

2. The ridge gives attachment to *posterior intercostal membrane*.
3. Upper area is related to *posterior intercostal membrane* but separated from it by *fatty tissue*. Lower area is related to *costal pleura*.

iv. *Posterior surface*
1. It is rough.
2. It receives attachment of *inferior costotransverse ligament*.

c. Tubercle
1. It is situated on the outer surface of rib at the junction of neck with the shaft.
2. It is divided into medial articular and lateral nonarticular parts.
3. Medial part articulates with the transverse process of corresponding vertebra to form *costotransverse joint*.
4. Lateral part gives attachment to *lateral costotransverse ligament*.

Note: *Remember there are three costotransverse ligaments, lateral, superior and inferior, which are attached to the regions as follows:*
Lateral-Lateral part of tubercle
Superior-Crest of neck
Inferior-Back of neck.

C. Shaft
1. It is the major part of rib which intervenes between the anterior and posterior ends of rib.
2. It is thin and flat.
3. A typical rib has three qualities:
    i. It is *curved*. This can be appreciated by the fact that it is never straight.
    ii. It is *angulated*. There is a bend in the rib about 5 cm in front of tubercle. This is called *'posterior angle'* or only 'angle' of rib. A similar bend 2 cm behind the anterior end of rib is called, *anterior angle* of rib (Fig. 21.8).
    iii. It is *twisted*. The twisting of the shaft can be appreciated by the fact that the inner surface faces slightly upwards behind the angle but it faces slightly downwards in the front of angle. Moreover due to twisting, the two ends of the rib can not touch a horizontal plane simultaneously.
4. The shaft has two borders (superior and inferior) and two surfaces (outer and inner).

a. Borders
    i. Superior border
        1. It is thick and rounded.
        2. It has outer and inner lips.

The Ribs | **187**

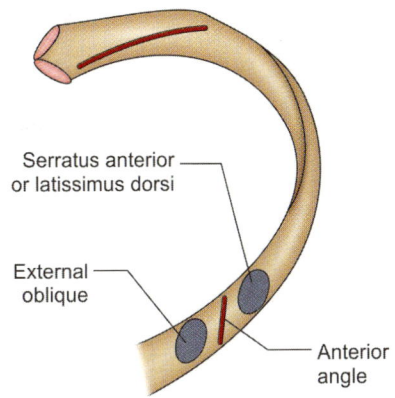

Fig. 21.8: Left typical rib: Anterior aspect

Note: *Remember that the upper border is for insertion whereas the lower border is for origin. Also that the external intercostal originates from the lower border of upper rib and gets inserted on the upper border of lower rib.*

3. Outer lip receives insertion of *external intercostal muscle*.
4. Inner lip receives insertion of *internal intercostal* and *intercostalis intimus* muscles.

ii. Inferior border
   1. It is sharp and forms the lower border of the costal groove.
   2. *External intercostal muscle* originates from the lower border.

b. Surfaces
   i. Outer surface
      1. It is smooth and convex.
      2. *Angle (posterior angle)* of rib is marked by a ridge which provides attachment to *posterior layer of thoracolumbar fascia*.
      3. *Levator costarum* and *sacrospinalis (erector spinae)* muscles are attached to outer surface, medial to the angle.
      4. Anterior angle is marked by an indistinct oblique line which separates the origin of external oblique (anterior to angle) from serratus anterior (in cases of middle 4 ribs) or latissimus dorsi (in cases of 9th and 10th ribs) (Fig. 21.9).

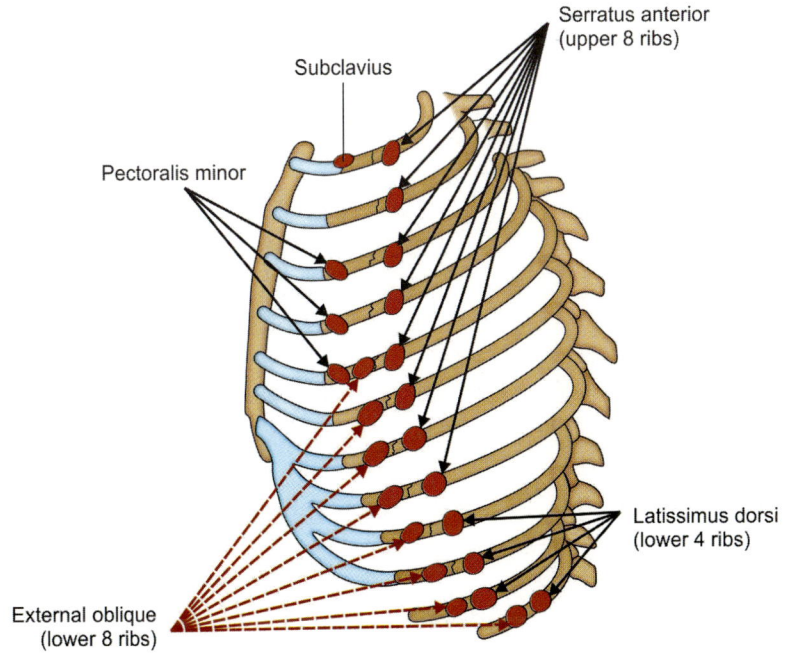

Fig. 21.9: The thoracic cage: Left lateral view

5. *Serratus anterior* (in cases of upper 8 ribs) or *latissimus dorsi* (in cases of 9th and 10th ribs) arises from the outer surface of rib just behind the anterior angle (Fig. 21.9).

ii. Inner surface

1. It is concave and smooth.
2. It has a *costal groove* in its lower part.
3. Costal groove lodges the following structures from above downwards:
   - Intercostal vein.
   - Intercostal artery.
   - Intercostal nerve.

Note: *Remember 'VAN' to consider the sequence of Vein, Artery and Nerve.*

4. *Internal intercostal muscle* originates from the floor of costal groove.
5. *Intercostalis intimus* originates from middle 2/4th of the upper lip of costal groove.

Note: *Remember that internal intercostal is internal in the costal groove, i.e. it is in the floor of the groove where as intercostalis intimus is intimately attached to the upper lip of costal groove.*

II. ATYPICAL RIBS

A. FIRST RIB

Distinguishing features

1. It is shortest.
2. It is broadest.
3. It is most curved.
4. It has no twisting.
5. Angle coincides with tubercle.
6. Head has got only single facet.
7. Costal groove is absent.
8. Neck is rounded and elongated.
9. It is flattened from above downwards and therefore has inner and outer borders and superior and inferior surfaces.

Side determination

1. Keep the larger end anteriorly and the smaller end posteriorly.
2. Keep the surface of the shaft having two grooves separated by a ridge, superiorly.
3. Keep the concave border towards inner side and convex border towards outer side.

Note: *Keep the rib on a flat surface considering its position in your own body. The rib belongs to the side on which both the ends touch the surface simultaneously. If the rib is placed on the wrong side then only the anterior end will be touching the table top.*

Anatomical position

1. Posterior end is nearer the midline than the anterior end.
2. Posterior end is 3.5 cm higher than the anterior end.
3. Upper surface faces upwards as well as forwards.

Features and attachments

Just like typical rib, the first rib is comprised of two ends (anterior and posterior) and a shaft.

a. Anterior end

1. It is larger end.
2. It meets with 1st costal cartilage.

b. Posterior end

It consists of head, neck and tubercle.

   i. Head

1. It is small and rounded.
2. It has a single rounded facet for articulation with the body of 1st thoracic vertebra to form *costovertebral joint*.
3. *Capsular ligament* of 1st costovertebral joint is attached to the margins of facet.
4. *Radiate ligament* is attached to the anterior margin of head.

   ii. Neck

1. It is rounded.

2. It is directed upwards, backwards and laterally.
3. *Inferior costotransverse ligament* is attached to its posterior surface.
4. Following structures form the anterior relations of the neck from medial to lateral (Fig. 21.11):
   - Sympathetic chain.
   - First posterior intercostal vein.
   - Superior intercostal artery.
   - First thoracic root (T_1) of brachial plexus.

Note: *Remember SVAN for the relations of anterior aspect of neck from medial to lateral in which S=Sympathetic chain, V=Vein, A=Artery and N=Nerve.*

iii. Tubercle
1. It is large and prominent.
2. It articulates with the transverse process of 1st thoracic vertebra.
3. *Lateral costotransverse ligament* is attached laterally to the tubercle.

c. Shaft
It consists of two borders (outer and inner) and two surfaces (upper and lower).

i. Outer border
1. It is convex.
2. It is thick posteriorly and thin anteriorly.
3. *1st Digitation of serratus anterior* arises from its middle.
4. It is related to scalenus posterior muscle in its posterior part while clavipectoral fascia and pectoralis major muscle in its anterior part.

ii. Inner border
1. It is concave.
2. *Scalene tubercle* is situated near its middle.
3. *Sibson's fascia* (suprapleural membrane) is attached to it.

iii. Upper surface (Figs 21.10 and 21.11)
1. It is rough and irregular.
2. It presents two shallow grooves separated by a ridge.
3. The ridge continues medially with the scalene tubercle along the inner border.
4. *Scalenus anterior* is inserted on the ridge and scalene tubercle.

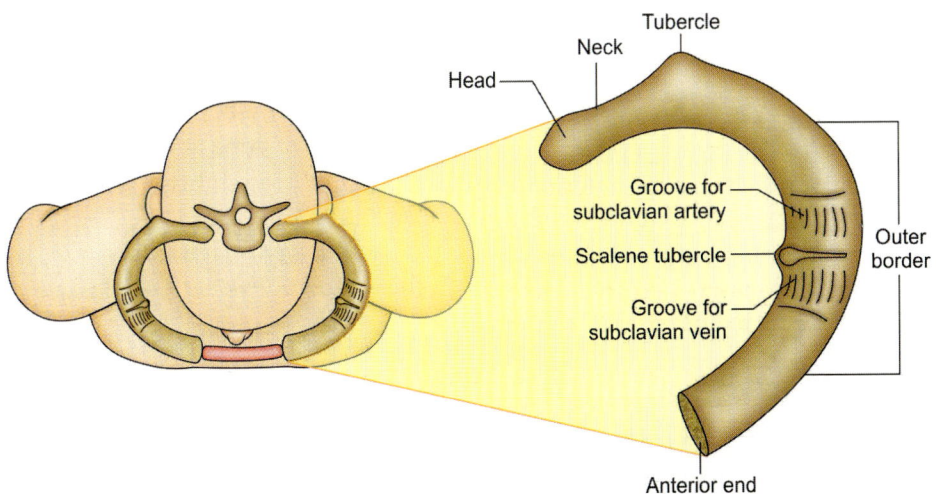

Fig. 21.10: First rib of left side. Superior aspect

190 Human Osteology

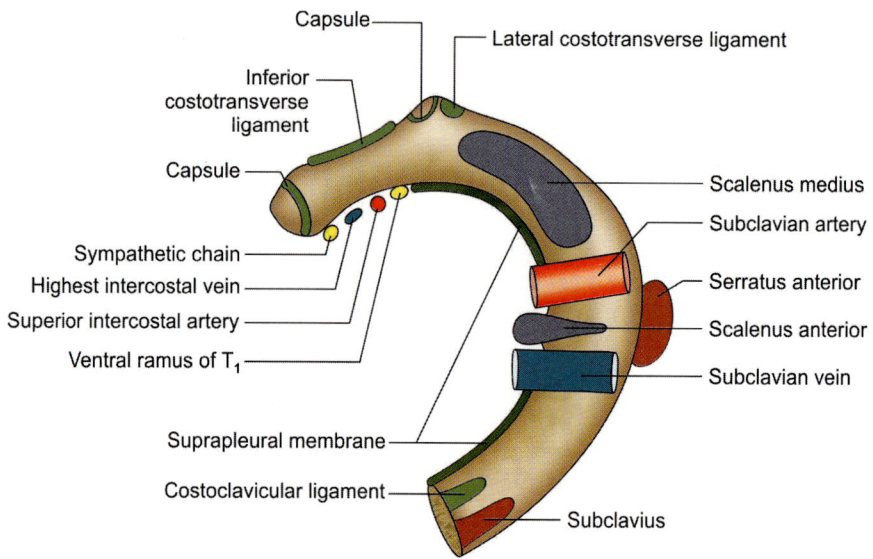

Fig. 21.11: First rib of left side: Superior view

5. *Subclavian vein* lies in the groove anterior to ridge.
6. *Subclavian artery* along with *lower trunk of brachial plexus* occupies the posterior groove.

Note: *Remember 'VAN' is the sequence of structures occupying the grooves on the superior surface from anterior to posterior, i.e. Vein, Artery and Nerve.*

7. Area anterior to groove for subclavian vein provides attachments to *subclavius muscle* (anteriorly) and *costoclavicular ligament* (posteriorly). These attachments are located near the anterior end because they also extend over the costal cartilage.
8. *Scalenus medius* is inserted on the rough area posterior to the groove for subclavian artery.

iv. Lower surface (Fig. 21.12)
1. It is smooth.
2. It is related to *costal pleura*.
3. *Intercostal muscles* are attached to this surface near its outer border.

4. *1st Intercostal nerve and vessels* are related to this surface mainly in its posterior part.

B. SECOND RIB (Fig. 21.13)
Distinguishing features
1. It is highly curved like first rib.
2. It is twice the length of 1st rib.
3. It has no twisting and therefore both the ends are in contact with the horizontal surface of table top.
4. Slight angle is present close to tubercle.
5. Like the 1st rib there is slight upward convexity of bone at the tubercle.
6. It has got a small head with two articular facets.
7. There is a *large rough muscular impression* on the outer convex surface of shaft.

Features and attachments
Second rib has the following additional features as compared to the typical ribs.
1. 2nd Rib is a transitional rib therefore outersurface faces more upwards than outwards and inner surface faces more downwards than inwards.

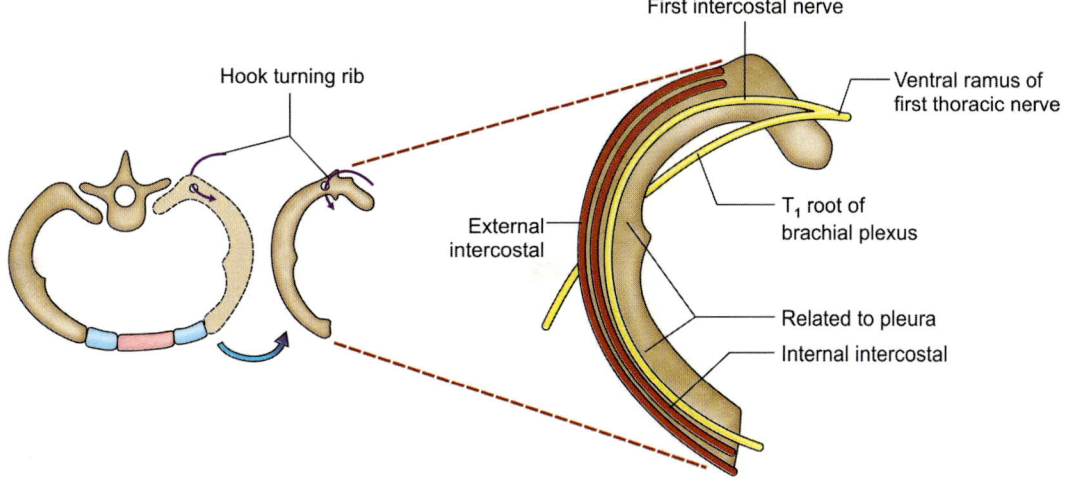

Fig. 21.12: First rib of left side: Inferior aspect

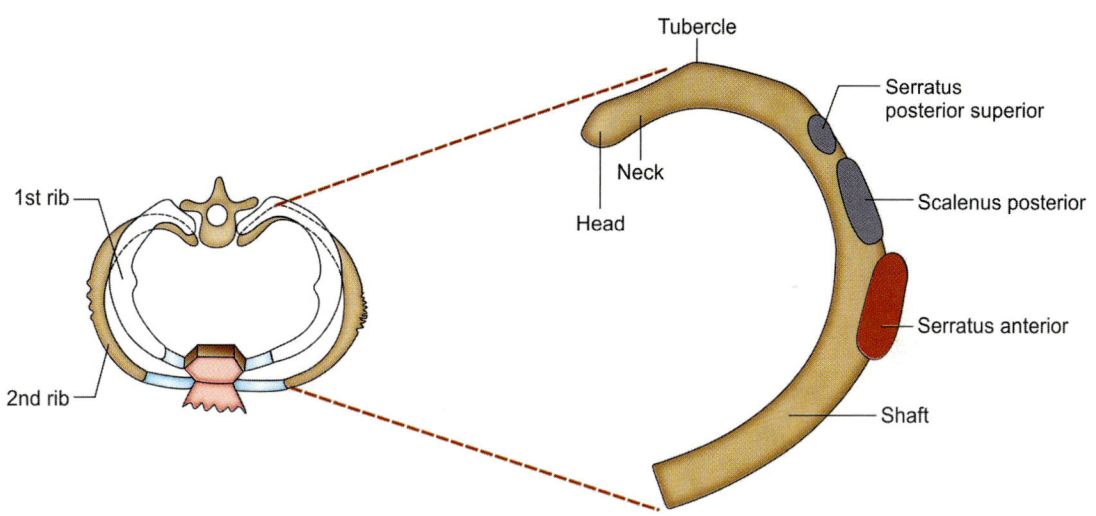

Fig. 21.13: Second rib of left side: Superior aspect

2. There is a *prominent rough impression* on the outer surface just behind its middle which gives origin to *serratus anterior muscle* (lower part of the 1st and whole of the 2nd digitations).
3. *Scalenus posterior* is attached to upper border and adjoining outer surface behind the rough impression.
4. 1st slip of *serratus posterior superior* is attached to the superior border further behind.
5. A short costal groove is visible in the posterior part of inner smooth concave surface.

C. TENTH RIB

It shows all the features of a typical rib except that it is shorter than the typical rib and head bears single facet to articulate with the body of corresponding (tenth) thoracic vertebra.

D. ELEVENTH RIB

The common features of eleventh and twelfth ribs differentiating them from typical ribs are as follows:
1. There is only one facet on the head.
2. There is no neck.
3. There is no tubercle.
4. Anterior ends are pointed.
5. They are quite shorter than typical ribs.

The features of eleventh rib which differentiate it from twelfth rib are as follows:
1. It is much longer than the twelfth rib.
2. A faint costal groove is observed on the inner surface.
3. Slight angle is present in the eleventh rib.

E. TWELFTH RIB

Identifying features
1. There is only one facet on the head.
2. There is no neck.
3. There is no tubercle.
4. Anterior end is pointed.
5. It is smaller than the eleventh rib.
6. There is no costal groove.
7. There is no angle.

Side determination
1. Keep the pointed end anterolaterally and broader end posteromedially.
2. Keep the slightly concave surface inwards and upwards (Fig. 21.14).
3. Keep the sharper border inferiorly.

Features and attachments

It has two ends (posterior and anterior), two surfaces (outer and inner) and two borders (upper and lower).

a. Ends
i. Anterior end
It meets with a small costal cartilage.

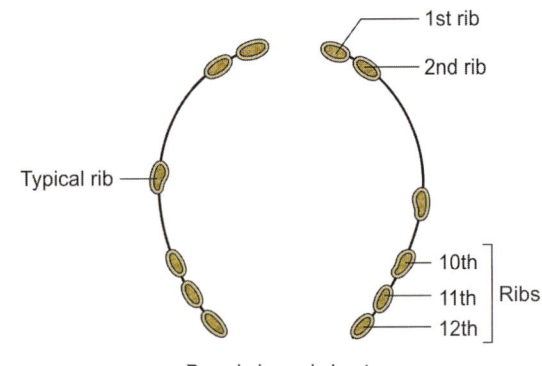

Fig. 21.14: Directions of surfaces of shafts of ribs

ii. Posterior end (Head)
Capsular and radiate ligaments are attached to the head.

b. Surfaces
i. Outer surface (Fig. 21.15)
Following structures are attached to the outer surface:
1. Close to head: *Costotransverse ligament* above and *lumbocostal ligament* below.
2. Near the tip: *Latissimus dorsi muscle* above and *external oblique muscle* below.
3. Rest of the surface: *Posterior lamella of thoracolumbar fascia* and *levator costae, erector spinae* and *serratus posterior inferior* muscles.

ii. Inner surface (Fig. 21.16)
1. An oblique line crossing the middle of this surface marks the *line of pleural reflection*.
2. *Quadratus lumborum* with *anterior lamella of thoracolumbar fascia* is attached to the lower part of the medial half.
3. *Internal intercostal muscle* is inserted near the upper border of its middle two fourth.
4. *Diaphragm* arises from the upper part of its anterior one fourth.

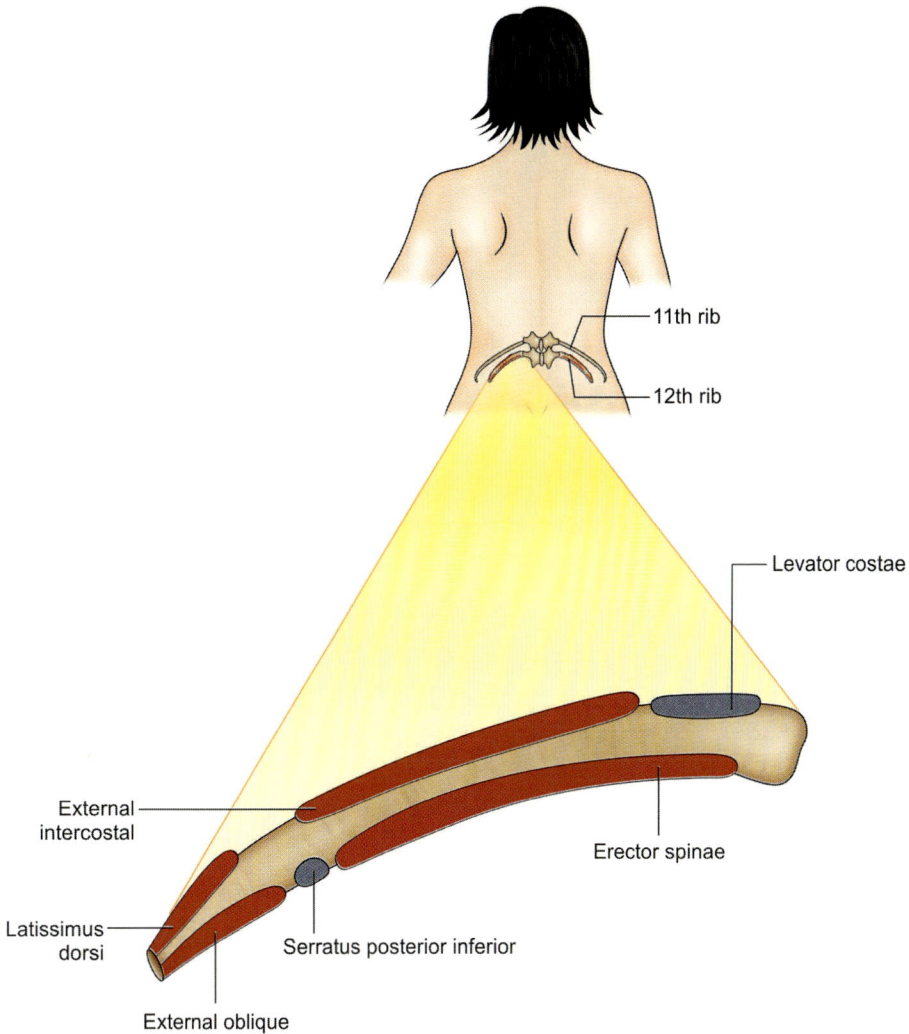

Fig. 21.15: Twelfth rib of left side: Posterior aspect

C. Borders

i. Upper border
External and internal intercostal muscles are inserted on this border.

ii. Lower border
1. Its medial half provides attachment to the *middle lamella of thoracolumbar fascia* which corresponds with the extent of quadratus lumborum.
2. Just beyond the lateral border of quadratus lumborum there is attachment of *lateral arcuate ligament*.
3. Lateral part of inferior border receives attachment of *posterior lamella of thoracolumbar fascia*.

OSSIFICATION OF RIBS

I. SECOND TO TENTH RIBS

Four ossification centres appear in total, one primary and three secondary.

A. Appearance
Primary centre
  1 for shaft: 8th week of intrauterine life.

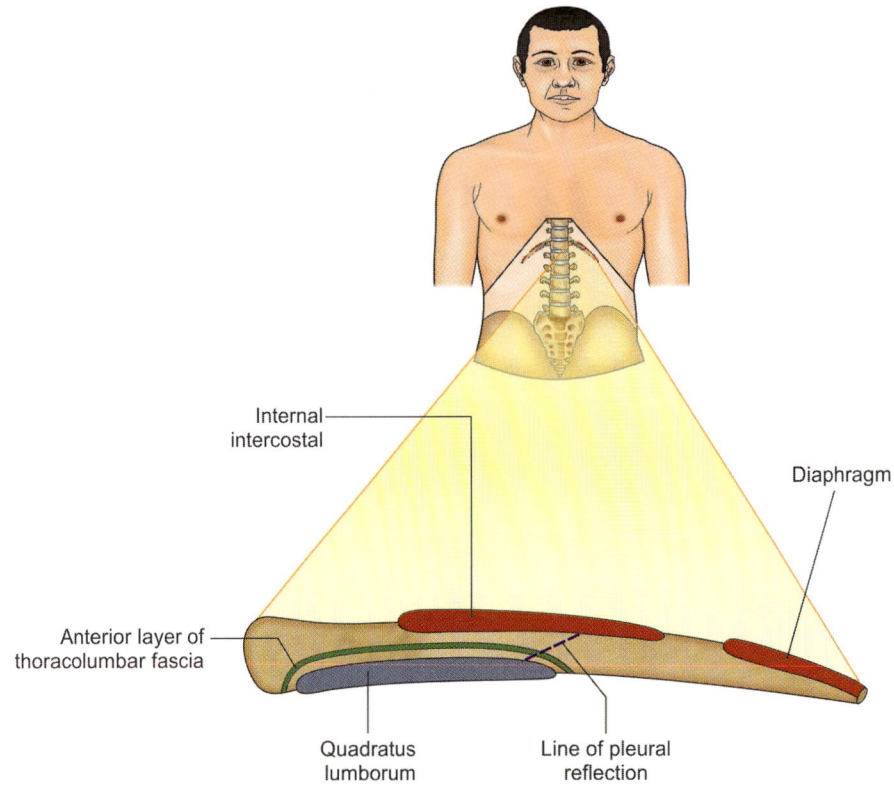

Fig. 21.16: Twelfth rib of left side: Anterior aspect

Secondary centres
  1 for head
  1 for articular part of tubercle
  1 for nonarticular part of tubercle
  All appear at puberty.
B. Fusion: 20 years

II. FIRST RIB

Three centres of ossification appear in total. One primary centre appears for shaft and two secondary centres appear one each for head and tubercle.

A. Appearance

Primary centre : 8th week of intrauterine life.

Secondary centres : Puberty

B. Fusion: 20 years.

III. ELEVENTH AND TWELFTH RIBS

Only two primary centres of ossification appear in total, i.e. one primary centre for shaft and one secondary centre for head.

A. Appearance

Primary centre : 8th week of intrauterine life.

Secondary centres : Puberty

B. Fusion: 20 years.

APPLIED ANATOMY

I. *Congenital anomalies of ribs*
  1. Congenital fusion of adjacent ribs or absence of one or more ribs is usually associated with congenital anomalies of vertebrae and severe scoliosis.

2. *Lumbar rib* is an additional rib at the level of 1st lumbar vertebra. The incidence is more common than the cervical rib. Lumbar ribs are clinically important because of following two reasons:
   i. It may misguide the level of 12th thoracic vertebra.
   ii. It may be confused with the fracture of transverse process of 1st lumbar vertebra.
3. Agenesis of rib reduces the total number of ribs. In Down's syndrome (trisomy 21) the person may have 11 pairs of ribs.
4. It is not very uncommon for the following abnormal behaviour of ribs:
   i. 7th rib behaving as false rib.
   ii. 8th rib behaving as true rib.
   iii. 10th rib behaving as floating rib.
5. *Bifid rib* is quite common in some races (Fig. 21.7).
6. *Thoracic outlet syndrome* is a varied clinical picture resulting from compression of neurovascular structures of the upper extremity between clavicle and 1st rib. Other terms used for this condition are cervical rib syndrome, *1st rib syndrome, shoulder arm syndrome,*

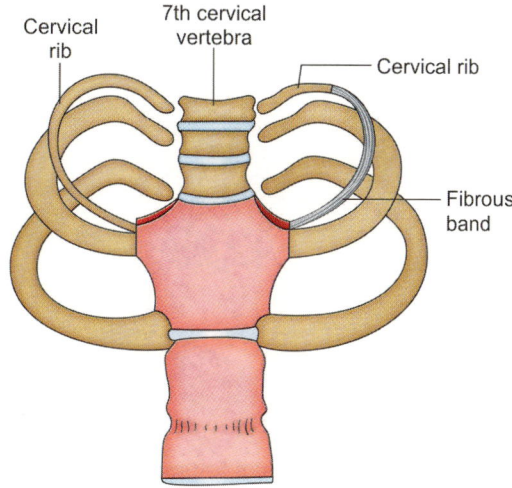

Fig. 21.18: Cervical rib

scalenus anticus syndrome or Naffziger's syndrome.

7. *Cervical rib* is a congenital overgrowth of the costal element of the 7th cervical vertebra. This condition may be unilateral or bilateral. The condition may or may not be associated with neurovascular symptoms. These symptoms are exaggerated by turning the chin to the affected side, hyperextending the neck and taking a deep breath (*Adson's sign*) (Fig. 21.18).

II. Fractures of ribs

1. The site of fracture and extent of visceral damage depends on mode of trauma. In cases of direct injury the rib is broken at the site of injury and the broken ends are directed inwards enhancing the chance of visceral damage (Fig. 21.19).

   During crush injuries the rib is usually fractured at its weak point, i.e. at its angle. Compare it with the junction of lateral 1/3rd and medial 2/3rd of clavicle. One can therefore conclude that junction of two curvatures is always a weak point (Fig. 21.20).

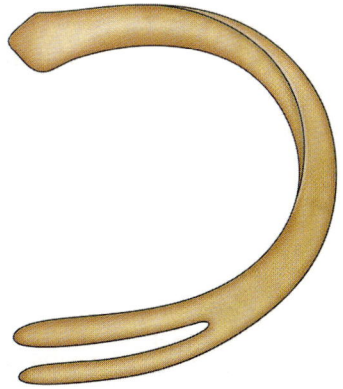

Fig. 21.17: A bifid rib

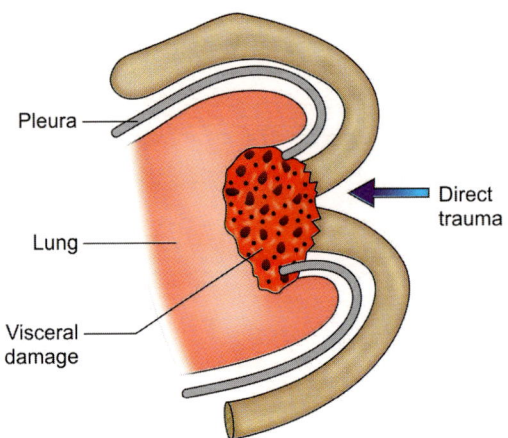

Fig. 21.19: Direct trauma of rib

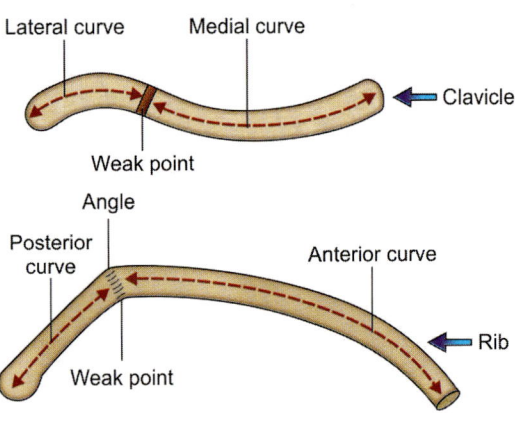

Fig. 21.20: Weak points of rib and clavicle

2. *Flail chest (Stove-in-chest)*
   This condition occurs when one or several ribs are fractured at multiple sites forming a 'flail segment'. On attempted inspiration the segment falls inwards and on attempted expiration the segment moves outwards. This is called *paradoxical respiration* (Fig. 21.21).
3. Ribs may be occasionally fractured from muscular strains as in violent coughing and heavy lifting.
4. Displacement of segment is minimal in single fracture.
5. In multiple fractures, the segments may perforate the pleura or lung.
6. Fractured ribs are very painful because fractured parts move during respiration.
7. Middle ribs are most commonly fractured.
8. Fracture of ribs may be associated with tearing of intercostal muscles.
9. Damage to pleura in case of rib fracture may lead to entery of air or blood into the pleural cavity. Aforementioned conditions are called *pneumothorax* or *hemothorax* respectively. Repeated radiographs are useful in such cases.

III. *Infections of ribs*
   1. *Osteomyelitis* of rib is usually haematogenous in origin.
   2. Ab scess in rib due to *tuberculosis (cold abscess)* usually originates from tuberculosis of lungs or lymph nodes of thorax.

IV. *Tumours of ribs*
   1. Tumours of chest wall most commonly originate from bone or cartilage of which approximately half are benign. *Chondromas* and *osteochondromas* are most common benign tumours involving the thoracic wall.
   2. *Tietze's syndrome* is a non-specific, non-suppurative condition that causes a

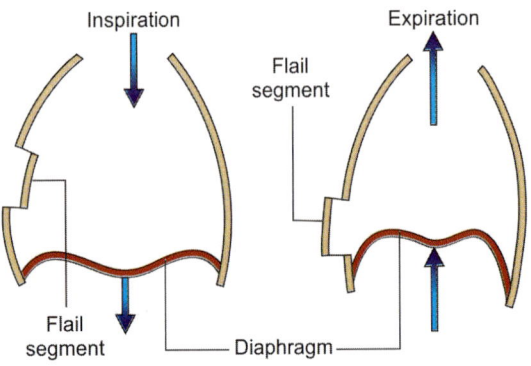

Fig. 21.21: Paradoxical respiration

painful swelling at the costochondral junction, usually involving the costochondral junction of 2nd rib.

3. *Chondrosarcoma* originating either in rib cartilage or in the sternum, is the most common malignant chest wall tumour.

4. *Ewing's tumour* destroys rib and produces a great widening with the characteristic "onion peel" radiographic appearance.

5. Metastatic tumours of ribs are usually derived from pulmonary and thyroid carcinoma.

V. *Miscellaneous conditions*

1. The ribs are some times chosen for bone grafting.

2. In *coarctation of aorta*, chest radiograph shows *rib notching* due to pressure by the intercostal collaterals (Fig. 21.22).

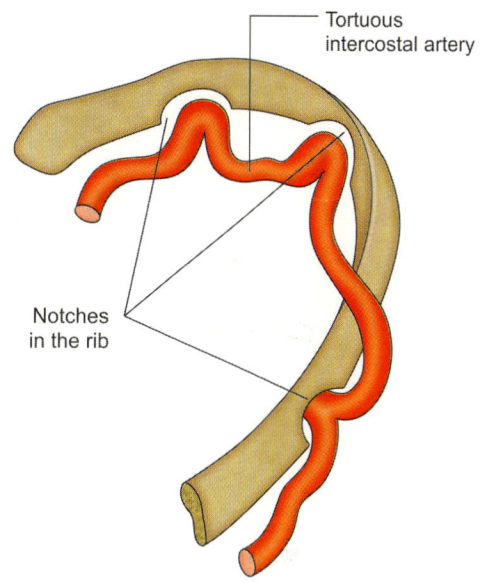

Fig. 21.22: Notching of rib by dilated and tortuous intercostal artery

CHAPTER

22 | The Hyoid

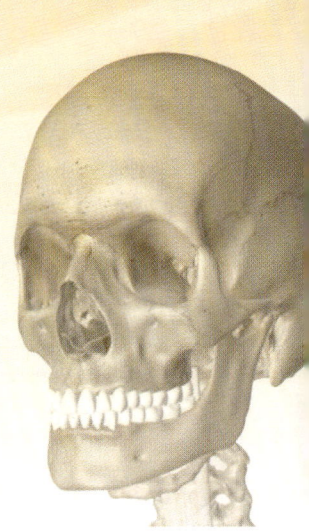

'Hyoid' is a Greek word which means 'U' shaped.

LEVEL

Hyoid lies at the level of 3rd cervical vertebra.

LOCATION (Fig. 22.1)

1. Hyoid is situated in the anterior midline of neck above the thyroid cartilage.
2. Its body (the bend of 'U') is the first resistant structure felt in the midline of neck, inferior to chin.
3. The tip of the greater cornu (the limb of 'U') of the hyoid can be palpated in the relaxed neck near the anterior border of sterno-cleidomastoid muscle midway between laryngeal prominence and mastoid process.

FEATURES AND ATTACHMENTS

Hyoid bone consists of a central body, a pair of greater cornua and a pair of lesser cornua.

I. BODY

It has two surfaces (anterior and posterior), two borders (upper and lower) and two lateral ends.

A. Surfaces

a. Anterior surface (Figs 22.2 and 22.3)

1. It is convex.
2. A median ridge divides it into two lateral halves.

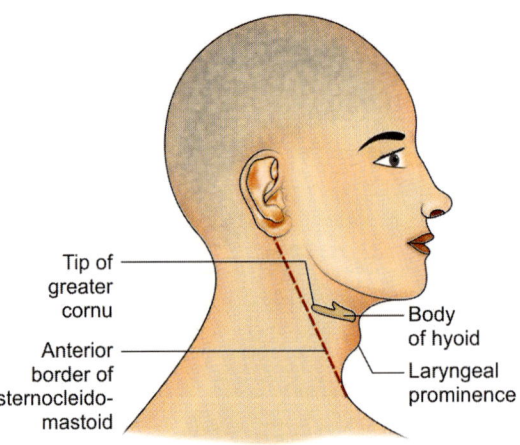

Fig. 22.1: Location of hyoid bone

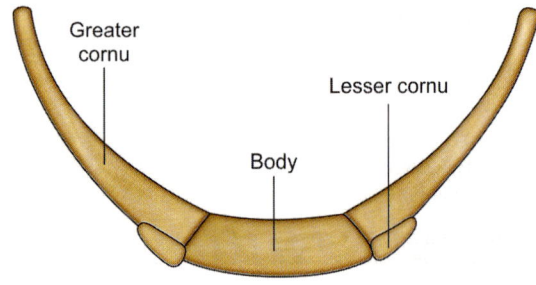

Fig. 22.2: The hyoid bone: Anterior aspect

The Hyoid | 199

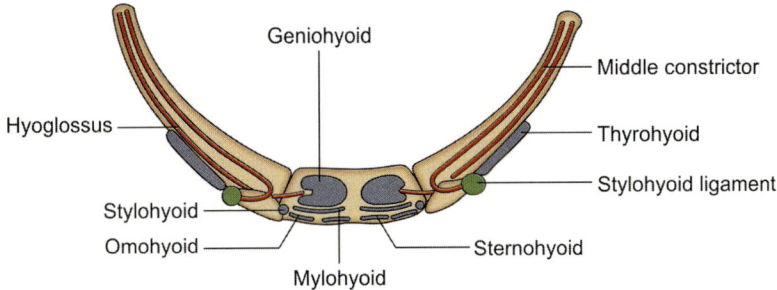

Fig. 22.3: The hyoid bone: Anterior aspect

3. *Geniohyoid* and *mylohyoid muscles* are inserted on this surface in its upper and lower parts respectively.
4. *Hyoglossus* partly originates from anterior surface.
5. *Investing layer of cervical fascia* is attached below the insertion of mylohyoid.

b. Posterior surface
1. It is concave.
2. It is related to following structures (Fig. 22.4).
    i. *Bursa*
    ii. *Thyrohyoid membrane*
    iii. *Epiglottis*

B. Borders
a. Upper border
It provides attachment to 3 structures from anterior to posterior
1. *Genioglossus muscle*
2. *Hyoepiglottic ligament*
3. *Thyrohyoid membrane.*

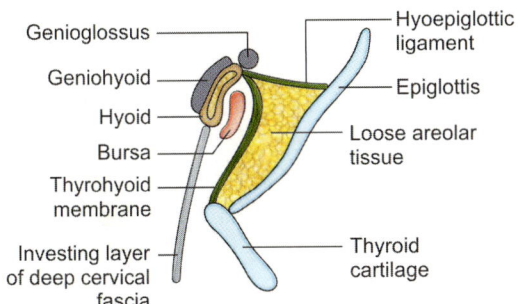

Fig. 22.4: Sectional view of hyoid

b. Lower border
Two muscles are mainly attached to this border on each side of midline from medial to lateral.
1. *Sternohyoid*
2. *Omohyoid*

C. Ends
1. Each end continues posteriorly as greater cornu.
2. Lesser cornu projects upwards at the junction of the body and greater cornu.

II. GREATER CORNUA (SINGULAR: GREATER CORNU)

Greater cronu has two surfaces (upper and lower), two borders (medial and lateral) and a tubercle (at the posterior end).

A. Surfaces
a. Upper surface
It has following attachments from medial to lateral.
1. *Middle constrictor* – along the whole length.
2. *Hyoglossus* – along the whole length.
3. *Stylohyoid muscle* – at the junction of lesser and greater cornua.
4. *Fibrous loop of digastric muscle* - lateral to attachment of stylohyoid muscle.

b. Lower surface
Fibroareolar tissue separates this surface from the thyrohyoid membrane.

B. Borders

a. Medial border

It receives attachment of *thyrohyoid membrane*.

b. Lateral border

Thyrohyoid muscle is attached to this border anteriorly.

III. LESSER CORNUA (SINGULAR: LESSER CORNU)

1. It is a small conical projection attached to the bone at the junction of the body and greater cornu by fibrous tissue.
2. It may form a synovial joint with the greater cornu.
3. It has following attachments:
   i. *Stylohyoid ligament at the tip.*
   ii. *Middle constrictor – posterolaterally.*

OSSIFICATION

1. The hyoid ossifies from ventral portions of the cartilages of 2nd and 3rd arches.
2. Lesser cornua and upper part of the body are developed from the 2nd arches.
3. Greater cornua and lower part of the body are developed from 3rd arches.
4. *Appearance of centres* – 6 centres of ossification appear, 2 for body and 1 for each cornu, as follows:
   Greater cornu – Just before birth
   Body – Just after birth
   Lesser cornu – Puberty
5. The cartilage at the tip of each greater cornu persists upto 3rd decade.

APPLIED ANATOMY

1. Some congenital anomalies associated with developing thyroid are commonly observed adjacent to the hyoid, e.g. suprahyoid thyroid, infrahyoid thyroid and thyroglossal cyst (Fig. 22.5).
2. Some times a muscular band connects the body of hyoid with isthmus or pyramidal lobe of thyroid gland. Thus is called *levator glandulae thyroideae* (Fig. 22.6).
3. Lingual artery arises from external carotid artery postero-inferior to the tip of the greater cornu. The latter thus forms an important surgical landmark for locating the lingual artery which is ligated essentially in radical surgery of tongue.
4. The hyoid bone is of great medicolegal importance. In suspected cases of death, fracture of hyoid bone suggests death by throttling or strangulation.

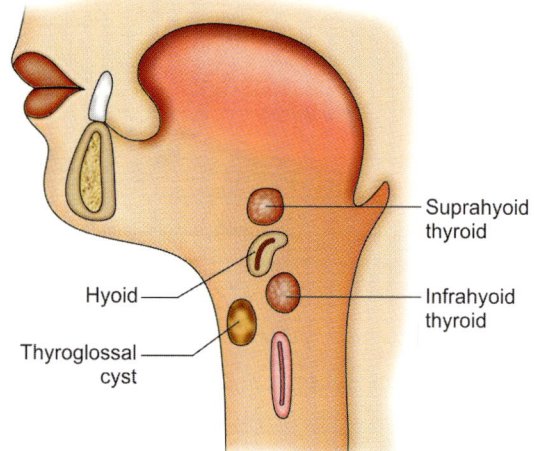

Fig. 22.5: Congenital anomalies close to hyoid bone

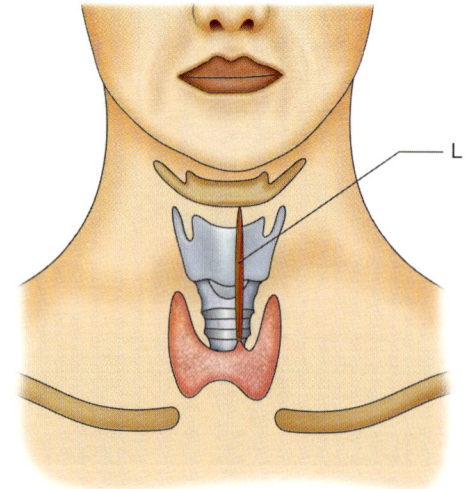

Fig. 22.6: Levator glandulae thyroideae (L)

CHAPTER
23 | # The Mandible

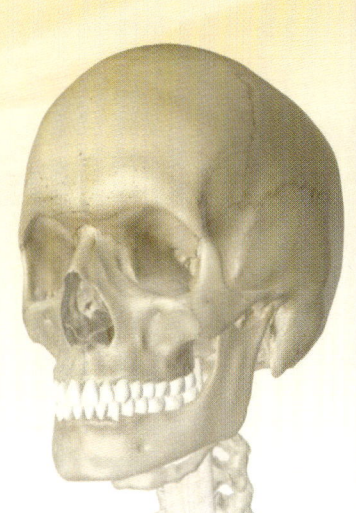

TERMINOLOGY

The word 'mandible' is derived from Greek word 'mandere' which means to masticate or chew. The Latin word 'mandibula' means lower jaw.

PECULIARITIES (Fig. 23.1)

1. It is a 'U' shaped bone.
2. It is also called 'lower facial skeleton'.
3. Mandible is the largest and strongest bone of the face.
4. It forms the skeleton of lower jaw.

FEATURES AND ATTACHMENTS

The mandible has a body and two rami.

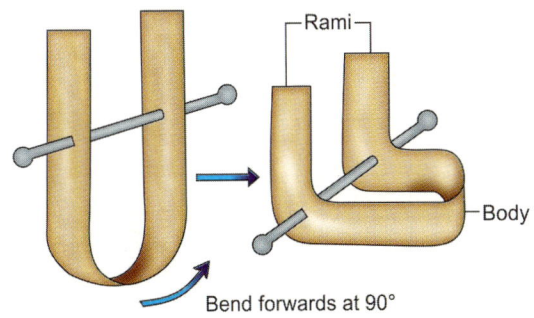

Fig. 23.1: Resemblance of mandible with 'U'

I. BODY

It is shaped like a horse shoe and has 2 surfaces (external and internal) and 2 borders (upper and lower).

A. Surfaces

a. External surface (Figs 23.2 and 23.3)

It has following features:

1. Symphysis menti

It is a faint ridge on the upper part of midline indicating the fusion of two halves of mandible.

2. Mental protuberance

It is triangular area in the lower part of midline. The upper angle of triangle marks the lower end of symphysis menti.

3. Mental tubercles

The lower angles of the triangular mental protuberance are marked by tubercles called mental tubercles.

Note: *Remember that mental protuberance is characteristic of human jaw.*

4. Mental foramen

It is located below the 2nd premolar or junction between two premolar teeth. Mental nerve and vessels pass through it.

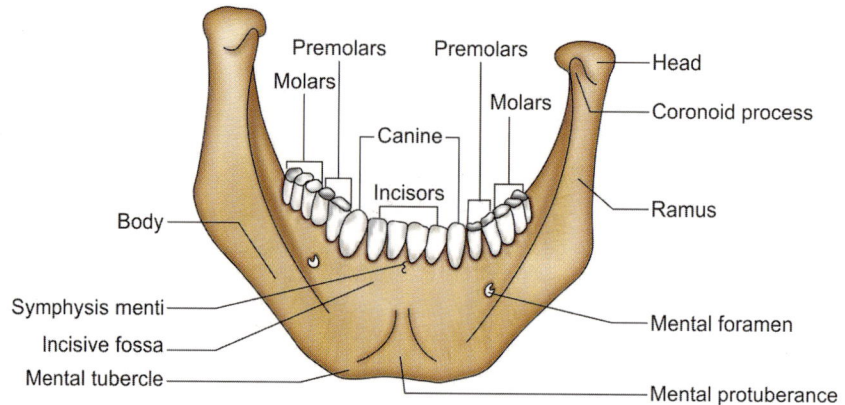

Fig. 23.2: Mandible : Anterior view

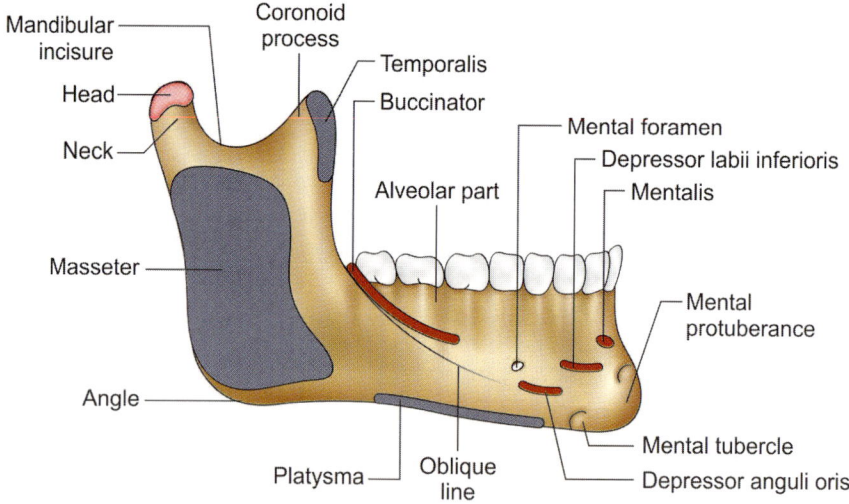

Fig. 23.3: Right half of mandible: External aspect

5. Incisive fossa

It is a shallow fossa below the incisor teeth. *Mentalis* and *orbicularis oris* originate from this fossa.

6. Oblique line

It is continuation of anterior border of ramus on the external surface of body. It is a faint ridge. It runs downwards and forwards to reach mental tubercle. Following muscles are attached to it from anterior to posterior:

   i. *Depressor labii inferioris.*
   ii. *Depressor anguli oris.*
   iii. *Buccinator (below the molar teeth).*

Note: *Junction of body and ramus is marked by the courses of facial artery and facial vein (Fig. 23.4).*

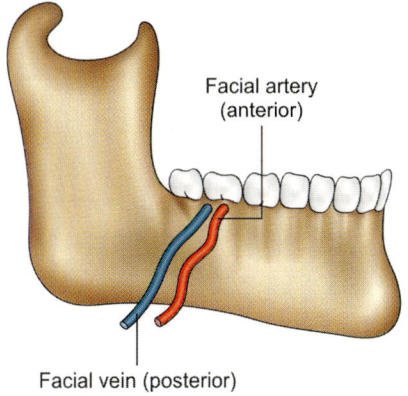

Fig. 23.4: Junction of body and ramus of mandible

ii. Facial artery.
iii. *Submandibular lymph nodes.*

3. Sublingual fossa

It is an area above the anterior part of mylohyoid line. It lodges the *sublingual salivary gland*.

4. Genial tubercles

These are irregular elevations on either side of midline just above the anterior ends of mylohyoid lines. Upper genial tubercle provides attachment to *genioglossus muscle* while lower genial tubercle gives origin to *geniohyoid muscle*.

> **Note:** *Genial tubercles are for genial muscles, since the tongue is higher as compared to the hyoid bone, the upper tubercle is for genioglossus and lower is for geniohyoid.*

b. Internal surface (Figs 23.5 and 23.6)

It has following features:

1. Mylohyoid line

It is an oblique ridge. It extends downwards and forwards from behind the 3rd molar tooth (1 cm below the alveolar border) to midline near the lower border between digastric fossae. *Mylohyoid muscle* is attached to it.

2. Submandibular fossa

It is present below the posterior part of mylohyoid line. It lodges following structures:
i. Submandibular salivary gland.

5. Attachment of superior constrictor of pharynx

Superior constrictor originates from the area above the posterior end of mylohyoid line.

6. Attachment of pterygomandibular raphe

This raphe is attached to inner surface of body in continuation with the origin of superior constrictor just behind the 3rd molar tooth.

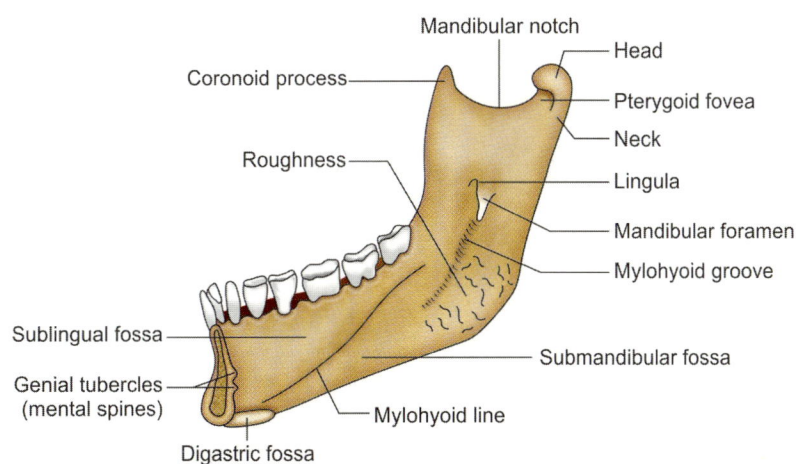

Fig. 23.5: Right half of mandible: Internal aspect

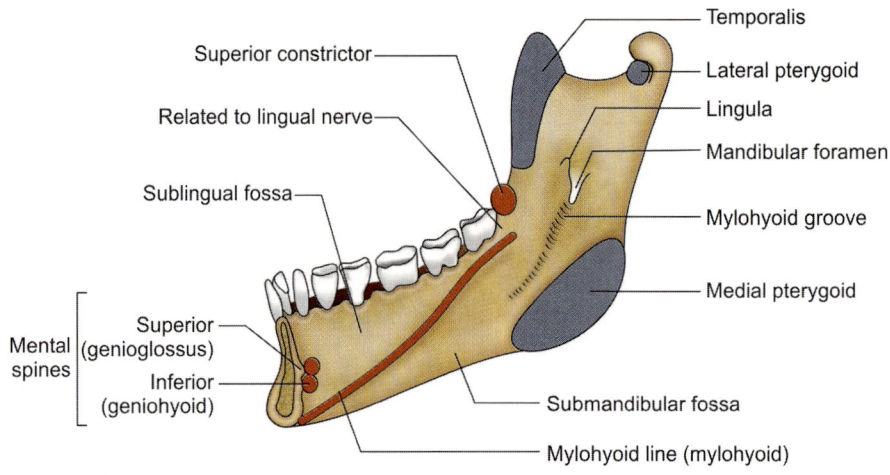

Fig. 23.6: Right half of mandible: Internal aspect

7. Relation of lingual nerve

Lingual nerve is related to mandible between the origin of superior constrictor and posterior end of mylohyoid line.

B. Borders

a. Upper border (Fig. 23.7)

1. It is also called alveolar part of mandible.
2. It is hollowed out by sixteen sockets for the roots of permanent teeth.
3. The sockets vary in size and depth.
4. The sockets may be single or subdivided by septa according to the teeth which they contain.

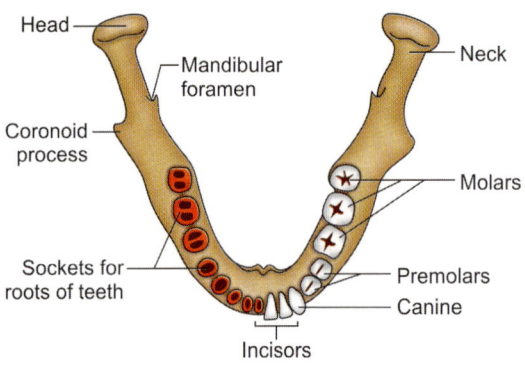

Fig. 23.7: Alveolar part of mandible: Superior view

b. Lower border

1. It is also called as the *base* of mandible.
2. *Digastric fossa* is a depression at its anterior (mesial) end on each side of the midline. It receives attachment of *anterior belly of digastric*.
3. *Investing layer of deep cervical fascia* is attached to the whole length of the base.
4. *Platysma* is inserted to the lower border near the outer surface.

II. RAMUS

Ramus of mandible has 2 surfaces (lateral and medial), 4 borders (upper, lower, anterior and posterior) and two processes (coronoid and condylar).

A. Surfaces

a. Lateral surface (Fig. 23.3)

1. A small posterosuperior area is related to *parotid gland*.
2. Remaining major area provides attachment to *masseter*.

> **Note:** Remember, house of Prime Minister is located on the lateral area. P stands for Parotid and M stands for Masseter.

b. Medial surface (Figs 23.5 and 23.6)

1. *Mandibular foramen and canal* – Mandibular foramen is located a little above the centre of medial surface. It leads into mandibular canal which curves downwards and forwards into the body, to open on the external surface at the mental foramen. *Inferior alveolar nerve and vessels* enter the mandibular canal through the mandibular foramen.
2. *Lingula* – It is a tongue shaped projection near the anterior margin of mandibular foramen. *Sphenomandibular ligament* is attached to the lingula.
3. *Mylohyoid groove* – It begins at the lower end of mandibular foramen behind the lingula and continues downwards and forwards to reach the inner surface of body. *Mylohyoid nerve* and *vessels* occupy the mylohyoid groove.
4. Medial surface of ramus between mylohyoid groove and angle of mandible is marked by ridges. This area is meant for the attachment of *medial pterygoid*.
5. Area in front of mylohyoid groove is related to *lingual nerve*.

B. Borders
a. Upper border
1. It is thin.
2. It forms *mandibular notch* or *incisure*.
3. *Masseteric nerve* and *vessels* cross the mandibular notch.

b. Lower border
1. It is backward continuation of base of mandible.
2. It meets with the posterior border of ramus to form *angle of mandible*.

c. Anterior border
1. It is continuous above with the coronoid process and below with alveolar border of body.
2. *Temporalis* muscle is inserted on this border and adjoining medial surface.

d. Posterior border
1. It is continuous above with the condylar process.
2. It meets with the lower border to form *angle of mandible*.
3. It is related to *parotid gland*.

C. Processes
a. Coronoid process
1. It is triangular upward projection from the anterosuperior part of ramus.
2. Its anterior border is continuous with the anterior border of the ramus and its posterior border bounds the mandibular notch.
3. *Temporalis muscle* gets inserted on the medial surface, apex and margins of coronoid process.

b. Condylar process
It is an upward projection from the poterosuperior part of ramus. It consists of an upper part (*head*) and a lower part (*neck*).

i. Head
1. It is side to side expanded part of condylar process.
2. It articulates with the temporal bone to form *temporomandibular joint*.

ii. Neck
1. It is constricted part below the head.
2. It provides attachment to *capsule* in its upper part.
3. *Lateral ligament of temporomandibular joint* is attached to its lateral part.
4. *Pterygoid fovea* is a depression on its anterior aspect. *Lateral pterygoid muscle* is inserted on the pterygoid fovea.
5. Medially the neck is related to *auriculotemporal nerve* above and *maxillary artery* below.

OSSIFICATION

1. Mandible is intramembranous as well as endochondral in origin.
2. The membrane involved is the mesenchymal sheath on the lateral aspect of both Meckel's cartilages. A centre appears on each side in this sheath during 7th week of intrauterine life.
3. Cartilages contributing to the mandible are as follows:
   i. *Anterior ends of Meckel's cartilages*
      These are invaded by bone from parent centres at 10th week of intrauterine life.
   ii. *Coronoid cartilages*
      These appear at 10th week of intrauterine life and disappear before birth.
   iii. *Condylar cartilages*
      These appear at 10th week of intrauterine life and persist till 3rd decade.
   iv. *Cartilaginous nodules*
      One or two of these nodules appear on each side of the symphysis menti at about 10th week of intrauterine life. These ossify to form mental ossicles at about the 7th month of intrauterine life and fuse with the body at the age of one year.
4. Parts of the mandible which are derived from cartilage are:
   i. Incisive part below the incisor teeth.
   ii. Coronoid and condylar processes.
   iii. Part of ramus above the mandibular foramen.

Note: *Remember that the names of all the parts of mandible which ossifying from cartilage start with C, i.e. Coronoid process, Condylar process, Cranial part of ramus and Chin part of body related to Cutting or incisor teeth.*

5. At birth mandible consists of two halves connected at *symphysis menti*. Bony union starts from below upwards during 1st year of age and is completed at the end of 3rd year.

AGE CHANGES IN MANDIBLE

Some of the differentiating features in different age groups are as follows:

I. Children (Fig. 23.8)

1. The body of mandible is more like a shell having sockets for both deciduous and permanent teeth.
2. The angle of mandible measures about 140°.
3. Coronoid process is above the level of condylar process.
4. The mandibular canal and mental foramen are close to the lower border of body.

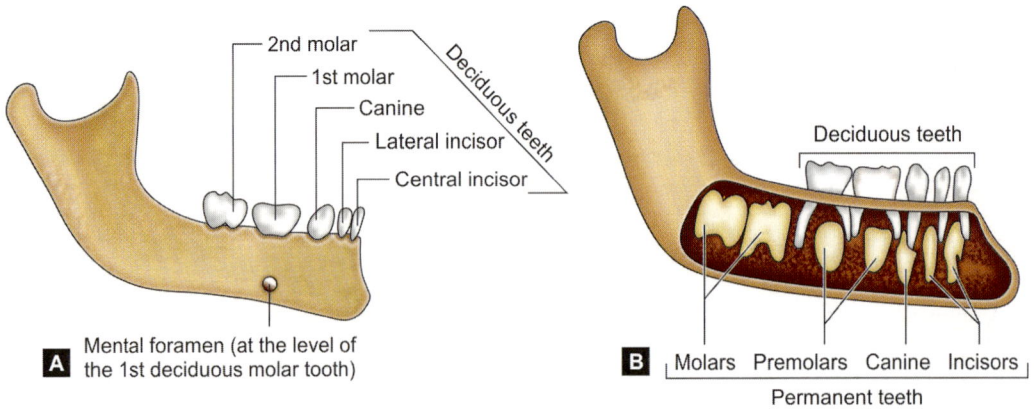

Fig. 23.8: Right lateral view of the mandible of a child between 2–6 years. (A) Surface features; (B) Body dissected

II. Adult (Fig. 23.9)

1. The alveolar and subalveolar parts of body are of equal depths.
2. The angle of mandible measures about 110°.
3. Condylar process projects above the level of coronoid process.
4. Mandibular canal runs parallel to the mylohyoid line.
5. The mental foramen is situated midway between upper and lower borders of body.

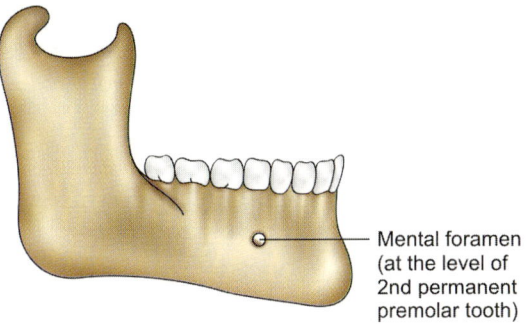

Fig. 23.9: Adult mandible: Right lateral view

III. Old age (Fig. 23.10)

1. Loss of teeth is a usual feature.
2. Alveolar part is absorbed.
3. Angle of mandible measures about 140°
4. Neck of mandible is bent backwards making the level of coronoid process higher than condylar process.
5. Mandibular canal and mental foramen are close to the upper border of body.

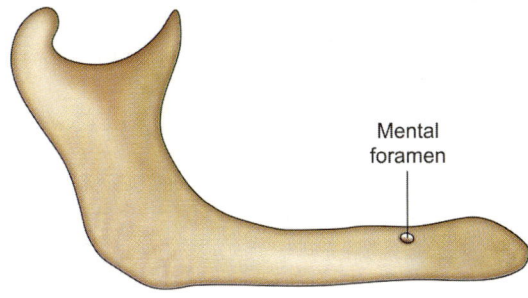

Fig. 23.10: The mandible at old age. Right lateral view

APPLIED ANATOMY

1. The mandible occupies a prominent and exposed position in the facial skeleton and therefore forms a common site of violent injuries.
2. Slender neck of the mandinble is liable to fracture as a result of violence received at the mental prominence (Fig. 23.11).

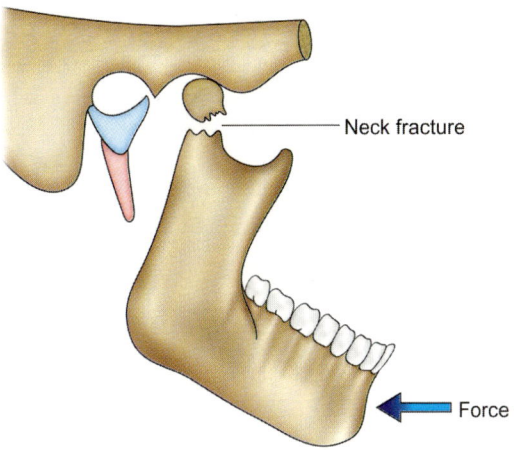

Fig. 23.11: Fracture of mandibular neck

3. Alveolar process is weaker than the rest of the mandible and therefore an independent alveolar fracture may occur.
4. Tendency of mandible to fracture with advancing age is due to resorption of alveolar portion of bone when the teeth are lost.
5. Elongated root of canine tooth reduces the bony substance and makes the mandible weaker at this site. Canine region is, therefore, the commonest site of fracture.
6. Thick periosteum over the mandible prevents gross displacement of fractured bones after fracture.
7. Impacted 3rd molar, mental foramen and missing teeth also contribute to the weakness in the mandible.
8. Strong muscles attached to the mandible play very important role in displacement of fractured segments of mandible. Such muscles are divided into 3 groups (Fig. 23.12).

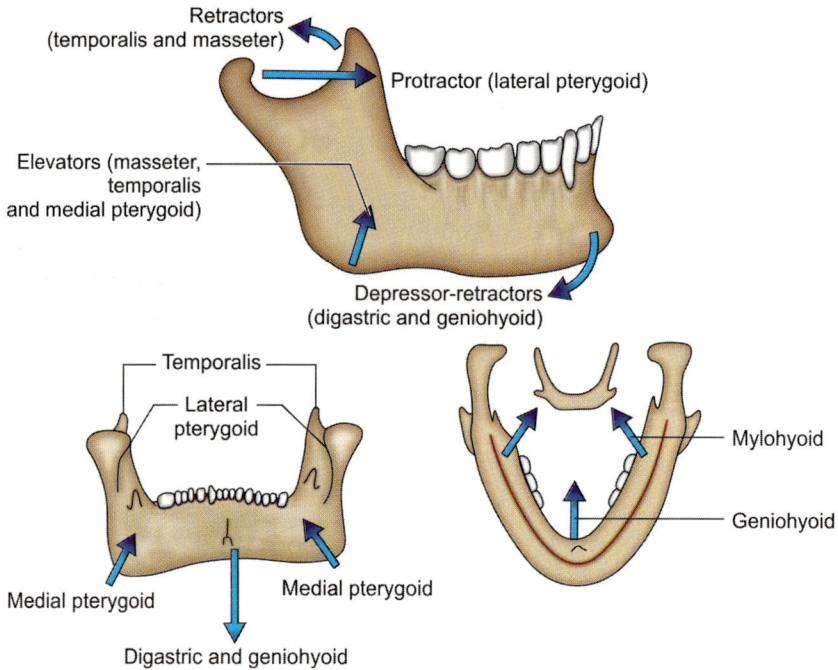

Fig. 23.12: Direction of composite forces of the mandibular muscles

i. *The depressor group*

It includes *geniohyoid* and *digastric muscles*. They cause posterior and inferior displacement of fractured anterior mandibular segment.

ii. *The elevator group*

The *masseter, temporalis* and *medial pterygoid muscles* belong to this group. Contraction of these muscles cause upward displacement of fractured segment if the fracture occurs in the region of angle.

iii. *The protrusor group*

It includes *lateral pterygoid muscle* which causes forward displacement of head in cases of fracture of mandibular neck.

9. Following is the general classification of mandibular fractures (Fig. 23.13):

i. *Simple*

Single fracture without exposure to exterior.

ii. *Compound*

Fractured site is exposed to exterior.

iii. *Comminuted*

It is multiple fractures of mandible at the same site. It may be both simple or compound.

iv. *Complicated*

It is fracture associated with injury of teeth, nerves or vessels.

v. *Impacted*

In this fracture one fragment has been driven into the substance of other fragment.

vi. *Greenstick*

In this, fractured site bends without displacement.

vii. *Pathological*

Fracture is due to underlying diseases like osteomyelitis or tumours.

10. Clinical classification of mandibular fractures (Fig. 23.14).

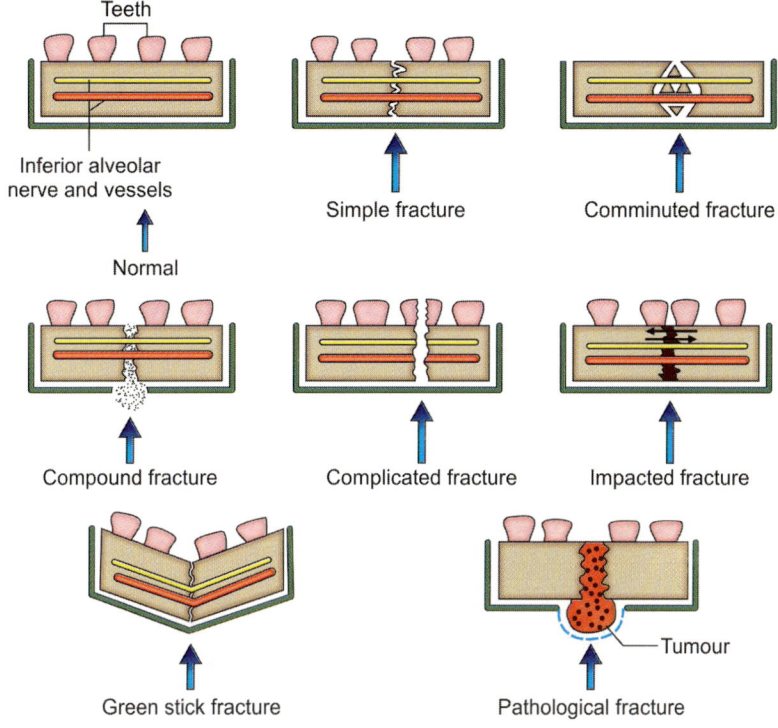

Fig. 23.13: Different types of fractures of mandible

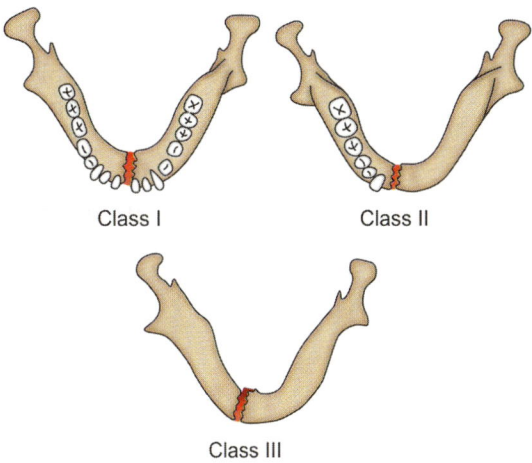

Fig. 23.14: Three classes of mandibular fractures

i. *Class I*
   Teeth present on both sides of fractured line.
ii. *Class II*
   Teeth present on one side of fractured line.
iii. *Class III*
   Fragments are edentulous (without teeth)
11. Depending upon the number of sites, mandibular fractures may be of following types (Fig. 23.15):
   i. *Single unilateral*
   ii. *Double unilateral*
   iii. *Bilateral*
   iv. *Multiple*
12. The mandible can be divided into following regions to simplify the sites of lesions, e.g. fractures (Fig. 23.16):
   i. *Condylar*
   ii. *Coronoid*
   iii. *Ramus*
   iv. *Angle*

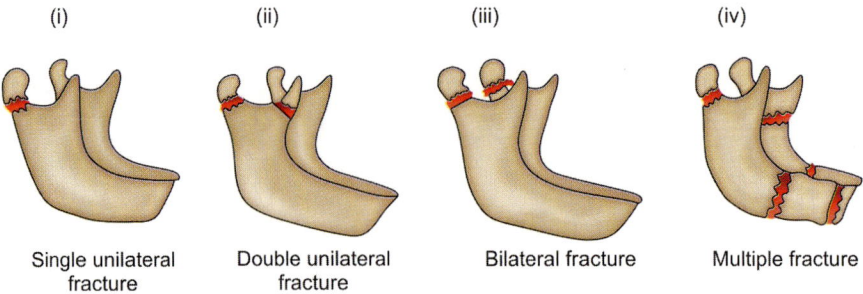

Fig. 23.15: Number of fractured sites as criterion for types of fractures

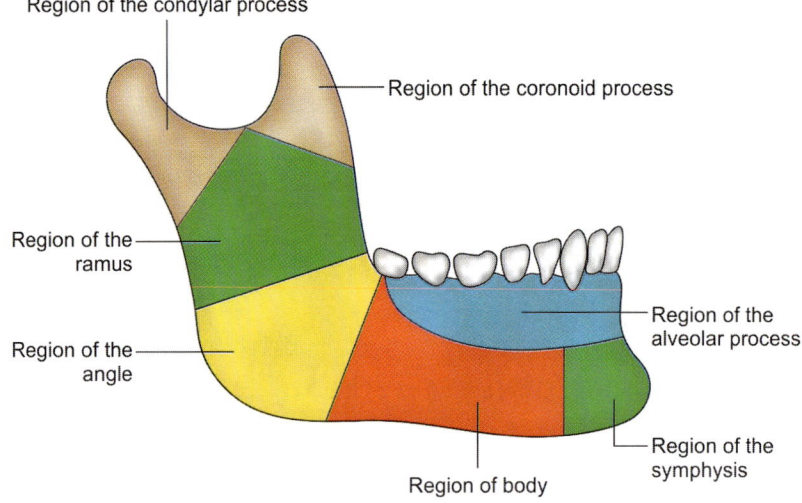

Fig. 23.16: Mandibular regions

    v. *Alveolar.*
    vi. *Body.*
    vii. *Symphysis.*
13. Tumours of the hard tissue of lower jaw can originate in teeth (*odontogenic tumours*) or mandible (*osteogenic tumours*)

A. Odontogenic tumours

These can be of following two types:

a. Odontoma

Arising from teeth proper. Odontomas may be of following three types according to their structures:
    i. *Calcified odontoma*
        It has dentine.
   ii. *Simple enamel pearl.*
        It has enamel.
   iii. *Cementoma*
        It has cementum.

b. Ameloblastoma

Arising from the embryonal (ameloblast) cells of developing teeth.

B. Osteogenic tumours

Following are the common osteogenic tumours:
    i. *Osteoma*
   ii. *Fibro-osteoma*
  iii. *Myxoma*
  iv. *Chondroma*
   v. *Sarcoma*
  vi. *Ewing's tumour*
 vii. *Multiple myeloma.*
viii. *Central giant cell tumour*

CHAPTER 24

The Maxillae

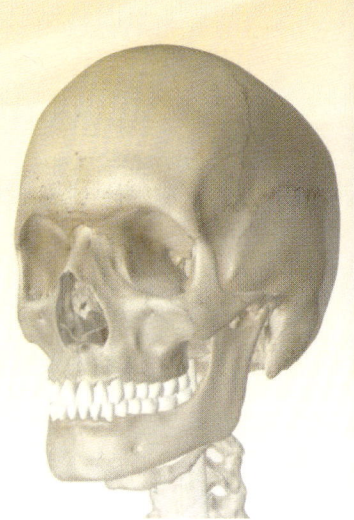

TERMINOLOGY

Maxilla is a Latin word meaning 'cheek' or 'jaw'. The word is commonly used in reference to upper jaw.

LOCATION

1. There are two maxillae which form major part of upper facial skeleton.
2. Whole of the upper jaw is formed by two maxillae.
3. Junction of two maxillae is marked by intermaxillary suture visible in the hard palate and face in midline.

FEATURES AND ATTACHMENTS

Each maxilla consists of a body and four processes (zygomatic, frontal, alveolar and palatine).

I. BODY (Figs 24.1 and 24.2)

It has 4 surfaces (anterior, infratemporal, orbital and nasal).

A. Anterior surface

1. It is directed forwards and laterally.
2. There is a vertical elevation at the site of socket for canine root. This is called *canine eminence*.
3. Medial to canine eminence is a depression called *incisive fossa* which gives origin to *depressor septi*.
4. The anterior surface below the incisive fossa gives attachments to *incisivus superior* and *orbicularis oris*.
5. Just above the incisive fossa there is attachment of *nasalis muscle*.
6. Lateral to canine eminence is another fossa called *canine fossa*. *Levator anguli oris* originates from the canine fossa.
7. Above the canine fossa is a foramen called *infraorbital foramen*. It transmits *infraorbital nerve and vessels*.
8. Above the infra-orbital foramen is sharp infra-orbital margin which gives origin to *levator labii superioris*.
9. Its upper part is limited medially by a deep notch called *nasal notch*.

B. Infratemporal surface

1. It faces backwards and laterally.
2. It forms anterior wall of *infratemporal fossa*.
3. It shows 2–3 openings of *alveolar canals* which transmit *posterior superior alveolar nerves and vessels*.
4. Its inferoposterior part is marked by *maxillary tuberosity* which articulates with the pyramidal process of palatine bone.

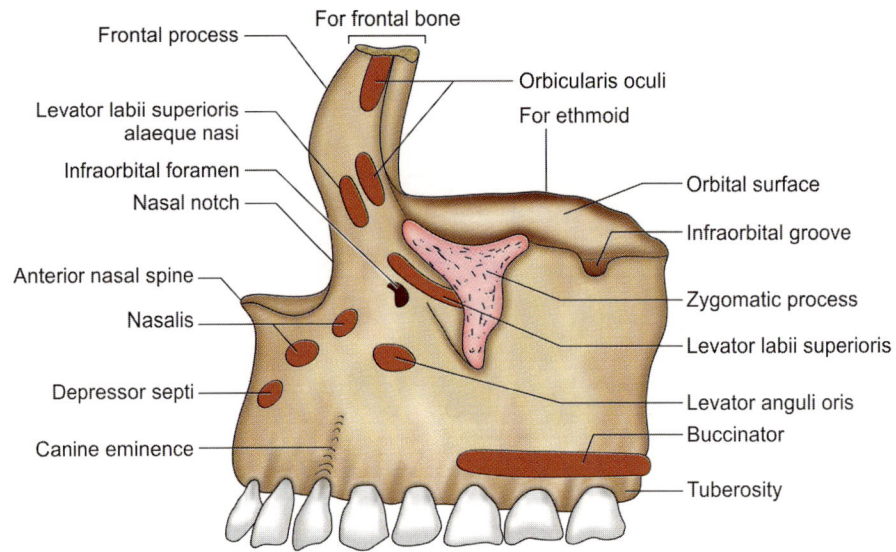

Fig. 24.1: Left maxilla : Lateral aspect

C. Orbital surface

1. It forms floor of orbit.
2. Running forwards is *infraorbital groove* in the middle of its posterior part. The groove continues with *infra-orbital canal* which opens on the anterior surface as *infraorbital foramen*. It is meant for *infraorbital nerve and vessels*.
3. Anteromedially it gives origin to *inferior oblique muscle*.
4. It has 3 borders (medial, posterior and anterior).

a. Medial border

It is marked anteriorly by *lacrimal notch*. Behind this notch this border provides attachments to lacrimal bone, orbital plate of ethmoid and orbital process of palatine bone from before backwards.

b. Posterior border

It forms anterior border of inferior orbital fissure.

c. Anterior border

It contributes to the medial part of infra-orbital margin.

D. Nasal surface (Fig. 24.2)

1. It forms the lateral wall of nasal cavity.
2. A large opening (*maxillary hiatus*) is the most prominent feature of this surface.
3. Maxillary hiatus leads into *maxillary sinus*, a large air space within the body of maxilla.
4. Maxillary hiatus is greatly reduced in size in articulated skull by ethmoid (uncinate process) and lacrimal bone above, inferior concha below and perpendicular plate of palatine bone behind.
5. Below the hiatus this surface forms inferior meatus of nasal cavity.
6. Posterior part of nasal surface has got an *oblique groove* which is converted into *greater palatine canal* by perpendicular plate of palatine bone. Greater palatine nerve and vessels pass through this canal.
7. In front of hiatus is *nasolacrimal groove*. This is converted into *nasolacrimal canal* by lacrimal bone and inferior concha. This canal is meant for *nasolacrimal duct*.
8. An oblique ridge called *conchal crest*, is present in front of nasolacrimal groove. It articulates with inferior concha.

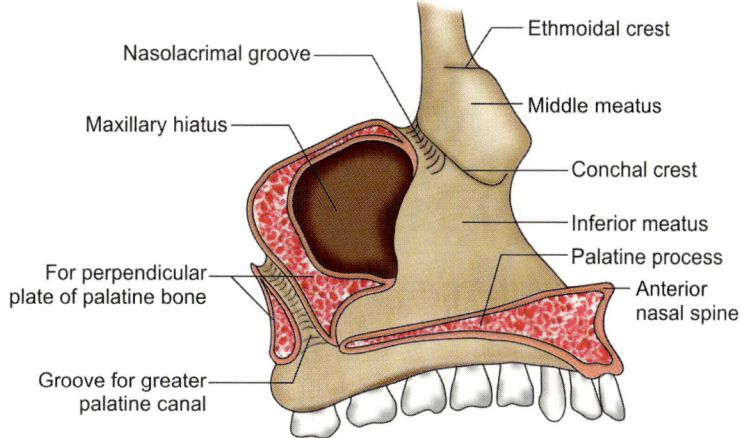

Fig. 24.2: Left maxilla: Medial aspect

II. PROCESSES

A. Zygomatic process
It has three surfaces, anterior, posterior and superior. The latter is rough for articulation with zygomatic bone.

B. Frontal process
It possesses an upper end, 2 surfaces (lateral and medial) and 2 borders (anterior and posterior).

a. Upper end
It articulates with the nasal notch of frontal bone.

b. Surfaces
i. Lateral surface (Fig. 24.1)
1. It has a vertical ridge (*anterior lacrimal crest*) in the middle for the attachment of *medial palpebral ligament*.
2. Area in front of crest gives attachments to *orbicularis oculi* and *levator labii superioris alaeque nasi*.
3. Area behind the lacrimal crest contributes to the anterior half of lacrimal groove.

ii. Medial surface (Fig. 24.2)
1. It has got a horizontal ridge (*ethmoidal crest*) in its middle. It articulates with middle nasal concha.
2. A roughened area above the crest articulates with ethmoid to complete anterior ethmoidal air cells.
3. The area below the ethmoidal crest forms *atrium* of middle meatus.

c. Borders
i. Anterior border
It articulates with nasal bone.

ii. Posterior border
It articulates with lacrimal bone.

C. Alveolar process
1. It is arched lower border of body.
2. It has sockets for upper teeth.
3. *Buccinator* originates from the posterior part of outer surface over the sockets for permanent molars roots.

D. Palatine process
It is a horizontal bracket like projection from the lower part of medial surface of body. It

forms anterior 3/4th of hard palate. It has two surfaces (superior and inferior) and three borders (medial, posterior and lateral).

a. Surfaces

i. Superior surface
1. It is concave and smooth.
2. It forms floor of nasal cavity.

ii. Inferior surface
1. It has *depressions* for palatine glands.
2. It has several *nutrient foramina* for nutrient vessels.
3. *Greater palatine groove* for greater palatine nerve and vessels is present in its posterolateral part.
4. When two maxillae meet, *incisive fossa* is noticed behind the incisor teeth.
5. *Incisive canal* is communication between incisive fossa and nasal cavity. It transmits *greater palatine artery* and *nasopalatine nerve*.

b. Borders

i. Medial border
1. It meets with the similar border of opposite maxilla to form *intermaxillary suture*.
2. This border is raised into a ridge called *nasal crest*. Nasal crests of two sides enclose a groove to receive the vomer.
3. Its anterior end is prolonged and meets with the similar prolongation of opposite side to form *anterior nasal spine*.

ii. Posterior border
It articulates with the anterior border of horizontal plate of palatine bone to form *palatomaxillary suture*.

iii. Lateral border
It fuses with the body.

OSSIFICATION

1. The maxilla is intramembranous in origin.
2. It develops in the mesenchyme just superficial to nasal capsule.
3. Three centres of ossification appear:
    i. One centre appears for the main mass just above canine fossa at about 6th week of intrauterine life.
    ii. Two centres appear for os incisivum (premaxillary part).

> **Note:** *Remember that premaxilla is that part of maxilla which holds incisor teeth and is a separate bone in most mammalian upper jaws.*

4. Maxillary sinus appears on the nasal aspect as a groove at about 4th month of intrauterine life.

AGE CHANGES IN MAXILLA

I. At birth
1. Vertical diameter is lesser than both the transverse and anteroposterior diameters.
2. Body is mainly occupied by sockets for the teeth.
3. Maxillary sinus is seen as a shallow groove on the nasal aspect.

II. Adult
1. Vertical diameter is greater than the transverse and anteroposterior diameters.
2. Maxillary sinus has greatly developed within the body.

III. Old age
1. Due to falling of teeth and resorption of alveolar margin, the vertical diameter is again greatly reduced.
2. Alveolar margin is reduced in thickness at the expense of the labial wall.

APPLIED ANATOMY

1. **Maxillary sinus (antrum of Highmore)**
    It is the air space in the body of maxilla. It is pyramidal in shape with base towards nasal cavity and apex towards zygomatic process. Its height and anteroposterior measurements are 1.5 inches each while width is 1 inch only. It is very important clinically due to following facts:

i. It is largest paranasal sinus and commonly involved during inflammation process (maxillary sinusitis).
ii. It drains into middle meatus which is higher than its floor. The latter is about 1.25 cm below the floor of nasal cavity. To facilitate the drainage of pus in maxillary sinus an opening is made in inferior meatus by operative procedures like *antral puncture* or *antrostomy* (Fig. 24.3).
iii. *Maxillary tumours* can produce a bulging in adjacent related surroundings, i.e. superiorly in the floor of orbit, inferiorly in the roof of oral cavity, anteriorly in the face, posteriorly in the infratemporal fossa and medially in the lateral wall of nasal cavity.

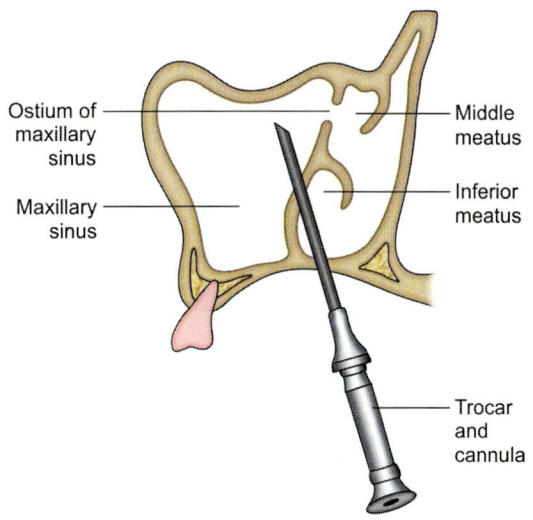

Fig. 24.3: Antral puncture

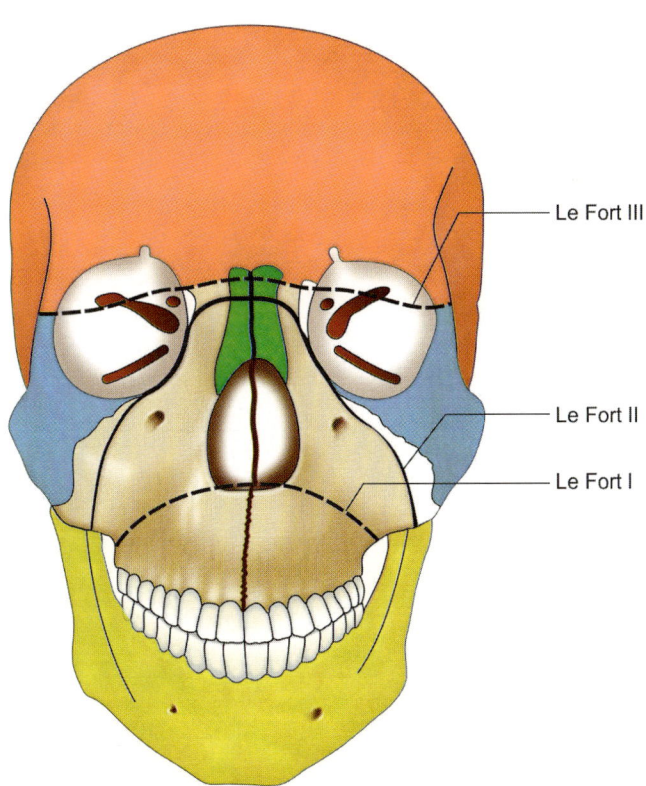

Fig. 24.4: Common fractures of maxillae and other bones

2. **Maxillary fractures (Fig. 24.4)**

    A. Unilateral fracture of maxilla usually involves its alveolar process.

    B. Bilateral maxillary fractures are classified into following three types:

    a. Le Fort I (Guerin's fracture)

    It is a horizontal fracture along the floor of nose and below the zygomatic bone.

    b. Le Fort II

    In this fracture line passes through orbits then runs medial to and below the zygomatic bones towards the alveolar margins.

    c. Le Fort III

    In this, the fracture line runs through nasal bones and orbits above the zygomatic bone. This fracture is also called craniofacial disjunction as the face separates from cranium.

CHAPTER
25

The Parietal Bones

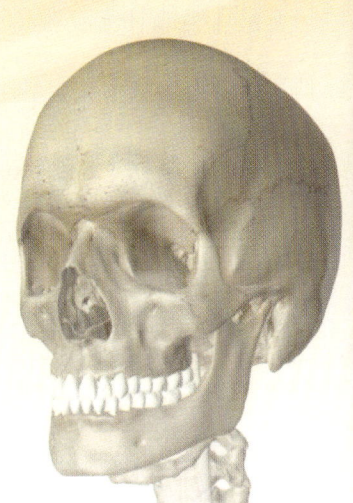

TERMINOLOGY

The word parietal is derived from Latin word 'paries' which means 'wall', because two parietal bones form large part of walls of calvaria.

SIDE DETERMINATION

1. Keep the bone by the side of your own cranial vault in such a way that outer surface is convex and inner surface is concave.
2. Inferior (squamosal) border is concave.
3. Anteroinferior angle is prominent and has got a vascular and narrow groove on its inner aspect.
4. The posteroinferior angle has got a shallow and wide groove for sigmoid sinus on its inner aspect.

FEATURES AND ATTACHMENTS

I. Surfaces

It has two surfaces, external and internal.

A. External surface (Fig. 25.1)

1. It is relatively smooth.

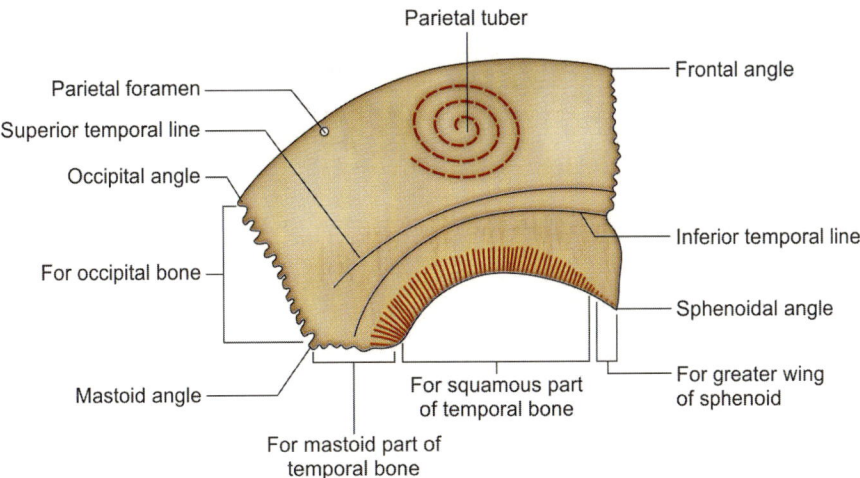

Fig. 25.1: Right parietal bone: External surface

2. Most prominent part of this surface is called parietal *tuberosity* or *eminence*.
3. There are two curved lines running anteroposteriorly. These are called *superior and inferior temporal lines*. Superior temporal line gives attachment to *tempral fascia* while area below inferior temporal line gives attachment to *temporalis muscle*.
4. Area above the superior temporal line is covered by *galea aponeurotica*.
5. A foramen may be present near the posterior part of sagittal border. This is called *parietal foramen*. It transmits *emissary vein*.

B. **Internal surface** (Fig. 25.2)
1. It is concave and exhibits elevations and depressions for cerebral sulci and gyri respectively.
2. Near the sagittal border there is a longitudinal half groove (to be completed with that of opposite side) for *superior sagittal sinus*. The margins of groove provide attachment to *falx cerebri*.
3. Grooves for the branches of *middle meningeal vessels* are present at the anteroinferior angle and at the middle of the lower border of the bone.
4. Adjacent to groove for superior sagittal sinus there are deep irregular pits (*granular foveolae*) produced by *arachnoid granulations*.
5. The bone is grooved near the posteroinferior angle by *sigmoid sinus*.

II. **Borders**

It has four borders, superior, inferior, anterior and posterior.

A. **Superior border**
1. This is also called sagittal border.
2. It articulates with the similar border of opposite side to form sagittal suture.

B. **Inferior border**
1. This is also called squamosal border.
2. It articulates with following 3 bones from anterior to posterior:
   i. Greater wing of sphenoid.
   ii. Squamous part of temporal.
   iii. Mastoid portion of temporal.

C. **Anterior border**
1. This is also called frontal border.
2. It articulates with the frontal bone to form *coronal suture*.

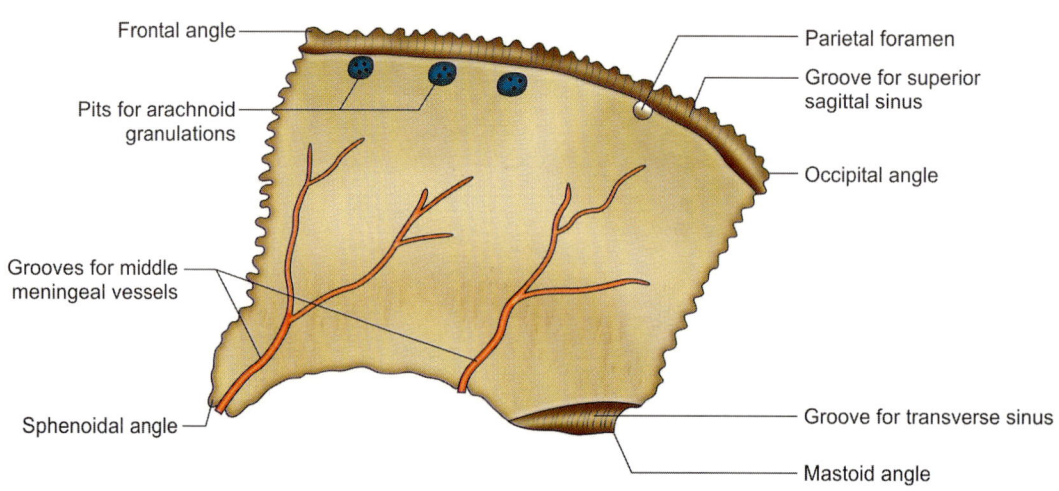

Fig. 25.2: Right parietal bone : Internal surface

D. Posterior border
1. This is also called occipital border.
2. It articulates with the squamous part of occipital bone to form *lambdoid suture*.

III. Angles
Parietal bone has four angles (frontal, sphenoidal, occipital and mastoid).

A. Frontal angle
1. This is also called anterosuperior angle.
2. It corresponds to *bregma*, i.e. the junction of coronal and sagittal sutures.

B. Sphenoidal angle
1. This is also called anteroinferior angle.
2. It correspsonds to *pterion*, i.e. a small area enclosing four bones (frontal, temporal, parietal and greater wing of sphenoid).

C. Occipital angle
1. This is also called posterosuperior angle.
2. It corresponds to *lambda*, i.e. junction of sagittal and lambdoid sutures.

D. Mastoid angle
1. This is also called posteroinferior angle.
2. It corresponds to *asterion*, i.e. small area enclosing three bones, parietal, temporal and occipital.

OSSIFICATION
1. Parietal bones ossify in membrane.
2. Each ossifies from two centres which appear at parietal tuberosity at about 7th week of intrauterine life.
3. The centres soon fuse with each other and then the ossification spreads radially.
4. Angles are the parts last to be ossified explaining the existence of a fontanelle at each angle before the ossification is completed.

AGE CHANGES
1. At birth
Temporal lines are present at quite a lower level.
2. Adult
A higher and permanent positions of temporal lines are reached only after the eruption of permanent molar teeth.

APPLIED ANATOMY
1. Occasionally the parietal bone is divided into upper and lower parts by an anteroposterior suture. The condition may be confused with fracture radiologically. The latter can be ruled out easily because the anomalous parietal suture is usually bilateral.
2. Parietal bones are loosely attached to the adjacent bones at sutures during intrauterine period allowing moulding (change in shape of calvaria) at the time of child birth. Calvaria returns to normal shape within few days after birth.
3. Parietal bones undergo remodelling to allow enlargement of calvaria during childhood. This is only possible because of their loose attachments to the adjacent bones.
4. *Granular foveolae* are more numerous and marked in aged parietal bones. This fact is of great medicolegal importance.
5. Regenerating capacity of the parietal bone is negligible due to lack of cambium layer in periosteum.
6. In neonates the parietal bone is pliable and soft and therefore a *depressed fracture (pond fracture)* is like a dimple. In adults such fractures are produced by direct blows and always show an irregular line of fracture at the periphery of depressed area (Fig. 25.3). The depression of the inner table forms the

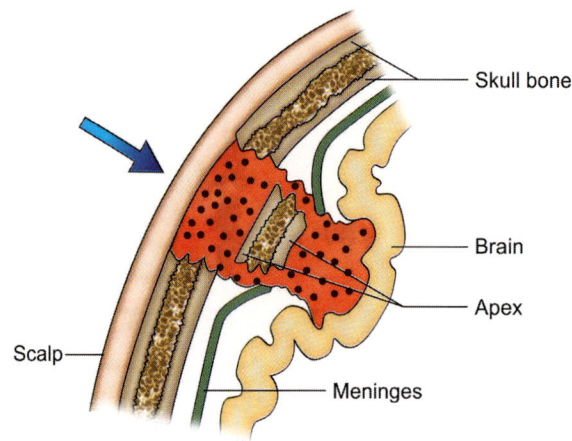

Fig. 25.3: A depressed fracture of parietal bone in adult

lowest limit of the depressed area also known as apex.

7. A crack in the inner table of parietal bone may damage a large diploeic vein and produce small epidural haematoma.

8. Almost invariably all fractures of the parietal bone in children are associated with rupture of dura mater.

9. In adult the parietal bone shows a fissured or linear fracture if the force is transmitted to this bone from frontal or occipital blows.

CHAPTER 26 | The Frontal Bone

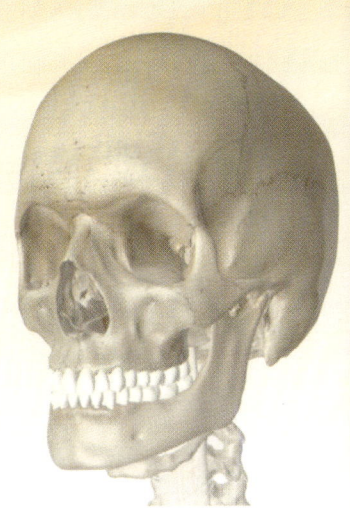

TERMINOLOGY

The term 'frontal' is derived from Latin word 'frons' which means 'brow' or 'forehead'.

LOCATION

Frontal bone forms the forehead, greater part of the roof of each orbit and most of the floor of anterior cranial fossa.

FEATURES AND ATTACHMENTS

Frontal bone has got a main part (frontal squama) and orbital parts.

I. Frontal squama (main part)

It has got an external surface, right and left temporal surfaces, an internal surface, a nasal part and a margin (parietal or posterior).

A. Surfaces

a. External surface (Figs 26.1 and 26.2)

i. *Supra-orbital margins.*
  1. These are lower limits of external surface on each side.
  2. They form upper borders of the orbital openings.

ii. *Supra-orbital notch or foramen*
  1. The junction of lateral two third of supra-orbital margin (sharp) with the medial one third (rounded) is marked by supra-orbital notch (some times foramen).
  2. This is meant for the passage of *supra-orbital nerve, supra-orbital artery* and *a communicating vein* between angular and superior ophthalmic veins.

iii. *Superciliary arch*
   This is an arched prominence just above the supra-orbital margin.

iv. *Glabella*
   It is the median prominence between superciliary arches.

v. *Frontal eminence*
  1. On each side, about 3 cm above the supra-orbital margin, there is an elevated area called frontal eminence or tuberosity.
  2. It is usually more marked in female.

vi. *Metopic suture*
   Frontal bone is bilateral in origin and the junction of the two halves is called frontal or metopic suture. Its remains can be seen even in adult in the reigon of glabella.

vii. *Zygomatic process*
  1. Supra-orbital margin extends laterally on each side into a zygomatic process.
  2. Zygomatic process articulates with frontal process of zygomatic bone.

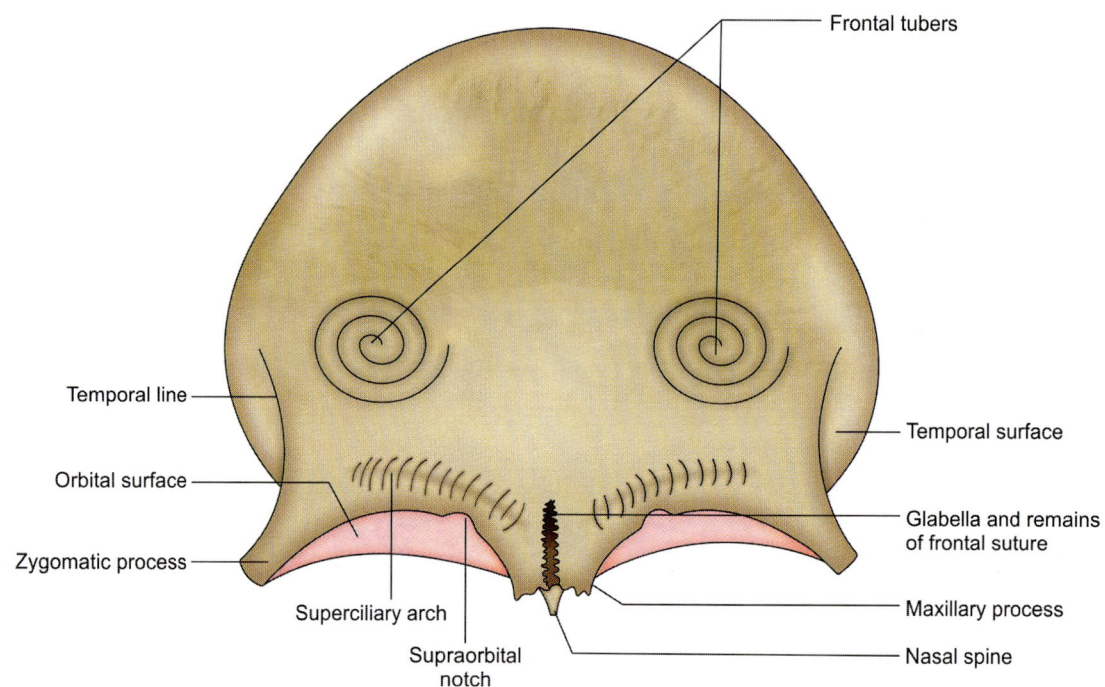

Fig. 26.1: Frontal bone : Anterior aspect

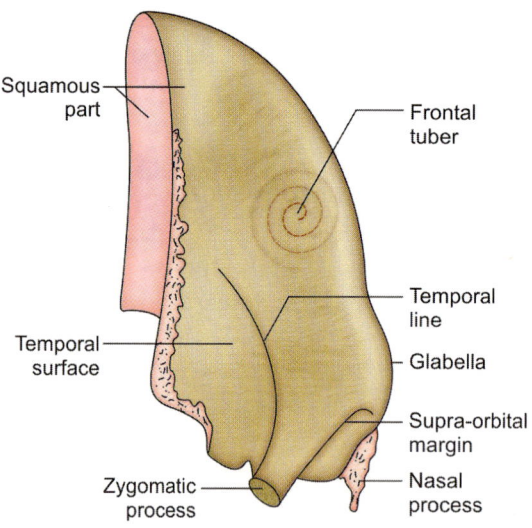

Fig. 26.2: Frontal bone : Right lateral aspect

viii. A line curves upwards and backwards from the zyomatic process. The line soon divides into two lines called *superior and inferior temporal lines*.

b. Temporal surfaces

1. An area on each side below and behind the temporal lines is called temporal surface.
2. It contributes to the anterior part of *temporal fossa* on the lateral aspect of skull (norma lateralis).
3. Superior temporal line gives attachment to *temporal fascia*.
4. Inferior temporal line and temporal surface of frontal bone give origin to *temporalis muscle*.

c. Internal surface (Fig. 26.3)

  i. This surface shows depressions and elevations for cerebral gyri and sulci respectively.

 ii. *Sagittal sulcus*

   1. It is a midline sulcus in the upper part of internal surface.

The Frontal Bones

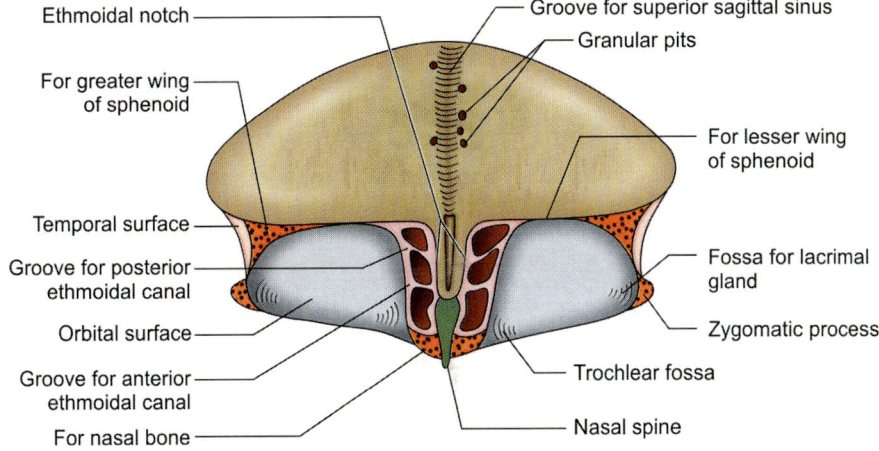

Fig. 26.3: Frontal bone: Inferior aspect

2. Its margins provide attachments to *falx cerebri*.
3. Sulcus itself lodges *superior sagittal sinus*.

iii. Frontal crest
1. Margins of sagittal sulcus meet in the midline in the lower part and continue as frontal crest.
2. This also gives attachment to *falx cerebri*.

iv. A notch below the frontal crest is converted into *foramen caecum* by articulation with ethmoid bone. An *emissary vein* passing through it connects the vein of nose with superior sagittal sinus.

v. Several depressions (*granular foveolae*) on each side of sagittal sulcus are produced by *arachnoid granulations*.

B. Nasal part

1. It is a downward projection of frontal bone between two supra-orbital margins.
2. Its lower serrated part is known as *nasal notch*.
3. Each half of the nasal notch articulates with the following three bones from anterior to posterior:

  i. Nasal bone.
  ii. Frontal process of maxilla.
  iii. Lacrimal bone.
4. Nasal spine is a midline downward continuation of the nasal part.
5. On each side of nasal spine there is a grooved area which froms the roof of nasal cavity.
6. Nasal spine itself articulates with crest of the nasal bone anteriorly and perpendicular plate of ethmoid posteriorly.

C. Posterior margin

1. This is also called parietal margin because its major part articulates with *parietal bones*.
2. The lower part of this margin is triangular and rough for articulation with *greater wing of sphenoid*.

II. Orbital parts

Orbital parts consist of two triangular laminae (*orbital plates*) separated by a gap called ethmoidal notch.

A. Orbital plate

It possesses two surfaces, orbital and internal.

a. Orbital surface
1. It faces downwards.
2. It forms *roof of the orbit*.
3. Its anterolateral part has got a *fossa for the lacrimal gland*.
4. Its anteromedial part (*trochlear fovea*) provides attachment to *fibrocartilaginous pulley* for tendon of superior oblique muscle.

b. Internal surface (Fig. 26.4)
1. It faces upwards.
2. It contributes to anterior cranial fossa.
3. It has impressions for gyri of frontal lobe of cerebral hemisphere.
4. It has grooves for meningeal vessels.

B. Ethmoidal notch (Figs 26.3 and 26.4)
1. It is 'U' shaped gap occupied by *cribriform plate of ethmoid*.
2. Under surfaces of its lateral margins possess several incomplete air cells which complete the ethmiodal air cells when ethmoid bone is in position.
3. Two grooves on the under surface of each margin are converted into *anterior and posterior ethmoidal canals* by similar grooves on the superior surface of ethmoidal labyrinth. These canals are meant for passages of *anterior and posterior ethmoidal nerves and vessels*.

4. The under surface of the anterior margin of the notch possesses openings for frontal sinuses (one on each side of the nasal spine).

III. Frontal sinus
Each frontal sinus is an irregular cavity of variable size. It is situated between outer and inner tables of frontal bone. They are separated from each other by a bony septum which is usually deviated to one side.

OSSIFICATION
1. Frontal bone ossifies in membrane.
2. Two primary centres appear, one for each half of frontal bone, in the region of frontal tuberosity.
3. Primary centres appear during 8th week of intrauterine life.
4. Ossification extends upwards to form frontal squama, backwards to form orbital part and downwards to form nasal part.
5. At birth frontal bone is made up of two halves separated by *frontal* or *metopic suture* (Fig. 26.5).
6. Union between two parts begins at 2nd year and completes at 8th year.

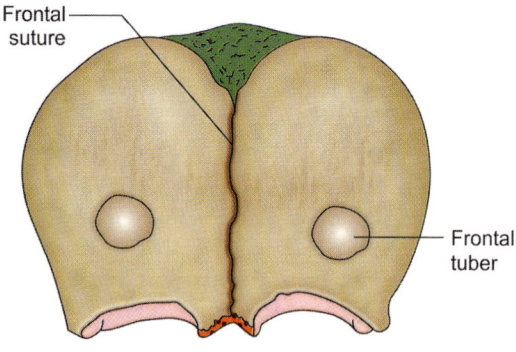

Fig. 26.5: Frontal bone at birth

APPLIED ANATOMY
1. Frontal squama is soft and pliable in neonates which can withstand considerable amount of compression and moulding, a fact clinically important during child birth.

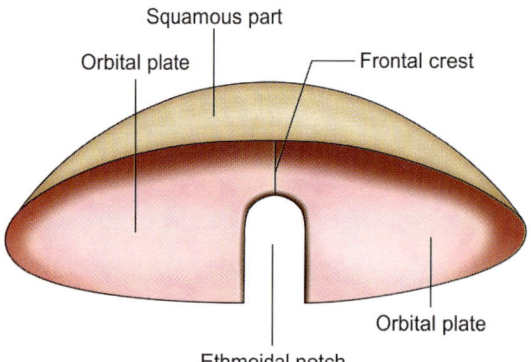

Fig. 26.4: Frontal bone: Superior aspect (diagrammatic)

2. Frontal squama is prone to depressed or fissured fractures. In neonates and infants, the depressed fracture is often like a dimple in the bone. In adults a depressed fracture is always associated with irregular line of fracture.
3. A severe impact at the root of the nose leads to fractures of frontal sinus walls (Fig. 26.6). If the fracture involves inner table forming the posterior wall of frontal sinus, then the air may enter into the cranial cavity (*aerocele*) causing meningitis and brain abscess.
4. *Fracture of orbital plate of frontal bone* causes haemorrhages into the orbit. The haemorrhage aquires a triangular shape under the conjunctiva whose apex is towards the corneoscleral junction and base towards the orbital margin (Fig. 26.7).

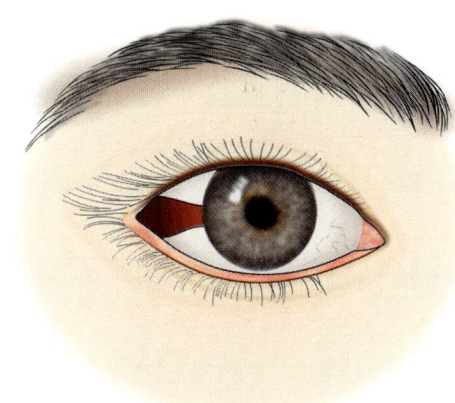

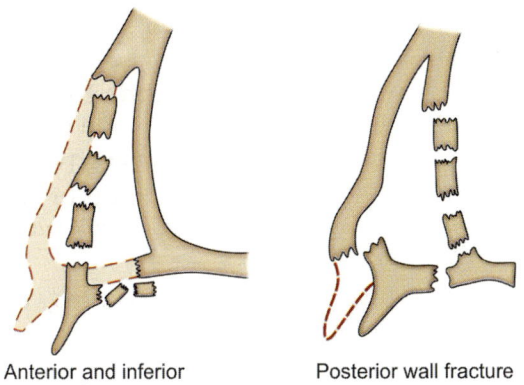

Anterior and inferior wall fracture   Posterior wall fracture

Fig. 26.6: Fracture of frontal sinus walls

Fig. 26.7: A triangular haemorrhagic appearance whose exact peripheral limit is not visible (orbital plate fracture)

5. A crack in the inner table of frontal squama may damage a large diploeic vein and produce small *epidural haematoma*.
6. Almost invariably the fractures of frontal squama in children are associated with rupture of dura mater.
7. A gap in frontal squama will not be regenerating and has to be filled with tantalum or titanium, a procedure called *cranial prosthesis*.

CHAPTER

27 | The Temporal Bones

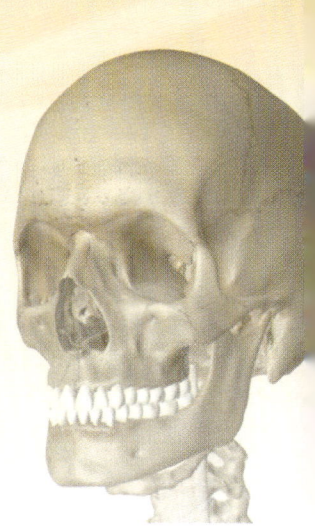

TERMINOLOGY

Temporal bone is so named because of its contribution to temporal region.

SIDE DETERMINATION

I. To distinguish superior and inferior, following features are to be noted:
   1. Thin plate like squamous part is directed upwards and lies in parasagittal plane.
   2. Styloid and mastoid processes occupy the lower part of the bone and are directed downwards.
II. To distinguish external and internal aspects, one should consider following features:
   1. The outer surface of squamous part is very smooth.
   2. Zygomatic process is present on the external aspect of bone.
   3. External acoustic meatus (present below the posterior part of zygomatic process) opens externally.
   4. Apex of petrous temporal is directed medially and a little forwards.
III. To distinguish anterior from posterior, following criteria should be taken into account:
   1. Zygomatic process is directed forwards.
   2. Mandibular fossa and external acoustic meatus are present below the posterior part of zygomatic process. Relatively, mandibular fossa is anterior to external acoustic meatus.

FEATURES AND ATTACHMENTS

Morphologically temporal bone is divided into four parts.
   1. Squamous part.
   2. Petromastoid part.
   3. Tympanic part.
   4. Styloid process.

For descriptive purpose, the petromastoid part is further subdivided into mastoid part and petrous part.

I. SQUAMOUS PART

It is thin and plate like and occupies anterior and superior part of temporal bone. It has two surfaces (temporal and cerebral) and two borders (superior and anteroinferior).

A. Surfaces

a. Temporal surface (Fig. 27.1)
   1. It is outer surface.
   2. It is smooth and slightly convex.

The Temporal Bones

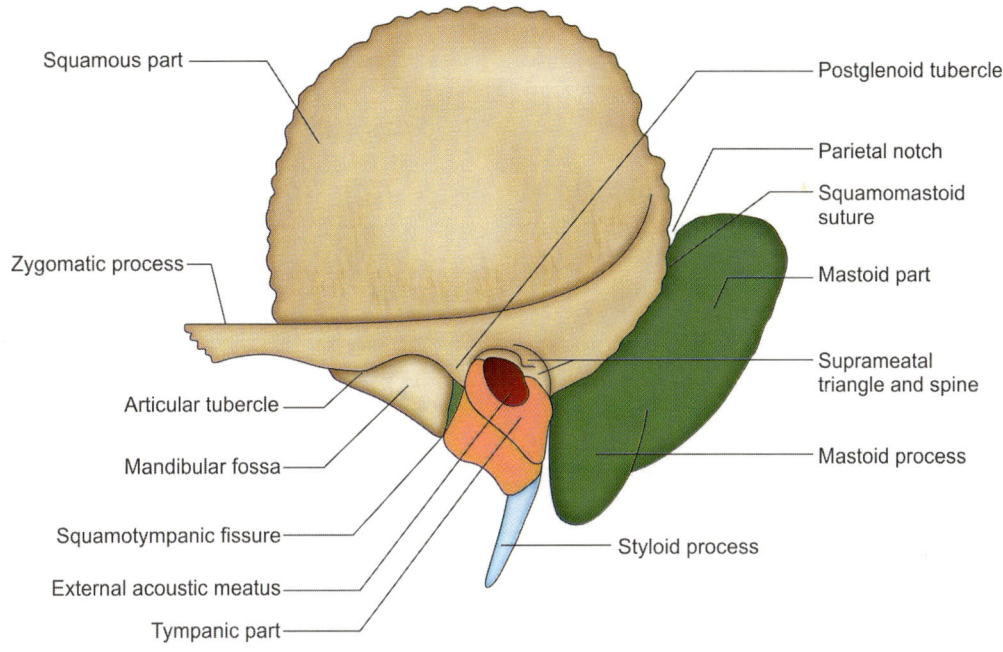

Fig. 27.1: Left temporal bone : External aspect

3. It contributes to the temporal fossa meant for the origin of *temporalis muscle.*
4. *Middle temporal artery* grooves the surface, just above the external acoustic meatus.
5. *Supramastoid crest* runs backwards and upwards across its posterior part. Temporal fascia is attached to this crest.
6. *Squamomastoid suture* marks the junction between squamous and mastoid parts. It is situated 1.5 cm. below the supramastoid crest.
7. Macewen's triangle (Suprameatal triangle) (Fig. 27.2)
   i. It is a triangular depression posterosuperior to external acoustic meatus.

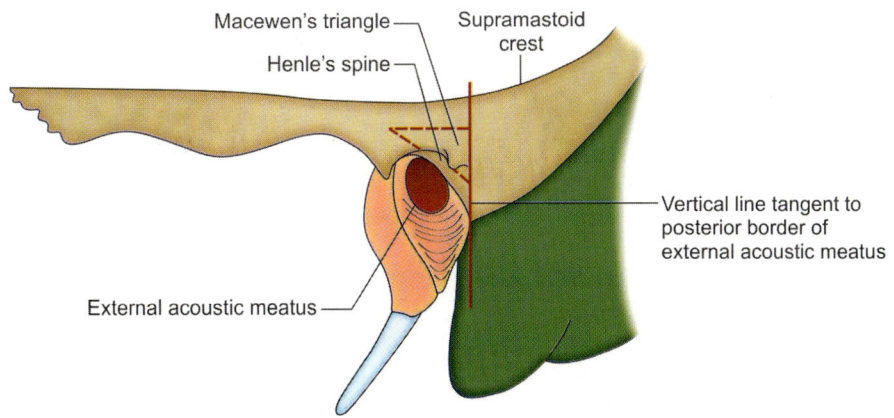

Fig. 27.2: Macewen's triangle of left side

ii. It is bounded by posterosuperior margin of external acoustic meatus, supramastoid crest and a vertical line tangent to posterior border of external acoustic meatus.
iii. *Spine of Henle* is sharp, spur like projection in the suprameatal triangle.
iv. Mastoid antrum is situated 12.5 mm deep to the surface of suprameatal triangle in adult.

8. Zygomatic process
   i. It is a forward projection from the lower part of temporal surface.
   ii. Its anterior end articulates with the temporal process of zygomatic bone to complete the zygomatic arch or zygoma.
   iii. Anterior part of zygomatic process has two surfaces (lateral and medial) and two borders (superior and inferior). *Masseter* originates from its medial surface and inferior border. *Temporal fascia* is attached to its superior border. Its lateral surface is subcutaneous.
   iv. Its posterior part is triangular having superior and inferior surfaces.
   v. Inferior surface of the posterior part of zygomatic process is bounded by two roots (anterior and posterior) which converge at the *tubercle of the root of zygoma*. Lateral *ligament of temporomandibular joint* is attached to this tubercle.
   vi. Anterior root extends medially from tubercle of the root of zygoma and is also called *articular tubercle*.

9. Mandibular fossa
   i. It is situated behind the articular tubercle.
   ii. Only anterior part of mandibular fossa is articular and contributed by squamous part of temporal bone.
   iii. Articular tubercle and anterior part of mandibular fossa is related to the superior surface of *articular disc* of temporomandibular joint.
   iv. Posterior part of mandibular fossa is non-articular and contributed by tympanic part of temporal bone. This part is related to the *parotid gland*.

10. Squamotympanic fissure
    i. It is situated in the mandibular fossa and marks the junction of squamous and tympanic parts of temporal bone.
    ii. Medial part of this fissure is divided into *petrosquamous and petrotympanic fissures* by the projection of *tegmen tympani* of petrous part of temporal bone.
    iii. Three structures pass through petrotympanic fissure, i.e. *chorda tympani nerve, anterior tympanic artery* and *anterior ligament of malleus*.

Note: *To remember the structures passing through petrotympanic fissure think of a 'CAT' in which C=Chorda tympani nerve, A=Anterior ligament of malleus and T=Tympanic artery.*

   iv. Petrotympanic fissure leads into middle ear.

b. Cerebral surface
1. It is inner surface.
2. It is grooved by *middle meningeal vessels*.
3. It has impressions for sulci and gyri of the temporal lobe of cerebrum.

B. Borders
a. Superior border
It articulates with parietal bone.

b. Anteroinferior border
It articulates with greater wing of sphenoid bone.

II. MASTOID PART
It forms the posterior part of the temporal bone. It consists of two surfaces (outer and inner), two borders (superior and posterior) and a downward projecting part called mastoid process.

A. Surfaces

a. Outer surface
1. *Auricularis posterior* and *occipital belly of occipitofrontalis* are attached to this surface.
2. *Mastoid foramen* is an infrequent opening near the posterior border. When present this foramen transmits an *emissary vein* from sigmoid sinus and a *branch from occipital artery*.

b. Inner surface
1. *Sigmoid sulcus* is a deep groove on the inner surface. It is meant for *sigmoid sinus*.
2. *Mastoid foramen* opens in the upper part of sigmoid sulcus.

B. Borders

a. Superior border
It articulates with the parietal bone at *parietomastoid suture*.

b. Posterior border
It articulates with the occipital bone at *occipitomastoid suture*.

C. Mastoid process
It possesses a lateral and a medial surface.

a. Lateral surface
It gives insertions to following three muscles from above downwards:
1. *Sternomastoid*.
2. *Splenius capitis*.
3. *Longissimus capitis*.

b. Medial surface
1. It is marked by a deep groove called *mastoid notch*, from which originates the *posterior belly of digastric*.
2. *Occipital groove* is observed medial to mastoid notch. This groove lodges the *occipital artery*.

III. PETROUS PART

Petrous is a Latin word which means strong or rock like. It is strong part of temporal bone and protects internal ear within it. Petrous part is comprised of a base, an apex, three surfaces (anterior, posterior and inferior) and three borders (superior, anterior and posterior).

A. Base
1. It is directed laterally.
2. It fuses with squamous part at petrosquamosal suture which disappears soon after birth.
3. Base also fuses with mastoid part.
4. Base is separated from the squamous and mastoid parts by an air filled space called *mastoid antrum*.

B. Apex
1. It projects medially and slightly forwards.
2. It is situated between greater wing of sphenoid and basilar part of occipital bone.
3. It forms posterolateral boundary of foramen lacerum.
4. It possesses anterior orifice of carotid canal.

C. Surfaces

a. Anterior surface (Fig. 27.3)
1. It contributes to middle cranial fossa.
2. This surface shows following features if one goes from apex to base:
    i. *Trigeminal impression*: It is a depression for trigeminal ganglion adjacent to apex.
    ii. *Roof of internal acoustic meatus*: It is another depressed area behind the ridge.
    iii. *Arcuate eminence*: It is a prominent elevation produced by superior semicircular canal. Its posterior sloping lies over lateral and posterior semicircular canals.

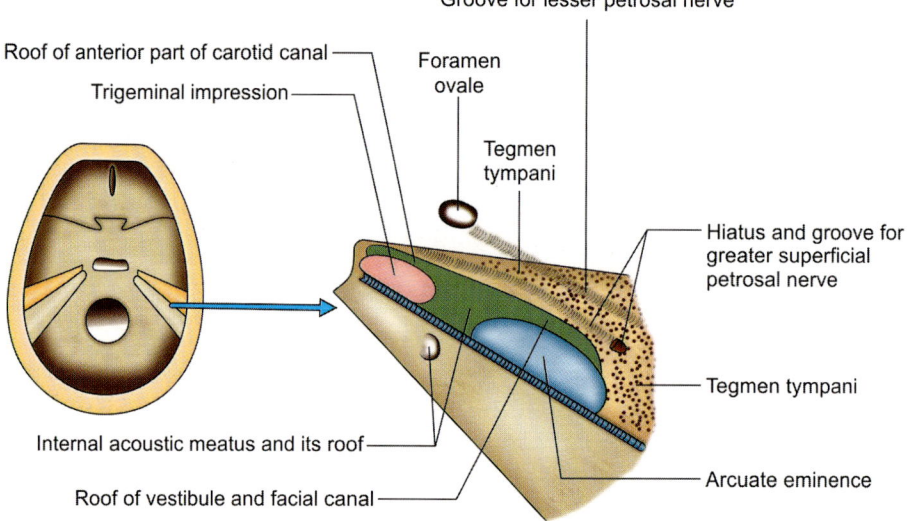

Fig. 27.3: Anterior surface of petrous part of right temporal bone

3. Area anterolateral to trigeminal impression forms the roof of *anterior part of carotid canal*.
4. Area anterolateral to arcuate eminence forms the roof of vestibule and beginning of *facial canal*.
5. Thin plate of bone between squamous part (cerebral surface) of temporal bone and features described above is called *tegmen tympani*. It forms roof of mastoid antrum, middle ear and canal for tensor tympani from posterior to anterior. Tegmen tympani projects downwards to form lateral walls of canal for tensor tympani and bony Eustachian tube and appears in the squamotympanic fissure.
6. A hiatus (opening) lateral to arcuate eminence leads into a *groove for greater superficial petrosal nerve* which runs towards the foramen lacerum on the tegmen tympani.
7. Lateral to groove for greater superficial petrosal nerve is present a *groove for lesser petrosal nerve* which runs towards the foramen ovale.

b. *Posterior surface* (Fig. 27.4)

1. It contributes to posterior cranial fossa.
2. *Internal acoustic meatus* is present in the centre of this surface. It transmits *facial and vestibulocochlear nerves* and *labyrinthine vessels*. It is about 1 cm in length.
3. *Fundus* of internal acoustic meatus is a plate of bone at its lateral end. This plate is divided into upper and lower areas by a transverse ridge called *crista falciformis*. The upper area is further divided into anterior and posterior areas by a vertical crest called *Bill's bar*. Anterior area shows *facial canal* for facial nerve. Posterior area is called *superior vestibular* area which presents number of small openings for the nerve fibres supplying utricle and superior and lateral semicircular ducts (Fig. 27.5).

Below the transverse crest, anteriorly is the *cochlear area* (which possesses number of foramina called *tractus spiralis foraminosus*) and posteriorly is the *inferior vestibular* area. Fibres of cochlear nerve

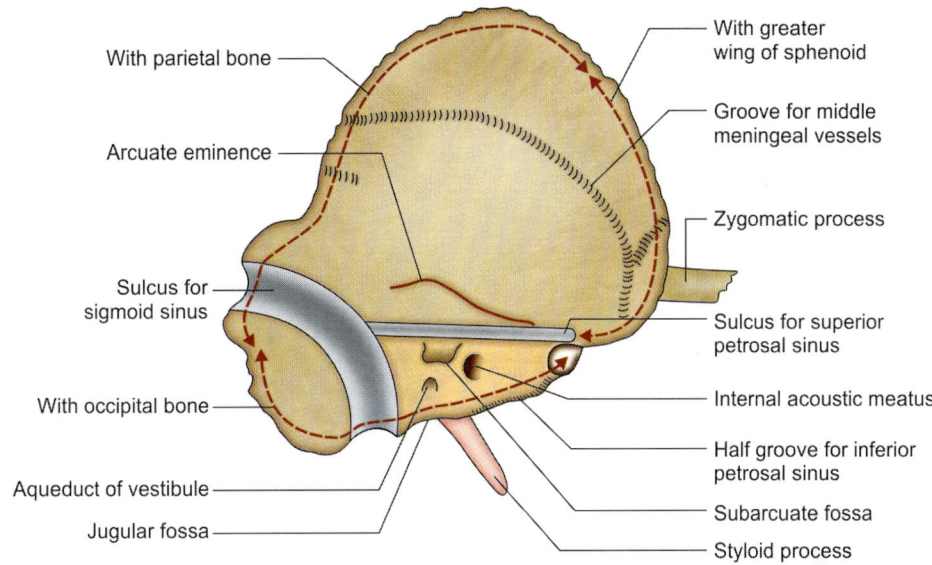

Fig. 27.4: Left temporal bone : Internal aspect

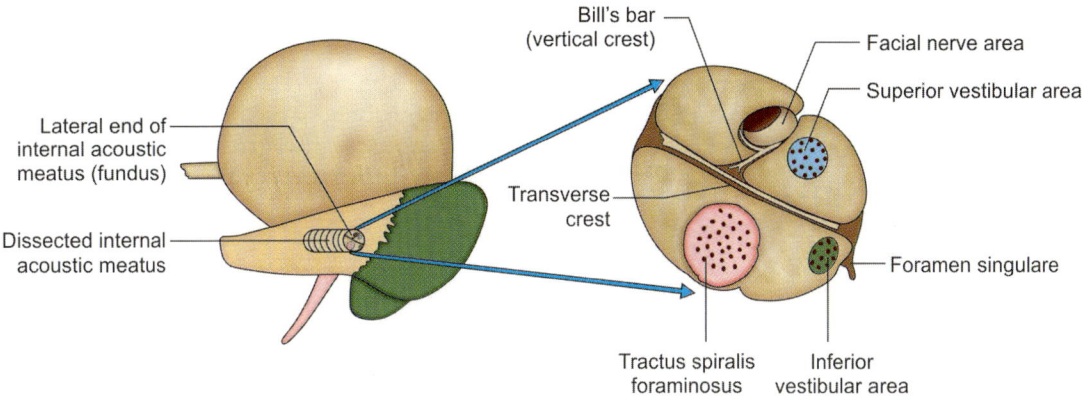

Fig. 27.5: Fundus of right internal acoustic meatus

enter the cochlear area while nerve fibres supplying the saccule enter the inferior vestibular area. Below and behind the inferior vestibular area is *foramen singulare* for the passage of nerve to posterior semicircular duct.

4. A slit behind the internal acoustic meatus leads into *aqueduct of vestibule* which contains saccus and ductus endolymphaticus along with small artery and vein.

5. An irregular depression called *subarcuate fossa* is located above and between the openings of internal acoustic meatus and aqueduct of vestibule. It lodges a process of dura mater.

c. *Inferior surface* (Fig. 27.6)

1. It is rough and triangular.
2. It is divided into four areas from apex to base.

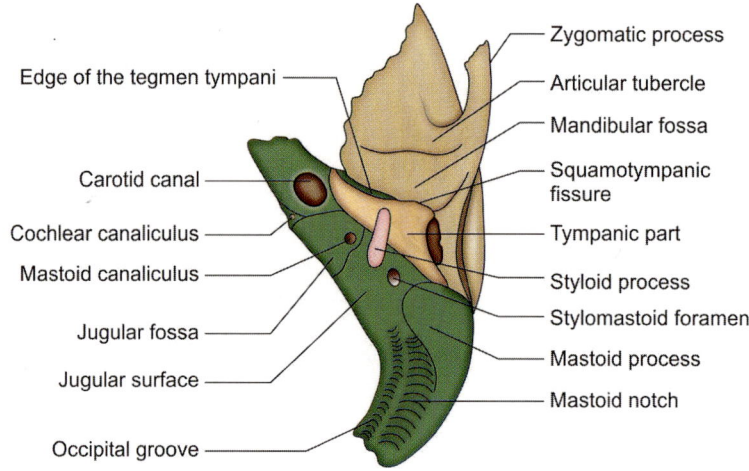

Fig. 27.6: Left temporal bone : Inferior aspect

i. *Quadrilateral area* near the apex provides attachment to *levator palati muscle*.

ii. *Carotid canal* (lower opening) is present behind the quadrilateral area. It transmits *internal carotid artery* along with its *sympathetic* and *venous plexuses*.

iii. *Jugular fossa* is a depression behind the carotid canal. It lodges *superior bulb of internal jugular vein*.

iv. *Jugular surface* is a quadrilateral area behind the jugular fossa. It articulates with jugular process of occipital bone.

3. A triangular depression in front of the medial part of the jugular fossa lodges the *inferior ganglion of glossopharyngeal nerve*. The apex of this triangular depression is marked by an opening leading into *cochlear canaliculus* which is traversed by:

   i. *Perilymphatic duct*
   ii. *Prolongation of dura mater*
   iii. A *vein* from cochlea which drains into internal jugular vein.

4. The *canaliculus for tympanic nerve* (a branch of glossopharyngeal nerve) is situated on the bony ridge between carotid canal and jugular fossa.

5. The *mastoid canaliculus* is present in the lateral wall of jugular fossa. It transmits the *auricular branch of vagus*.

D. Borders

a. Superior border

1. It is grooved by *superior petrosal sinus*.
2. Margins of the groove provide attachment to *tentorium cerebelli*.

b. Anterior border

1. It is divided into medial and lateral parts.
2. Medial part articulates with greater wing of sphenoid.
3. Lateral part joins the squamous part at *petrosquamosal suture* which disappears soon after birth.

c. Posterior border

1. It can be divided into medial and lateral parts.
2. Medial part has got a sulcus which with similar sulcus on the occipital bone forms a *groove for inferior petrosal sinus*.
3. Lateral part is occupied by larger *jugular fossa* laterally and smaller *glossopharyngeal notch* medially. Lateral part forms *anterior boundary of jugular foramen* whose posterior boundary is formed by jugular notch of occipital bone.

IV. TYMPANIC PART

It is curved bony plate situated below the squamous part and in front of mastoid part of temporal bone. It joins the squamous part at *squamotympanic fissure* and mastoid part at *tympanomastoid fissure*. Auricular branch of vagus emerges through the tympanomastoid fissure. Tympanic part has two surfaces (anterior and posterior) and three borders (lateral, upper and lower).

A. Surfaces

a. Anterior surface

1. It forms the posterior nonarticular part of the *mandibular fossa*.
2. It is related to the *parotid gland*.

b. Posterior surface

1. It forms the anterior wall, floor and the lower part of the posterior wall of the *external acoustic meatus*.
2. Its medial end is marked by a groove called *tympanic sulcus*. This sulcus provides attachment to the circumference of the *tympanic membrane*.

B. Borders

a. Lateral border

1. It is free.
2. It continues with cartilaginous part of external acoustic meatus.

b. Upper border

1. Laterally it fuses with the *postglenoid tubercle*.
2. Medially it forms posterior boundary of *petrotympanic fissure*.

c. Lower border

1. Medially it extends upto carotid canal.
2. Laterally it splits to form the veginal process which encloses the root of styloid process.

V. STYLOID PROCESS

1. Styloid process is divisible into two parts:
   a. Proximal or tympanohyal part

   It is surrounded by a bony sheath derived from lower border of tympanic part of temporal bone.

   b. Distal or stylohyal part

   It is visible lower part. It is this part which is described below.

2. Styloid process is a conical projection directed downwards, forwards and slightly medially.
3. It provides attachments to five structures (3 muscles and 2 ligaments):
   i. Medially - *Stylopharyngeus muscle*.
   ii. Anteriorly - *Styloglossus muscle*.
   iii. Posteriorly - *Stylohyoid muscle*.
   iv. Laterally - *Stylomandibular ligament*.
   v. At the tip - *Stylohyoid ligament*.
4. Some important relations are as follows:
   i. It is interposed between two important structures, the *parotid gland* (laterally) and *internal jugular vein* (medially).
   ii. *External carotid* artery crosses the tip of styloid process superficially.
   iii. *Facial nerve* crosses the base of styloid process laterally.
5. *Stylomastoid foramen* is situated behind its base (between it and the mastoid process). Following structures pass through this foramen:
   i. *Facial nerve*.
   ii. *Stylomastoid artery*.

SPACES AND CANALS

I. External acoustic meatus (Fig. 27.7)

1. Bony part of external acoustic meatus is about 16mm long. This contribution is about 2/3rd of the total length (24 mm).
2. It is directed medially, downwards and slightly forwards.
3. Tympanic part of the temporal bone contributes to its anterior wall, floor and lower part of the posterior wall.
4. Squamous part of the temporal bone forms its roof and upper part of posterior wall.

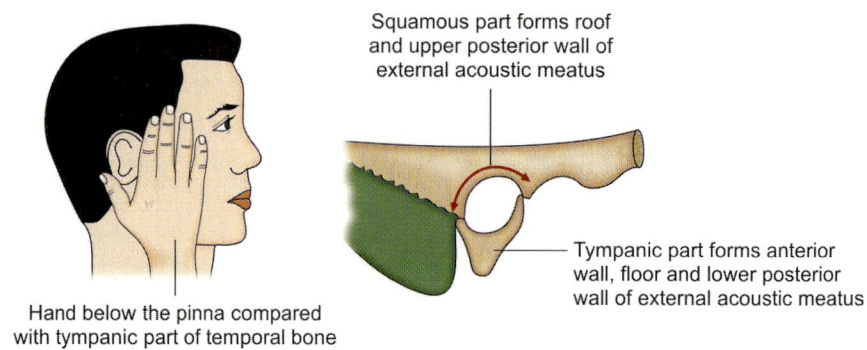

Fig. 27.7: Bony contributions to external acoustic meatus: Right lateral view

II. Middle ear space (tympanic cavity)

A. Parts

Tympanic cavity consists of three parts:
- a. *Tympanic cavity proper (mesotympanum):* Opposite the tympanic membrane.
- b. *Epitympanic recess (epitympanum):* Above the level of the tympanic membrane.
- c. *Hypotympanum:* Below the level of the tympanic membrane.

B. Measurements

1. Vertical diameter – 15 mm.
2. Anteroposterior diameter – 15 mm.
3. Transverse diameters:
   - i. Upper part – 6 mm.
   - ii. Lower part – 4 mm.
   - iii. Opposite the centre of tympanic membrane – 2 mm.

C. Boundaries

a. Roof
It is formed by *tegmen tympani* which separates the middle ear from middle cranial fossa.

b. Floor
It is formed by thin plate of bone which separates the cavity from *superior bulb of internal jugular vein*.

c. Lateral wall (Fig. 27.8)
1. It is formed mainly by *tympanic membrane*.
2. Close to circumference for tympanic membrane there are three small apertures:
   - i. *Petrotympanic fissure*: It is located anteriorly.
   - ii. *Anterior canaliculus for chorda tympani*: It is located at the medial end of petrotympanic fissure.
   - iii. *Posterior canaliculus for chorda tympani*: It is located posteriorly.

d. Medial wall (Fig. 27.9)
1. It is the lateral wall of internal ear.
2. It has a rounded elevation called *promontory* produced by the basal turn of cochlea.
3. Promontory is grooved by the nerves of tympanic plexus.
4. A depression behind the promontory, the *sinus tympani*, indicates the position of the *ampulla of the posterior semicircular canal*.
5. *Fenestra vestibuli* is a reniform opening posterosuperior to the promontory. It connects the tympanic cavity to the vestibule of internal ear.

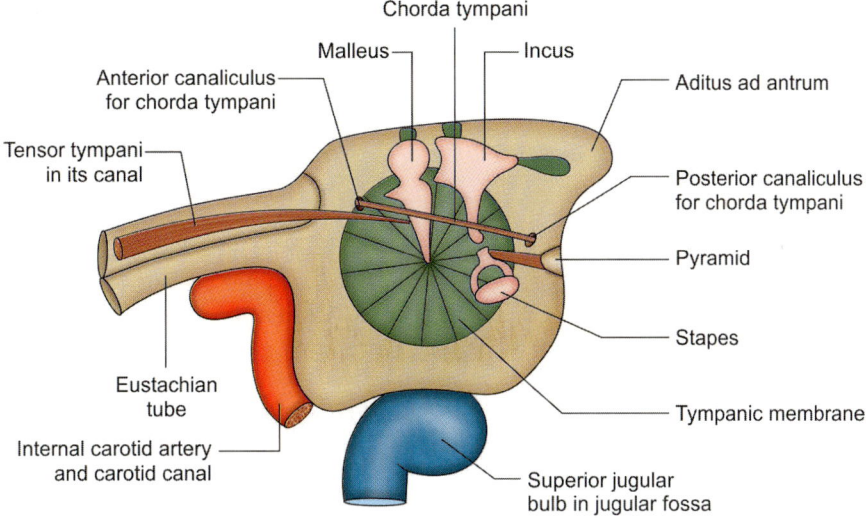

Fig. 27.8: Lateral wall of middle ear of right side

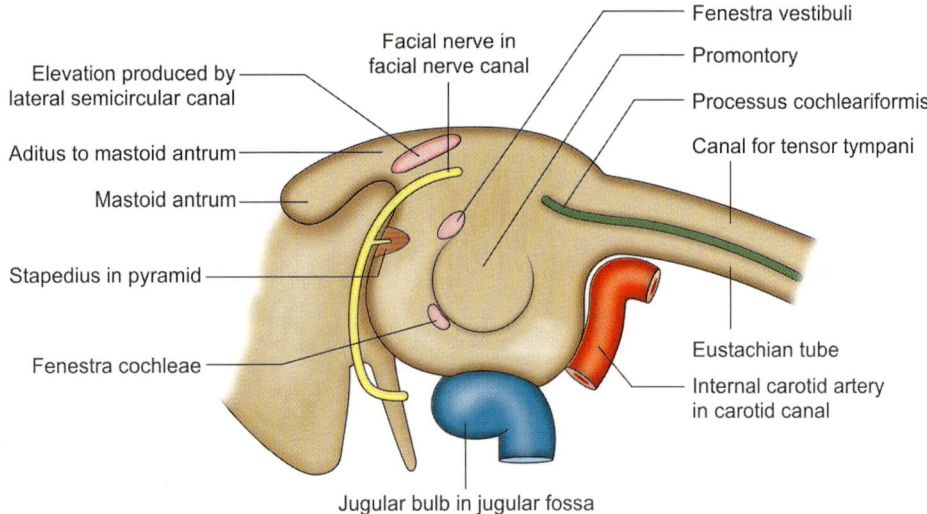

Fig. 27.9: Medial wall of middle ear of the right side

6. *Fenestra cochleae* is a rounded opening in the posteroinferior part of the promontory. It connects the tympanic cavity with the scala tympani of the cochlea.

7. Above and posterior to the fenestra vestibuli there is an elevation produced by *facial nerve canal*.

e. *Posterior wall*

1. *Aditus to the mastoid antrum* is an opening in the upper part of posterior wall. It connects epitympanic recess with the mastoid antrum.
2. The medial wall of the aditus to mastoid antrum shows an elevation produced by *lateral semicircular canal*.

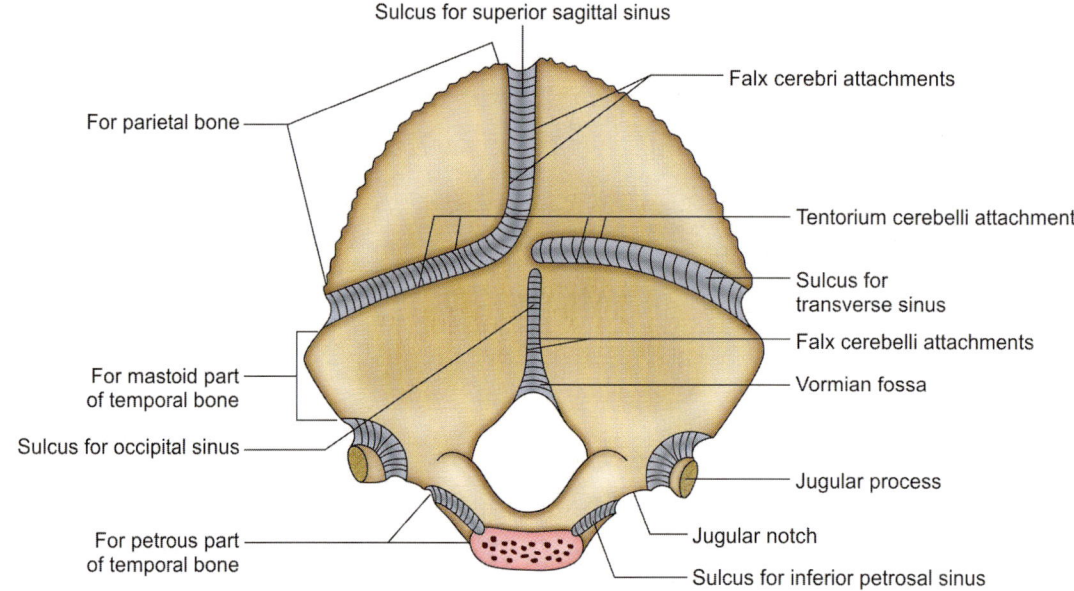

Fig. 29.3: Occipital bone : Internal aspect

9. Internal surface above the grooves for transverse sinuses is related to *occipital lobes of cerebrum*.

B. Angles

a. *Superior angle* reaches lambda which during intrauterine life is membranous (*posterior fontanelle*).

b. *Lateral angle* on each side meets with mastoid part of corresponding temporal bone to form *asterion*.

C. Borders

a. Lambdoid border

It extends on each side from superior angle to lateral angle and articulates with posterior margin of corresponding parietal bone to form *lambdoid suture*.

b. Mastoid border

It extends on each side from lateral angle to jugular process and articulates with mastoid part of corresponding temporal bone to form occipitomastoid suture.

OSSIFICATION

I. Origin

1. Part of the occipital bone above the highest nuchal line develops in membrane.
2. Rest of the occipital bone ossifies in cartilage.

II. Appearance of centres

Usually seven centres appear at 8th week of intrauterine life as follows:
4 for squamous part (one for each half of the membranous and cartilaginous parts).
2 for lateral parts.
1 for basilar part.

III. Fusion

1. Membranous and cartilaginous portions fuse with each other when the baby starts holding neck, i.e. 3rd month.

3. *Facial nerve canal* lies vertically in the posterior wall anterior to which is a *pyramidal eminence* projecting into the middle ear cavity.
4. Pyramidal eminence is occupied by *stapedius muscle*.
5. *Fossa incudis* is a small depression in the postero-inferior part of the epitympanic recess. It contains short process of incus.

f. Anterior wall
1. Its lower part is formed by thin plate of bone which separates middle ear from the *carotid canal*.
2. Its upper part is occupied by two openings. Upper opening leads into *canal for tensor tympani*. The lower opening leads into osseous part of *Eustachian tube*. These two canals are visible from the apex side of petrous temporal at petrosquamosal junction.
3. The septum between the afore-mentioned canals runs on the medial wall and just above the fenestra vestibuli its posterior end curves laterally to form *processus cochleariformis*.

III. Mastoid antrum
1. It is an air sinus in the petrous part of temporal bone.
2. It is well developed at birth and is almost of adult size.
3. Mastoid antrum is a spherical sinus.
4. In adult the mastoid antrum has a capacity of about 1 ml.
5. *Aditus ad antrum* is an opening in the upper part of anterior wall of mastoid antrum. It connects the antrum with epitympanic recess of middle ear.
6. Roof of antrum is formed by *tegmen tympani*.
7. Posteriorly the antrum is closely related to *sigmoid sinus*.
8. Medial wall is related to posterior semicircular canal.
9. Anteroinferiorly the antrum is related to canal for facial nerve.
10. Floor has multiple apertures which connect mastoid antrum with *mastoid air cells*.
11. The lateral wall of antrum corresponds to the *suprameatal triangle*. This wall is 1 mm thick at birth and increases at a rate of 1 mm per year until it reaches the adult thickness of about 12.5 mm.

IV. Mastoid air cells
1. These are very small intercommunicating spaces in the temporal bone continuous with mastoid antrum.
2. At birth neither mastoid air cells nor mastoid process are present. Only after birth mastoid air cells grow out of the mastoid antrum into the mastoid process.
3. The mastoid air cells are mainly seen in the mastoid process, but may extend into the surrounding bones like petrous or squamous parts of temporal bone or even zygomatic bone and jugular process of occipital bone.
4. Some common groups of air cells are as follows (Fig. 27.10):

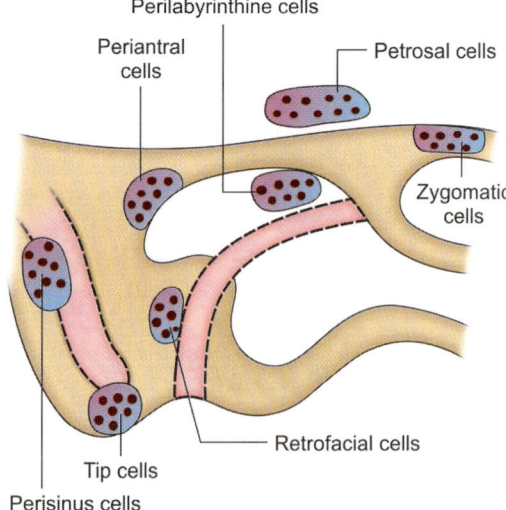

Fig. 27.10: Types of air spaces (air cells) in temporal bone

i. Tip cells.
   ii. Perisinus cells.
   iii. Retrofacial cells.
   iv. Periantral cells.
   v. Perilabyrinthine cells.
   vi. Petrous cells.
   vii. Zygomatic cells.
5. Depending upon the pneumatization, the mastoid process may be of three types (Fig. 27.11):
   i. Pneumatic or cellular.
   ii. Sclerotic or acellular.
   iii. Diploeic or mixed.

V. Bony labyrinth (osseous labyrinth) (Figs 27.12 and 27.13)

It consists of three parts, vestibule, semicircular canals and cochlea.

A. Vestibule

1. It is the central part of bony labyrinth.
2. In its lateral wall, there is an opening of *fenestra vestibuli* (oval window) occupied by foot plate of stapes in life.
3. Its medial wall corresponds to the fundus of internal acoustic meatus.

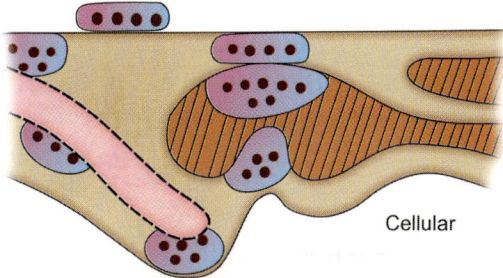
Cellular

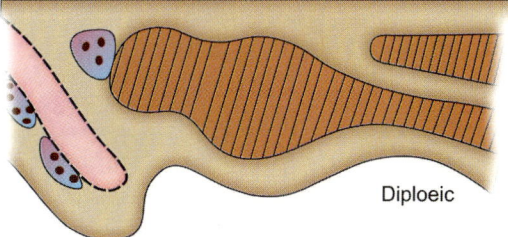
Diploeic

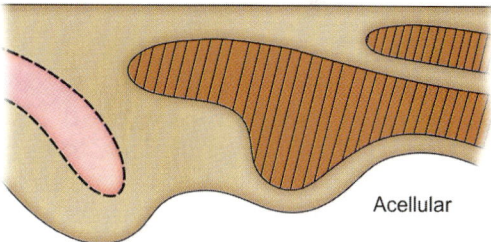
Acellular

Fig. 27.11: Types of mastoid

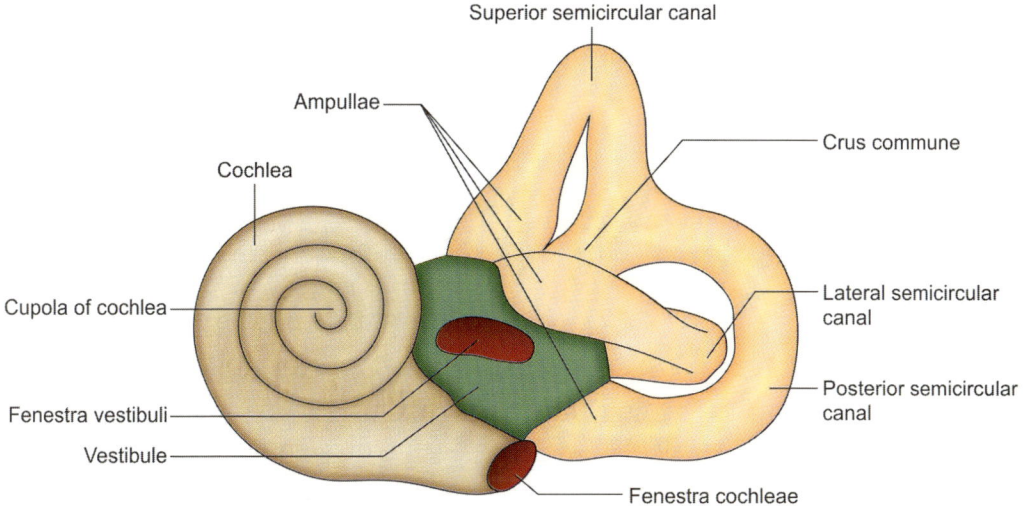

Fig. 27.12: The left bony labyrinth. Lateral aspect

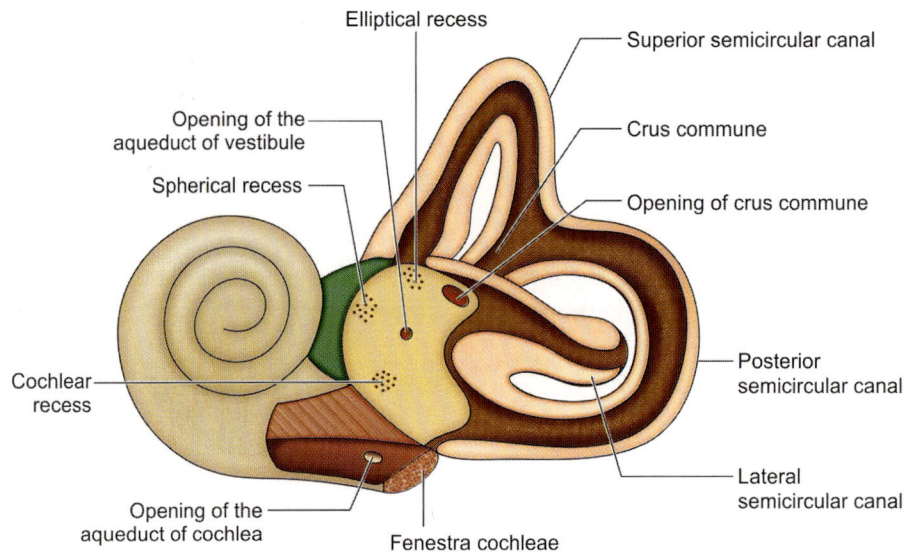

Fig. 27.13: The interior of the left osseous labyrinth

4. Anterior part of medial wall has a *spherical recess for saccule*. This recess has multiple perforations which correspond to the openings in inferior vestibular area of fundus of internal acoustic meatus.
5. Posterosuperior to spherical recess is an *elliptical recess* which lodges the *utricle*. This recess also has number of foramina which correspond to openings in the superior vestibular area of fundus.
6. Below the elliptical recess is the opening of aqueduct of vestibule through which passes ductus endolymphaticus.

B. Semicircular canals

1. They lie posterosuperior to the vestibule.
2. There are three semicircular canals.
   i. Anterior or superior.
   ii. Lateral or horizontal.
   iii. Posterior.
3. Ipsilateral semicircular canals lie in three planes at right angles to each other.
4. Each canal is about two-thirds of a circle.
5. Superior semicircular canal is placed in a vertical plane perpendicular to the long axis of the petrous bone at about 45° with sagittal plane.
6. Posterior semicircular canal is placed in a vertical plane in the long axis of the petrous bone. This also makes an angle of 45° with sagittal plane.
7. Lateral semicircular canal makes an angle of 30° with horizontal plane. This canal lies horizontally if the head is bent forwards for 30°.
8. One end of each canal is dilated called *ampulla*.
9. Both the ends of each canal open into vestibule. Since non-ampullated ends of superior and posterior semicircular canals have common opening in vestibule, thus only five openings connect the three canals with the cavity of the vestibule.

C. Cochlea

1. It is conical in shape and consists of two and three-quarter spiral turns of a tapering cylindrical canal.
2. The axial bone around which the canal spirals is called as *modiolus*.

3. The basal turn of cochlea produces *promontory* on the medial wall of middle ear.
4. From the modiolus a shelf of bone projects into the canal. Since the shelf follows the spiral path of canal, this is called as *spiral lamina*.
5. The spiral lamina forms a hook like structure (*called hamulus*) at the apex of modiolus.
6. Basal turn of cochlea shows two holes:
   i. *The fenestra cochleae*
      It is closed in life by *secondary tympanic membrane*.
   ii. *The opening of aqueduct of cochlea*
      It leads downwards to reach the apex of glossopharyngeal notch.
7. Base of modiolus is perforated by spirally arranged foramina. This area corresponds to the cochlear area of the fundus of internal acoustic meatus.

OSSIFICATION

1. Temporal bone ossifies partly in cartilage and partly in membrane.
2. Squamous and tympanic parts ossify in membrane.
3. Petromastoid part and the styloid process ossify in cartilage.
4. **Appearance of centres**
   i. *Squamous part*
      Single centre appears near the root of zygomatic process during 8th week of intrauterine life.
   ii. *Petromastoid part*
      As many as 14 centres may appear in the cartilaginous mass (otic capsule) around developing internal ear during 5th month of intrauterine life. These centres fuse by 6th month of intrauterine life.
   iii. *Tympanic part*
      Single centre appears during 12th week of intrauterine life. At birth, a tympanic ring represents the tympanic part.
   iv. *Styloid process*
      It develops from cranial end of 2nd arch cartilarge. It ossifies from two centres. Centre for tympanohyal appears before birth and for stylohyal appears after birth.
5. **Fusion**
   i. Squamous part fuses with tympanic part just before birth.
   ii. Petromastoid part fuses with the squamous part and tympanohyal during 1st year.
   iii. Stylohyal fuses with the tympanohyal after puberty.

APPLIED ANATOMY

1. At birth the tympanic cavity, tympanic membrane, mastoid antrum, ear ossicles and internal ear are all of adult size.
2. At birth the mastoid process is absent and the facial nerve lies on the surface at its exit from stylomastoid foramen. This makes the postauricular incision a risky procedure in newborns.
3. A very long styloid process may lead to multiple complications and in such cases it has to be removed by surgery.
4. In majority of the people the pneumatization of temporal bone is adequate. In 20% cases the pneumatization may be arrested in childhood. This is easily pointed out in X-ray and is called sclerolic or acellular mastoid, a condition which is prone to inflammation.
5. Infections of the middle ear (*otitis media*) invariably leads to the infections of the mastoid antrum and mastoid air cells.
6. Suprameatal triangle is clinically very important as it helps in localizing the mastoid antrum. Mastoid antrum is located 1.25 cm deep to the surface of this triangle.
7. Gross fractures of temporal bones are divided into longitudinal and transverse

in relation to the long axis of petrous temporal bone. Longitudinal fractures are common and are due to blows to the temporal or parietal areas. The transverse fractures are less common and are due to blows in occipital region (Fig. 27.14).

8. Zygomatic arches form the prominences of the face and therefore prone to facial injuries.
9. Fracture of zygomatic process of temporal bone may involve the lateral wall of orbit and injure the eye.
10. Squamous part of temporal bone contributes to vault and therefore prone to both fissured and depressed fractures. Petrous part contributes to base of skull and thus invariably shows a linear fracture.
11. Fracture of tegmen tympani might connect the subarachnoid space with middle ear leading to CSF leakage into the middle ear. If the tympanic membrane is also damaged then the CSF will appear as discharge through external acoustic meatus. This condition is called *CSF otorrhea*. The passage may also act as portal for sepsis of meninges and brain.
12. Since the petrous part of temporal bone is very strong, most fracture lines end here without making a tear in it.
13. The indications of the fracture of petrous part of temporal bone are as follows:
    i. CSF otorrhea.
    ii. Tear of tympanic membrane.
    iii. Collection of blood in the middle ear.
14. Discolouration and edema of the tissue over mastoid process (*Battle's sign*) is indication of sigmoid sinus damage.
15. Fracture of petrous temporal may damage the facial nerve and result into facial paralysis.
16. Involvement of vestibulocochlear nerve in petrous fracture will lead to hearing loss, vertigo and nystagmus.

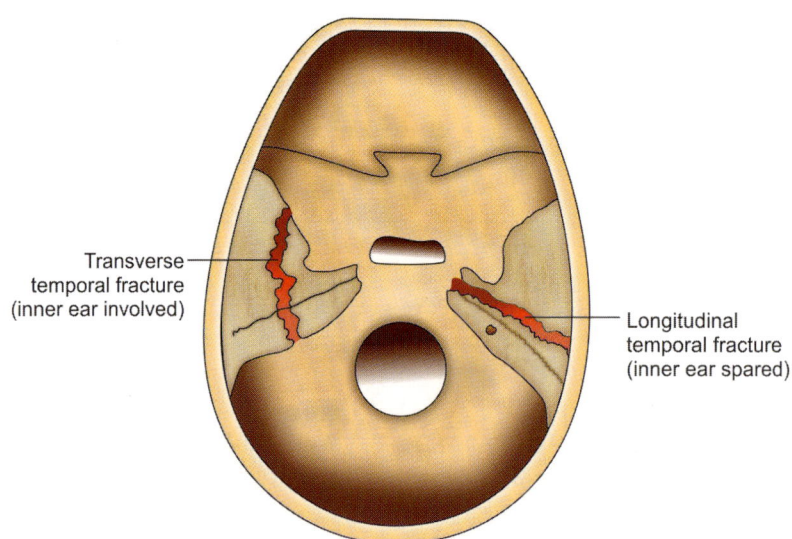

Fig. 27.14: Fractures of temporal bone

CHAPTER 28

The Auditory Ossicles

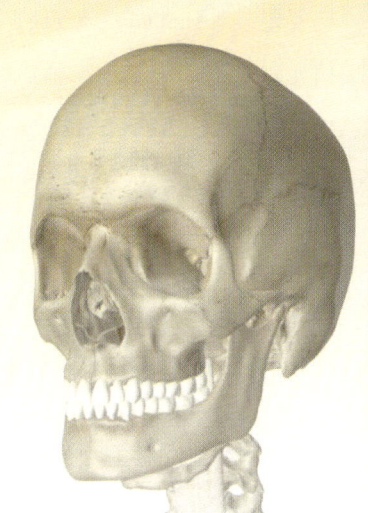

TERMINOLOGY

There are three ossicles named malleus, incus and stapes.

These names are Latin in origin, the meanings of which are as follows:

Malleus : Hammer

Incus : An anvil

Stapes : A stirrup

Note: *Remember that MIS is situated between tympanic membrane and the oval window where M = Malleus, I = Incus and S = Stapes.*

FEATURES AND ATTACHMENTS (Fig. 28.1)

I. Malleus

It consists of head, neck and handle.

A. Head

1. It is large upper end of the bone.
2. It is located within the epitympanic recess.
3. Its posterior surface articulates with the body of incus.

B. Neck

1. It is the constricted part below the head.
2. Its medial surface is crossed by *chorda tympani nerve*.

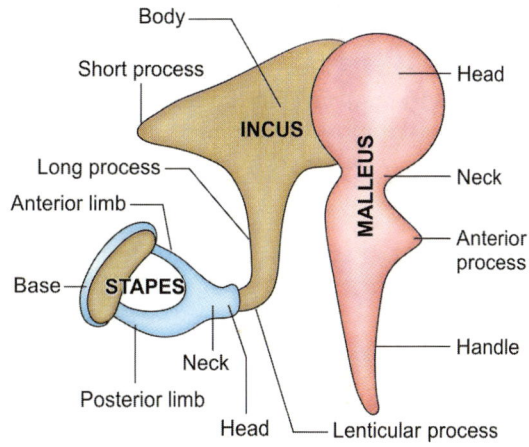

Fig. 28.1: Ossicles of the right ear : Lateral aspect

C. Handle

1. It is lower elongated part of malleus.
2. It is embedded in the tympanic membrane and moves with it.
3. Its upper end (root) shows following features:
   i. A slight projection on the medial aspect provides attachment to *tendon of tensor tympani*.
   ii. *Anterior process* projects forwards. *Anterior ligament of malleus* is attached to it. This ligament extends into the petrotympanic fissure.

iii. *Lateral process* projects laterally from where extend anterior and posterior malleolar folds to the ends of tympanic sulcus.

II. Incus

It has a large body and two processes (long and short).

A. Body

1. It is cubical in shape.
2. Its anterior surface is cancave and articulates with head of malleus.

B. Processes

a. Long process

1. It projects downwards parallel to handle of malleus.
2. Its lower end (*lenticular process*) bears an articular surface on the medial aspect for articulation with the head of stapes.

b. Short process

1. It is directed backwards.
2. It is attached by a ligament to the fossa incudis just below the aditus.

III. Stapes

It has a head, a neck, two limbs (anterior and posterior) and a foot plate (base).

A. Head

1. It is rounded
2. It articulates with the long process of incus.

B. Neck

1. It is constricted part adjacent to head.
2. *Tendon of stapedius* is attached to its posterior surface.

C. Limbs (crura)

1. Anterior and posterior limbs diverges from the neck.

2. These two limbs are attached to the foot plate.

D. Foot plate (base)

1. It is oval in shape.
2. It fits into the fenestra vestibuli.

OSSIFICATION

1. Malleus and incus develop from the dorsal end of Meckel's cartilage.
2. Stapes develops from the dorsal end of hyoid arch cartilage.
3. Malleus ossifies by two centres:
   i. One endochondral centre near the neck.
   ii. One centre for anterior process appears in dense connective tissue.
   Appearance
   4th month of intrauterine life.
   Fusion
   6th month of intrauterine life.
4. Incus ossifies by single endochondral centre in the upper part of long process. This centre appears at 4th month of intrauterine life.
5. Stapes ossifies by single endochondral centre which appears in the base at 4th month of intrauterine life.
6. At birth the auditory ossicles are of almost adult size.

FUNCTIONS

1. Malleus functions as a lever as it is attached to the tympanic membrane.
2. The base of stapes is considerably smaller than the tympanic membrane. Due to this fact, the vibratory force of the stapes is about 10 times that of tympanic membrane. Thus the auditory ossicles increase the force

but decrease the amplitude of vibrations transmitted from tympanic membrane.

APPLIED ANATOMY

1. *Treacher Collins' syndrome* is a condition in which there are abnormalities of ossicles and cranio-facial skeleton. This may be one of the causes of congenital conductive deafness.

2. Damage to ossicles in cases of head injury with fracture of temporal bone leads to very severe and permanent conductive deafness.

3. Late conductive deafness due to aseptic necrosis of the long process of incus can occur some years after head injury.

4. *Ankylosis of stapes* is a common occurrence in cases of *otosclerosis*.

CHAPTER

29 | The Occipital Bone

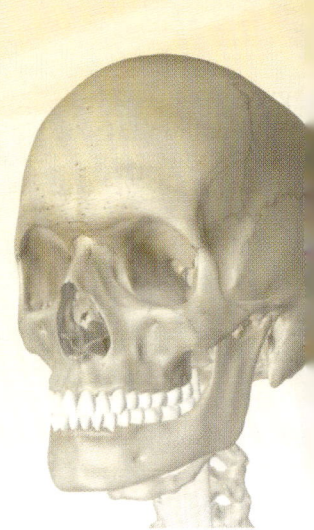

TERMINOLOGY

Word 'occipital' is derived from Greek words 'ob' (meaning back) and 'cipit' (meaning head). Hence referred to the back of head.

LOCATION

Occipital bone occupies the posterior part of skull and plays major role in the formation of posterior cranial fossa.

FEATURES AND ATTACHMENTS

The largest foramen of the skull called as *foramen magnum*, is located in the occipital bone. The components of occipital bone are better described in relation to this foramen. It consists of 1 *basilar part* (above and in front of foramen magnum), 2 *lateral parts* (lateral to foramen magnum) and 1 *squamous part* (above and behind the foramen magnum).

I. Foramen magnum

1. It is located in the floor of posterior cranial fossa.
2. It provides a communication between posterior cranial fossa and vertebral canal.
3. Its margins provide attachments to following structures:
    i. Anterior margin: *Anterior atlanto-occipital membrane.*
    ii. Posterior margin: *Posterior atlanto-occipital membrane.*
    iii. Lateral margins: *Alar ligament.*
4. Structures passing through the foramen magnum are as follows:

A. Anterior part
  i. *Apical ligament of dens.*
  ii. *Superior longitudinal band of cruciform ligament.*
  iii. *Membrana tectoria.*

B. Posterior part
  i. *Medulla oblongata.*
  ii. *Meninges.*
  iii. *Spinal roots of accessory nerves.*
  iv. *Meningeal branches of upper cervical nerves (c_{1-3})*
  v. *Vertebral arteries.*
  vi. *Sympathetic plexuses around vertebral arteries.*
  vii. *Anterior and posterior spinal arteries.*

II. Basilar part

It extends upwards and forwards to meet the body of sphenoid. Before 25 years of age a growth cartilage intervenes between sphenoid and basilar part of occipital bone but after this period the two bones fuse. Basilar part has got two surfaces (superior and inferior) and two lateral margins.

a. Superior surface
1. It is smooth.
2. It forms *clivus* with the body of sphenoid.
3. It is related to *medulla oblongata*.
4. Its lower part receives attachments of following structures from above downwards:
    i. Membrana tectoria.
    ii. Superior longitudinal band of cruciform ligament.
    iii. Apical ligament of dens.
5. Its lateral margins are grooved by *inferior petrosal sinuses*.

b. Inferior surface
1. Its middle is marked by a tubercle called *pharyngeal tubercle*. This tubercle is approximately 1 cm anterior to foramen magnum. Attached to this tubercle is the upper part of pharyngeal raphe (*pharyngeal ligament*).
2. Anterolateral to pharyngeal tubercle is the area for *longus capitis*.
3. Posterolateral to pharyngeal tubercle (just in front of condyle) is the attachment of *rectus capitis anterior*.

c. Lateral margins
These are rough and articulate with petrous parts of the temporal bones.

III. Lateral parts (right and left)
Each can be divided into broader medial portion (adjacent to foramen magnum) and narrower lateral portion (jugular process).

A. Medial portion
a. Inferior surface
1. It is marked by an articular *occipital condyle*.
2. The articular surface of occiptal condyle is oval and convex to articulate with concave superior articular process of atlas.
3. Occipital condyle is located lateral to anterior half of foramen magnum.
4. Behind the condyle is *condylar fossa* which may have *condylar canal* for emissary vein from sigmoid sinus.
5. Lateral to anterior part of condyle is the outer opening of *hypoglossal canal*.

b. Medial aspect
1. It has got a *tubercle* and a *foramen*.
2. The *tubercle* is situated on the medial aspect of condyle and provides attachment to *alar ligament*.
3. The foramen located just above the tubercle forms the inner opening of *hypoglossal canal*.
4. Following structures pass through hypoglossal canal:
    i. Hypoglossal nerve.
    ii. Meningeal branch of ascending pharyngeal artery.

c. Superior surface
1. It is marked by an oval eminence called *jugular tubercle*.
2. Jugular tubercle overlies the hypoglossal canal.
3. The posterior part of jugular tubercle often presents a shallow groove for IX, X and XI cranial nerves.

B. Jugular process
1. Its lateral end presents a rough area which joins the jugular surface of temporal bone by a growth cartilage. The cartilage ossifies at the age of 25 years.
2. Its anterior margin is notched and completes the *jugular foramen* with similar notch on the posterior border of petrous part of temporal bone.
3. Its superior surface is marked by a deep groove which lodges terminal part of *sigmoid sinus*.

4. Its inferior surface provides attachment to *rectus capitis lateralis*.

IV. Squamous part

It has two surfaces (external and internal), 3 angles (1 superior and 2 lateral) and 4 borders (2 lambdoid and 2 mastoid).

A. Surfaces

a. External surface (Figs 29.1 and 29.2)

1. The middle of the external surface is marked by a projection called *external occipital protuberance*.
2. Two lines extend laterally on each side from external occipital protuberance.
   i. A superior faint line is called *highest nuchal line*. This provides attachment to *occipital belly of occipitofrontalis*.
   ii. An inferior well defined line is called *superior nuchal line*. This receives attachments of *trapezius* and *sternomastoid* in its medial and lateral parts respectively.
3. A midline ridge extends from the external occipital protuberance to foramen magnum. This is called *external occipital crest*. It gives attachment to *ligamentum nuchae*.
4. Running laterally on each side from the middle of external occipital crest is another ridge called *inferior nuchal line*.
5. There are two muscles attached between superior and inferior nuchal lines on both the sides, i.e. *semispinalis capitis* (medially) and *obliquus capitis superior* (laterally).
6. Similarly, there are two muscles attached to each side of midline below the inferior nuchal line, i.e. *rectus capitis posterior major* (laterally) and *rectus capitis posterior minor* (medially).

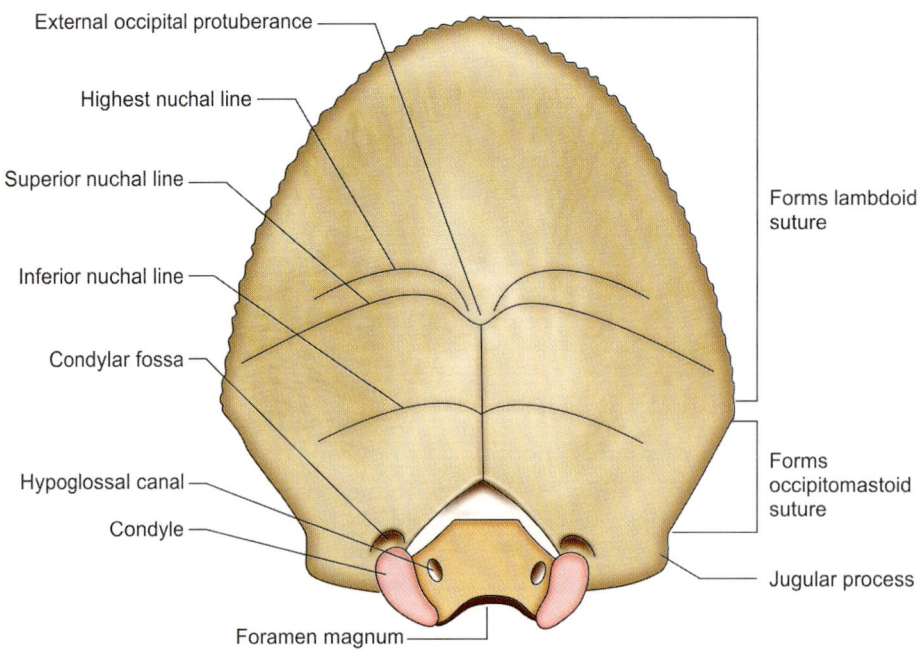

Fig. 29.1: Occipital bone: Posterior aspect

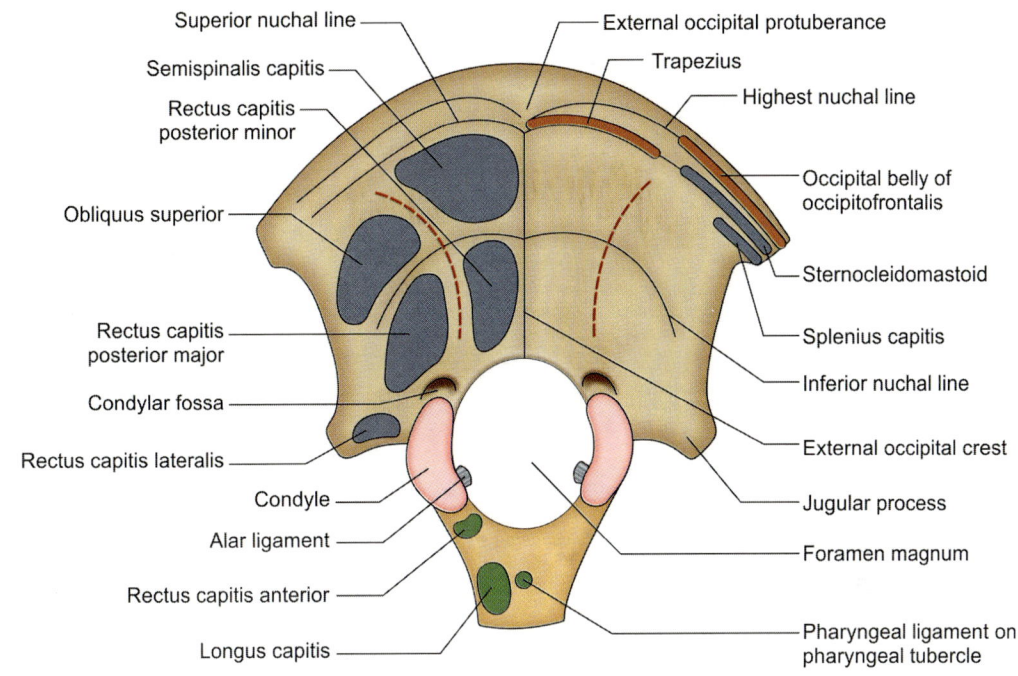

Fig. 29.2: Occipital bone: Inferior aspect

Note: *Remember that the rectus capitis muscles are named after their relations with occipital condyle. The one lying anterior to condyle is rectus capitis anterior. The muscle lying lateral to condyle is called rectus capitis lateralis. Rectus capitis posterior will naturally be located behind the condyle. Since the latter muscle is two in number, these are further qualified by adding 'major' and 'minor' to their names.*

It is interesting to note that rectus capitis anterior, lateralis and posterior are attached to three components of occipital bone, i.e. basilar part, lateral part and squamous part respectively.

b. Internal surface (Fig. 29.3)

1. Its middle is marked by an elevation called *internal occipital protuberance* which corresponds with the external occipital protuberance on the external surface.
2. Four grooves diverge from the internal occipital protuberance, one upwards, one downwards and two laterally whose margins provide attachments to *falx cerebri, falx cerebelli* and *tentorium cerebelli* respectively.
3. The groove running upwards is produced by *superior sagittal sinus*.
4. The groove running downwards is occupied by *occipital sinus*.
5. The groove extending laterally is produced by corresponding *transverse sinus*.
6. The internal surface is marked by a depression in the midline near the posterior margin of foramen magnum. This is *vermian fossa* related to inferior vermis of cerebellum.
7. Midline elevation extending from internal occipital protuberance to posterior margin of foramen magnum is called *internal occipital crest. Falx cerebelli* is attached to it.
8. On each side of internal occipital crest a hallow is related to *cerebellar hemisphere*.

2. Squamous part fuses with lateral parts when primary dentition completes, i.e. at 2 years.
3. Lateral parts fuse with basilar part when the permanent dentition begins, i.e. at 6 years.
4. Basilar part fuses with sphenoid and lateral part fuses with temporal bone at the age of 25 years.

Note: *Remember, the occipital condyle is contributed partly from lateral part and partly from basilar part of occipital bone.*

APPLIED ANATOMY

1. The squamous part of the occipital bone contributing to vault is prone to both fissured and depressed fractures but the portions lying in the base of skull always show linear fracture.
2. Margins of foramen magnum form a natural thick bony buttresses at the base of skull, therefore the fracture lines often converge towards the foramen magnum.
3. A crack in the inner table of the squamous part of occipital bone may damage the large diploeic vein and produce small epidural haematoma.
4. Almost invariably fractures of squamous part of occipital bone in children are associated with rupture of dura mater.
5. Basal fracture of skull involving hypoglossal canal will damage the hypoglossal nerve.
6. A gap in the squamous part of occipital bone forming cranial vault is usually filled with tantalum or titanium due to lack of regeneration in this part whose periosteum is devoid of cambium layer.

CHAPTER 30
The Zygomatic Bones

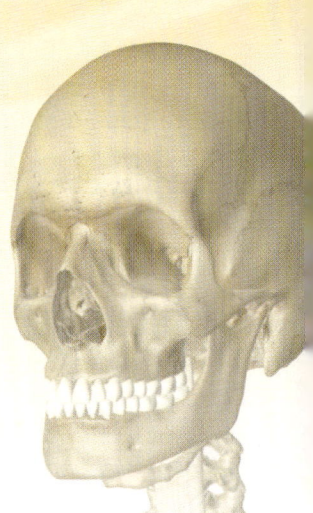

TERMINOLOGY

Term zygomatic is derived from Greek word 'zyg' which means 'yoke'. Hence the zygomatic refers to a bone which is shaped like a yoke uniting the frontal, maxilla and temporal bones.

Zygomatic bone is also called *'malar bone'* because it forms prominence of the cheek which is called 'mala' in Latin.

Term *'zygoma'* is used by clinitians which includes both 'zygomatic bone' and 'zygomatic arch'. Anatomists use the term 'zygoma' for 'zygomatic arch'.

The term *'zygomatic complex'* implies to zygomatic bone and other bones adjacent to it i.e. maxilla and zygomatic process of frontal bone.

LOCATION

Zygomatic bones are present in the upper and lateral parts of face.

FEATURES AND ATTACHMENTS

Each zygomatic bone has three surfaces (lateral, temporal and orbital), five borders (anterosuperior, anteroinferior, posterosuperior, posteroinferior and posteromedial) and two processes (frontal and temporal).

I. Surfaces

A. Lateral surface (Fig. 30.1)

1. It is convex.

2. *Zygomaticofacial foramen* is present near the orbital (anterosuperior) border. It transmits *zygomaticofacial nerve and vessels.*
3. Area below the zygomaticofacial foramen give origin to two muscles:
   i. *Zygomaticus major* (posteriorly)
   ii. *Zygomaticus minor* (anteriorly).

B. Temporal surface (Fig. 30.2)

1. Its anterior part is rough for articulation with maxilla.
2. Its posterior larger part is smooth and forms anterior boundary of temporal fossa.
3. Close to posteroinferior border this surface provides attachment to *masseter muscle.*
4. *Zygomaticotemporal foramen* present on this surface transmits *zygomaticotemporal nerve and vessels.*

C. Orbital surface

1. It partly contributes to the lateral wall and floor of the orbit.
2. It possesses *zygomatico-orbital foramina* which transmit:
   i. *Zygomaticotemporal and zygomaticofacial nerves.*
   ii. *Zygomatic branches of lacrimal artery.*

The Zygomatic Bones

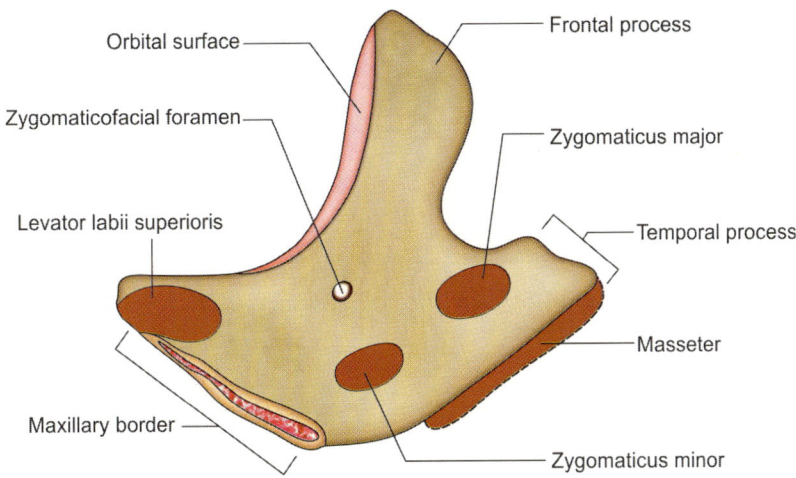

Fig. 30.1: Left zygomatic bone: Lateral aspect

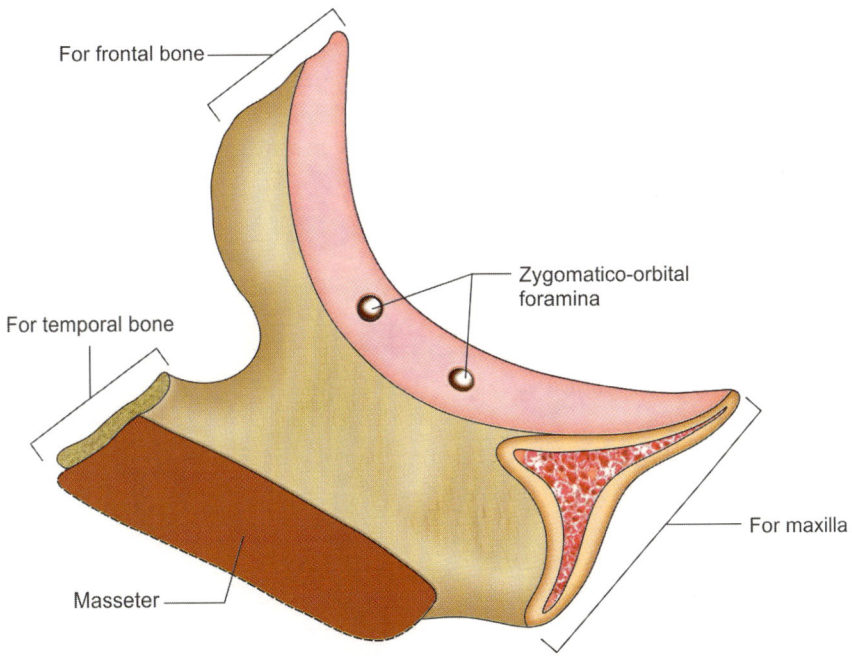

Fig. 30.2: Left zygomatic bone: Medial aspect

II. Borders

A. Anterosuperior border

1. This is also called *orbital border*.
2. It provides attachement to *orbital septum*.

B. Anteroinferior border

1. This is also called *maxillary border*.
2. *Levator labii superioris* arises partly from this border near the orbital border.

C. Posterosuperior border
1. It is also called *temporal border*.
2. *Temporal fascia* is attached to this border.

D. Posteroinferior border
Masseter muscle originates from this border.

E. Posteromedial border
It articulates with the greater wing of sphenoid above and maxilla below.

III. Processes
A. Frontal process
1. It articulates with the zygomatic process of frontal bone(to form *fronto-zygomatic suture*) superiorly and greater wing of sphenoid bone posteriorly.
2. *Whitnall's tubercle* is present on its orbital aspect about 1 cm below the frontozygomatic suture. Following structures are attached to this tubercle:
   i. *Lateral check ligament.*
   ii. *Lateral palpebral ligament.*
   iii. *Suspensory ligament of eye ball.*
   iv. *Aponeurosis of levator palpebrae superioris.*

B. Temporal process
1. It is directed backwards.
2. It articulates with zygomatic process of temporal bone to complete *zygomatic arch*.
3. Its inferior margin and medial surface provide attachment to *masseter muscle*.

OSSIFICATION
1. Zygomatic bone ossifies in membrane.
2. Usually single centre appears at the age of 8th week of intrauterine life.
3. Sometimes a horizonatal suture divides the bone into an upper larger and a lower smaller segments.

APPLIED ANATOMY
1. '*Malar flush*' is the redness of skin over zygomatic prominence. This is observed in tuberculosis, mitral stenosis (narrowing of left atrio-ventricular orifice) and rheumatic fever.
2. Zygomatic bone is of great clinical importance due to its functional significance
   i. It protects the globe of eye.
   ii. It gives origin to masseter muscle.
   iii. It transmits part of the masticatory forces to cranium
   iv. It absorbs the force of an impact before it reaches the brain.
3. When a rapidly moving object hits the zygomatic bone, a comminuted fracture results with displacement of bone fragments (Fig. 30.3).
4. '*Tripod*' fracture means fracture of zygomatic complex. Zygomatic bone is

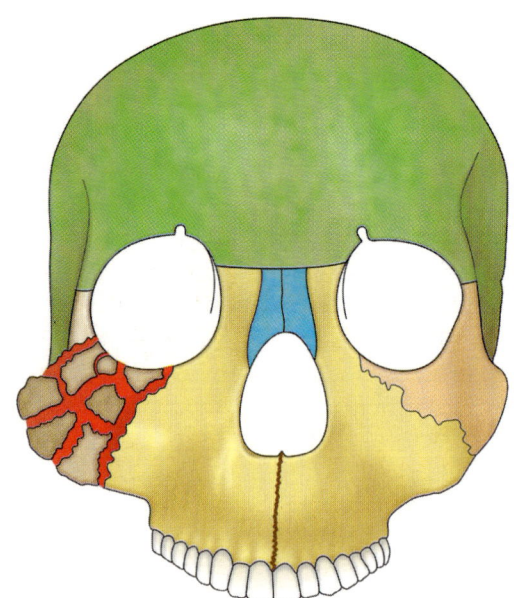

Fig. 30.3: Comminuted fracture of body of zygomatic bone and orbital floor

like three legged stool, the seat of stool is main portion of zygomatic bone while legs are frontal process, inferior orbital margin and zygomatic buttress.

5. Frontozygomatic suture, zygomatic prominence, the zygomatic buttress and 1st molar tooth, all lie in same vertical line. In majority of the cases, zygomatic complex fracture is associated with rotation along this axis (Fig. 30.4).

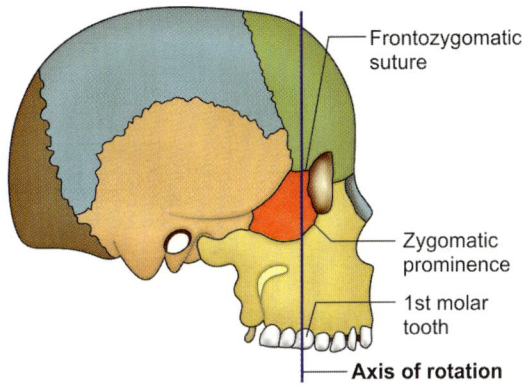

Fig. 30.4: Vertical axis of rotation during zygomatic complex fracture

6. Zygomatic bone forms one of the principal means by which occlusal stress is transmitted from the maxilla and spreads over the base of skull.
7. Fracture of zygoma (zygomatic arch and zygomatic bone) is second among the common fractures of the middle 3rd of the face.
8. The junctions of frontal and temporal processes of zygomatic bone form important landmarks in the treatment of maxillo-facial injuries.
9. The periosteum and attachment of strong temporal fascia limit the displacement of zygomatic bone following injury.
10. In depressed fracture of zygomatico-maxillary complex, there is displacement of zygomatic bone without its fracture (Fig. 30.5).

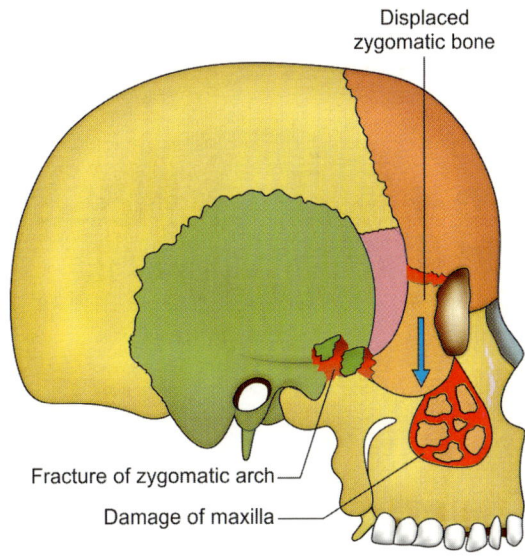

Fig. 30.5: Depressed fracture of zygomatico-maxillary complex

11. Le Fort III fracture of face is a horizontal fracture just below the base of skull. The fracture line passes laterally through frontozygomatic sutures. As there is a concurrent fracture of zygomatic arches, the maxillae and zygomatic bones are separated from rest of the skull (Fig. 30.6).

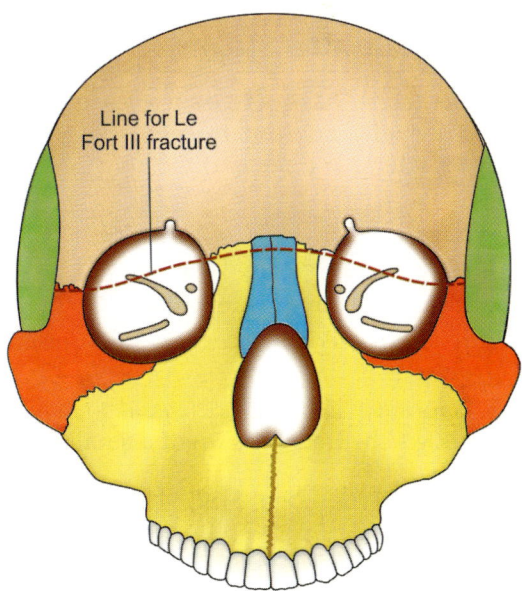

Fig. 30.6: Le Fort III fracture

CHAPTER

31 | The Nasal Bones

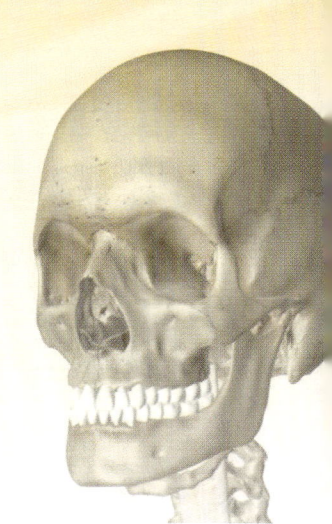

TERMINOLOGY

Nasal bone is so named because of its location. It forms the bridge of the nose.

LOCATION

Two nasal bones meet with each other in midline in the upper part of external nose. They are located below the nasal part of frontal bone and between the frontal processes of maxillae.

FEATURES AND ATTACHMENTS

Each nasal bone has got two surfaces (external and internal) and four borders (superior, inferior, lateral and medial).

I. Surfaces

A. External surface (Fig. 31.1)
1. It is convex from side to side.
2. It is covered by *procerus* and *nasalis* muscles.
3. A foramen in the centre (*vascular foramen*) allows the transmission of a small vein.

B. Internal surface (Fig. 31.2)
1. It is concave from side to side
2. It presents a *vertical groove* for the *anterior ethmoidal nerve*.

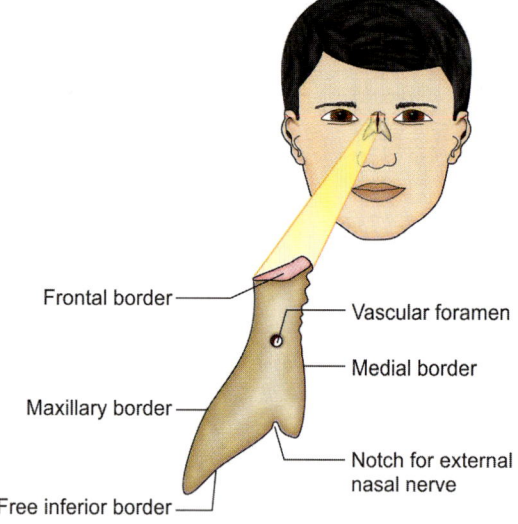

Fig. 31.1: Right nasal bone: External surface

II. Borders

A. Superior border
1. It is serrated.
2. It articulates with nasal part of frontal bone.

B. Inferior border
1. It is notched for the passage of *external nasal nerve*.
2. It is continuous with the lateral nasal cartilage.

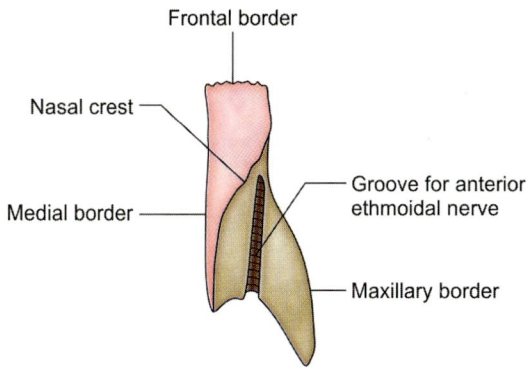

Fig. 31.2: Right nasal bone: Internal surface

C. Lateral border
It articulates with frontal process of maxilla.

D. Medial border
1. It is thick above than below.
2. It articulates with opposite nasal bone (*to form internasal suture*) and prolonged behind as *nasal crest*.
3. Nasal crest articulates with following structures from above downwards:
   i. *Nasal spine of frontal bone.*
   ii. *Perpendicular plate of ethmoid.*
   iii. *Septal cartilage.*

OSSIFICATION
1. Nasal bone ossifies in membrane overlying the anterior part of cartilaginous nasal capsule
2. Centre of ossification appears in its middle during 3rd month of intrauterine life.

APPLIED ANATOMY
1. Nasal bone is usually fractured due to direct hard blow.
2. The fractures of nasal bone are transverse in nature.
3. The common site for the fracture of nasal bone is ½ inch above its inferior border.
4. Slight mobility of anteroinferior part of the nasal bone protects the nose against mild injuries.
5. An impact directed in the anteroposterior plane will cause a depression of the nasal bridge due to fracture of nasal bone, frontal process of maxilla and septal cartilage.

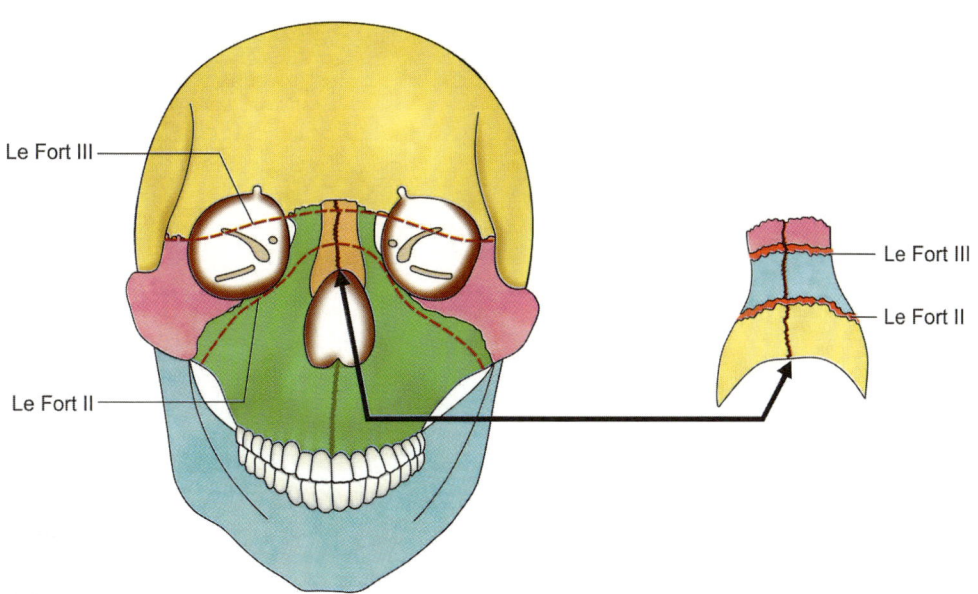

Fig. 31.3: Le Fort fractures

6. A force directed from the lateral aspect will result in a deviation of the nasal bridge to opposite side.
7. Traumatic alteration in the shape of nose because of fracture of nasal bones is of great clinical importance due to cosmetic reasons specially in young females.
8. In cases of Le Fort II and Le Fort III fractures of maxillae, nasal bones are also involved. Le Fort I fracture of maxillae spares the nasal bone.

CHAPTER 32

The Lacrimal Bones

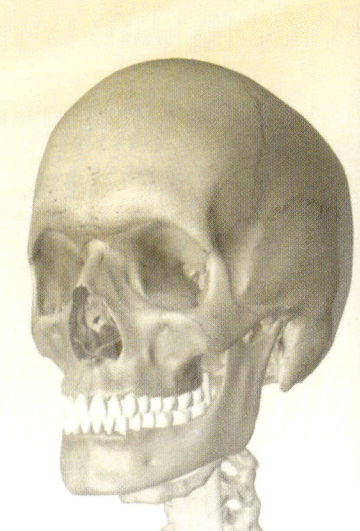

TERMINOLOGY

'Lacrimal' is a Latin word which means 'tear'. The bone is so named because of its relation with the tear sac.

PECULIARITIES

1. It is most fragile amongst the cranial bones.
2. It is the smallest of the cranial bones.

LOCATION

1. There are two lacrimal bones.
2. Each lacrimal bone is located in the anterior part of the medial wall of orbit.
3. It also contributes to the middle meatus of nose.

FEATURES AND ATTACHMENTS

Lacrimal bone is rectangular in shape. It has two surfaces (medial and lateral) and four borders (anterior, posterior, superior and inferior).

I. Surfaces
A. Medial surface (Fig. 32.1)
1. It is also called nasal surface.
2. Its anteroinferior part contributes partly to the middle meatus of nose.

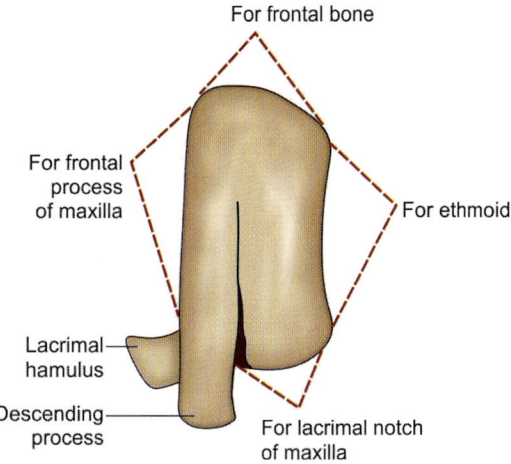

Fig. 32.1: Right lacrimal bone : Medial surface

3. Its posterosuperior part articulates with the ethmoid and completes few anterior ethmoidal air cells.

B. Lateral surface (Fig. 32.2)
1. It is also known as the orbital surface.
2. It is divided into anterior and posterior parts by a vertical crest called *posterior lacrimal crest*.
3. The anterior part is grooved and forms posterior half of the floor of the *lacrimal groove*. Anterior half of the lacrimal

258 | Human Osteology

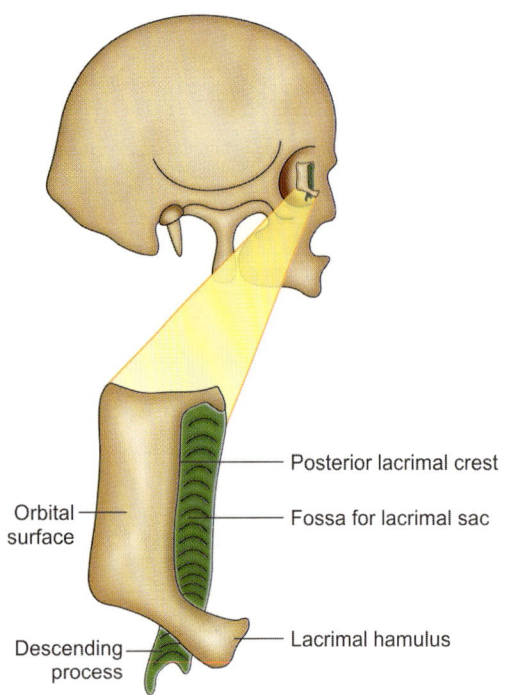

Fig. 32.2: Right lacrimal bone : Lateral surface

II. Borders

A. Anterior border
It articulates with the frontal process of maxilla.

B. Posterior border
It articulates with the orbital plate of ethmoid.

C. Superior border
It articulates with the nasal notch of frontal bone.

D. Inferior border
It articulates with the orbital surface of maxilla.

OSSIFICATION

1. Lacrimal bone ossifies in membrane.
2. Single centre of ossification appears in the mesenchyme around the cartilaginous nasal capsule.
3. The centre appears at about 12th week of intrauterine life.

groove is formed by frontal process of maxilla. The groove lodges *lacrimal sac*.
4. Portion behind the posterior lacrimal crest is smooth and forms part of medial wall of orbit.
5. Lower end of posterior lacrimal crest projects forwards as *lacrimal hamulus*. It articulates with maxilla to complete the *upper end of nasolacrimal canal*.
6. Posterior lacrimal crest provides attachment to *lacrimal fascia*.
7. The crest and small area of lateral surface immediately behind it give origin to *lacrimal part of orbicularis oculi muscle*.
8. The medial wall of groove projects downwards as *descending process*. This process articulates with the lips of nasolacrimal groove of the maxilla and lacrimal process of inferior concha to complete the bony canal for nasolacrimal duct.

APPLIED ANATOMY

1. A severe impact on the nasal bridge may involve the lacrimal bone and damage the lacrimal passage.
2. Lacrimal bone is included by clinicians in the central portion of middle 3rd facial skeleton. All the bones of middle 3rd facial skeleton receive adequate blood supply from periosteal arteries and therefore all the fragments of fractured bone retain a periosteal blood supply.
3. Lacrimal bone is involved in Le Fort III fracture.
4. Since the anteroinferior part of nasal surface of lacrimal bone is covered with nasal mucosa, the fracture of the bone may open into nasal cavity with potential risk of infection.
5. To reach the medial wall of optic canal during surgical procedure called *"optic*

nerve decompression", most of the bones of medial wall of orbit (including lacrimal bone) are infractured.

6. Lacrimal bone is very fragile, therefore an extraprecaution should be taken to avoid trauma during surgery of lacrimal system.

7. In some of the cases of obstruction of lacrimal sac or nasolacrimal duct, *'dacryocystorhinostomy'* is performed. In this operation an artificial passage is made for drainage into nasal cavity, by breaking the lacrimal bone.

CHAPTER

33 | The Ethmoid Bone

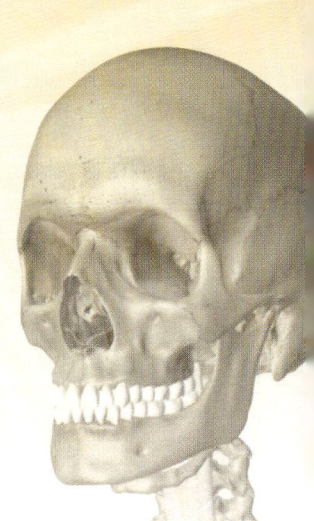

TERMINOLOGY

'Ethmoid' is a Greek word which means 'sieve like'. Ethmoid is so named because it possesses a perforated (sieve like) plate called cribriform plate.

LOCATION

Single ethmoid bone is situated in the anterior part of the base of the cranium between the orbits. It forms part of the medial wall of the orbits and part of the bony septum, roofs and lateral walls of the nasal cavities.

FEATURES AND ATTACHMENTS

Ethmoid bone consists of a cribriform plate, a perpendicular plate and two lateral masses called labyrinths.

I. Cribriform plate (Fig. 33.1)

1. It is the median part of the superior surface of ethmoid.
2. It contributes to the median portion of anterior cranial fossa (anterior part of the interior of base of skull).
3. It occupies the ethmoidal notch of the frontal bone.
4. It possesses a median triangular upward projection called *crista galli* (named because

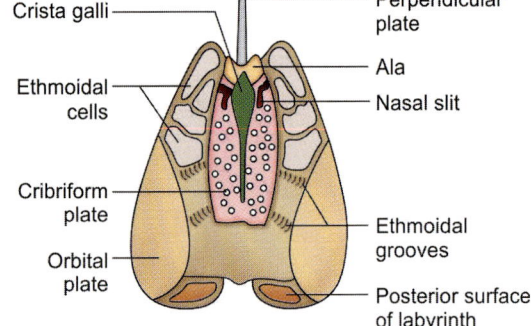

Fig. 33.1: Ethmoid : Superior aspect

of its resemblance to crown of a cock, zoological name of which is *Gallus domesticus*).

5. Posterior sloping border of the crista galli gives attachment to *falx cerebri*.
6. Anterior border of the crista galli has two alae which articulate with frontal bone to complete *foramen caecum. Emissary vein* passes through this foramen.
7. On each side of the crista galli, the cribriform plate shows a number of perforations through which pass about *15-20 filaments of the olfactory nerve*. This part is also related to olfactory bulb superiorly.
8. Just lateral to anterior part of crista galli there is a slit like passage for a *process of dura mater*.

9. Just lateral to the anterior end of slit there is a foramen for the passage of *anterior ethmoidal nerve*.

II. Perpendicular plate (Fig. 33.2)

1. It is a quadrangular flat plate projecting downwards from the midline of cribriform plate.
2. Its anterior border articulates with the nasal process of frontal bone and the crest of the nasal bones.
3. Its posterior border articulates with sphenoidal crest above and vomer below.
4. Its superior border is attached to the cribriform plate.
5. Its inferior border receives the attachment of septal cartilage.
6. Its surfaces are mainly smooth except in the upper parts where there are grooves for filaments of olfactory nerves.

III. Labyrinths

Large number of air filled spaces (*ethmoidal air cells*) constitute the labyrinth. These air cells are divisible into anterior, middle and posterior *ethmoidal sinuses* by bony plates. Many of these air cells open on the surface and completed only when articulating with the adjacent bones. Each labyrinth may be considered to have six surfaces.

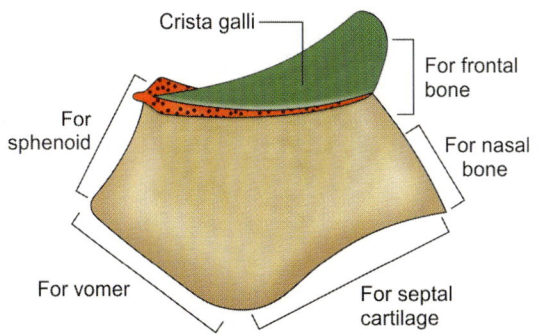

Fig. 33.2: Perpendicular plate of ethmoid : Right lateral aspect

A. Upper surface

1. It has several open air cells which are completed only after articulation with edges of ethmoidal notch.
2. It has two grooves which are converted into anterior and posterior ethmoidal canals by articulation with frontal bone.

B. Lower surface

It articulates with upper part of the nasal surface of maxilla to complete the ethmoidal air cells from below.

C. Anterior surface

It possesses half cut air sinuses which are completed by the frontal process of maxilla and lacrimal bone.

D. Posterior surface (Fig. 33.3)

It articulates with sphenoidal concha and orbital process of palatine bone to complete the posterior ethmoidal sinus.

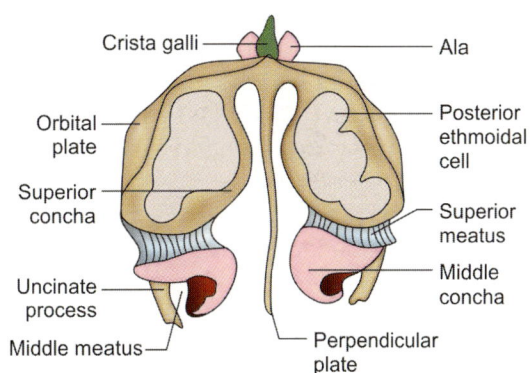

Fig. 33.3: Ethmoid : Posterior aspect

E. Lateral surface (Fig. 33.4)

1. It is thin and smooth plate called *orbital plate*.
2. It covers the middle and posterior ethmoidal sinuses.
3. It forms large part of medial wall of orbit.
4. It is quadrangular in shape and articulates as follows:

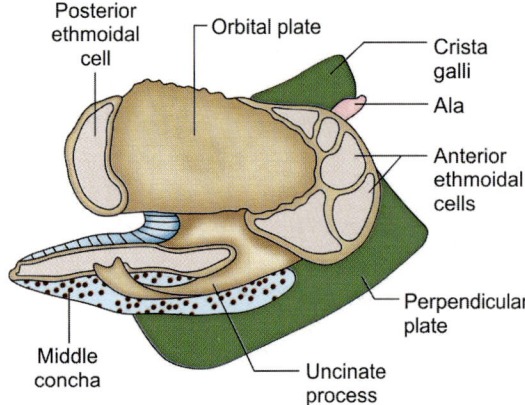

Fig. 33.4: Ethmoid :Right lateral aspect

    i. Superiorly with orbital plate of frontal bone.
    ii. Inferiorly with the maxilla and orbital process of palatine bone.
    iii. Anteriorly with lacrimal bone.
    iv. Posteriorly with sphenoid bone.

E. Medial surface

1. It forms part of the lateral wall of corresponding half of nasal cavity.
2. Its upper part is marked by numerous vertical grooves which lodge filaments of olfactory nerve.
3. Its posterior part is marked by an anteroposterior fissure called *superior meatus*.
4. Posterior ethmoidal sinus opens into superior meatus.
5. Superior meatus is bounded above by a curved plate called *superior nasal concha*.
6. Below and in front of superior meatus is another curved plate of bone called *middle nasal concha*.
7. Lateral surface of middle concha is concave and forms medial wall of *middle meatus*.
8. Lateral wall of middle meatus is marked by a swelling produced by middle ethmoidal air cells. This swelling is called *bulla ethmoidalis*.
9. Middle ethmoidal sinus opens on the surface of bulla or immediately above it.
10. A thin bar of bone called *uncinate process* projects downwards and backwards from the anterior part of the labyrinth.
11. The curved gap between uncinate process and bulla is called *hiatus semilunaris*.
12. The upper end of hiatus semilunaris is continuous with a curved canal called *ethmoidal infundibulum*.
13. Anterior ethmoidal sinus opens into the infundibulum.
14. In 50% cases the infundibulum continues superiorly as *frontonasal duct* to reach the frontal sinus.

OSSIFICATION

1. At the age of 3rd month of intrauterine life the walls of nasal cavity are marked by a cartilaginous framework called *cartilaginous nasal capsule*.
2. Cartilaginous nasal capsule consists of two lateral regions and a median nasal part.
3. Single centre appears for each labyrinth in the lateral region of nasal capsule at about 5th month of intrauterine life.
4. Perpendicular plate and crista galli ossify from single centre which appears in the median septal part of nasal capsule at the age of 1st year after birth.
5. The labyrinths fuse with perpendicular plate in the region of cribriform plate at about 2 years of age.
6. The ethmoid air cells begin to develop during intrauterine life and are present in the form of narrow pouches at birth.

APPLIED ANATOMY

1. A severe impact on the nasal bridge may involve frontal processes of maxillae and two orbital plates of ethmoid bones.
2. In case of head injury, a discharge of CSF from nose (*CSF rhinorrhea*) is indicative of

fracture of cribriform plate of ethmoid in the anterior cranial fossa.
3. If the basilar fracture involves the cribriform plate, it may result into *anosmia* (loss of smell sensation) due to damage of olfactory nerve filaments.
4. Fracture of cribriform plates may cause meningitis if it opens into the nasal cavity.
5. Bony septum of nose (perpendicular plate of ethmoid and vomer) is paper thin and does not resist much to forces responsible for fracture.
6. The ethmoid is spared in Le Fort I fracture while involved in Le Fort II and III fractures (Fig. 33.5).
7. Since the ethmoid bone is clothed in mucosa over large areas of its surfaces, its fractures open into nasal cavity or ethmoid air cells with potential risk of infection.
8. *Nasal ethmoidostomy* is performed in several operations involving the ethmoidal labyrinth. In this an artificial opening is made in the ethmoidal labyrinth to drain the sinuses, e.g. after removal of frontoethmoidal mucoceles or optic nerve decompression in optic canal.

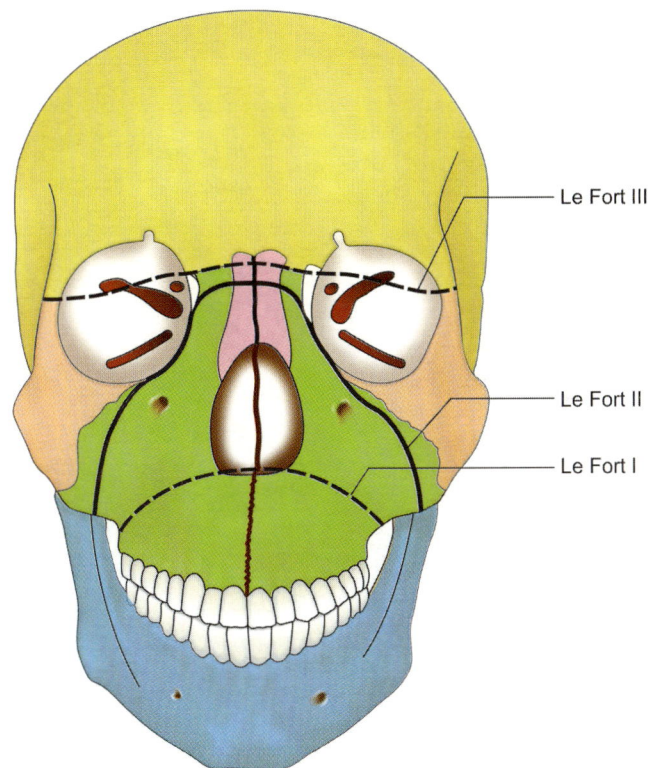

Fig. 33.5: Common fractures of maxillae and other bones of skull

CHAPTER 34

The Inferior Nasal Conchae

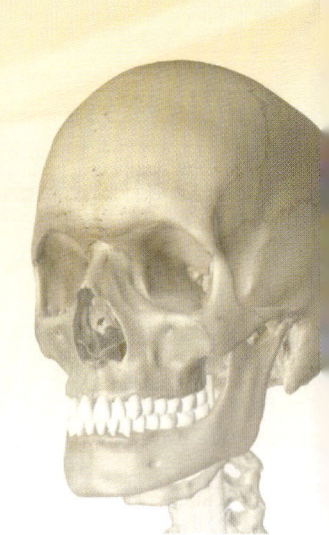

TERMINOLOGY

'Concha' is a Latin word which means 'shell'. Conchae (superior, middle and inferior) are bracket like projections of thin (like egg shell) bones from lateral wall of nose.

LOCATION

Inferior concha is an independent bone whose long axis occupies the whole length of the lower part of the lateral wall of each half of nasal cavity.

FEATURES AND ATTACHMENTS

Each inferior concha has two ends (anterior and posterior), two surfaces (medial and lateral) and two borders (superior and inferior).

I. Ends
A. Anterior end
It is pointed and directed forwards.
B. Posterior end
It is directed backwards and is more pointed and tapering.

II. Surfaces
A. Medial surface (Fig. 34.1)
1. It is convex.

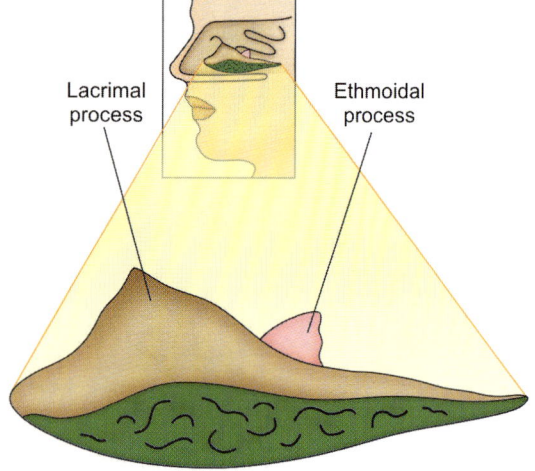

Fig. 34.1: Right inferior concha : Medial aspect

2. It has numerous apertures and grooves for vessels.

B. Lateral surface (Fig. 34.2)
1. It is concave.
2. It forms medial wall of the inferior meatus of nose.

III. Borders
A. Superior border
1. It is thin and irregular.
2. It is divided into three parts:

264

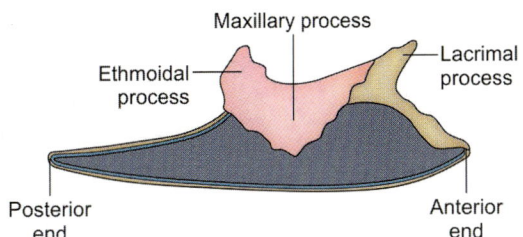

Fig. 34.2: Right inferior concha : Lateral aspect

a. Anterior part
This articulates with conchal crest of maxilla.

b. Posterior part
This articulates with conchal crest of palatine bone.

c. Middle region
This part possesses three processes which are as follows from anterior to posterior:

  i. Lacrimal process
  It is an upward projection to articulate with the descending process of lacrimal bone.

  ii. Maxillary process
  It is a curved downward projection which articulates with nasal surface of maxilla and lower part of anterior border of perpendicular plate of palatine bone.

  iii. Ethmoidal process
  It is an upward projection to articulate with uncinate process of ethmoid.

B. Inferior border
1. It is free.
2. It is thick.

OSSIFICATION

1. It develops from the lowest part of lateral region of the cartilaginous nasal capsule.
2. The centre of ossification appears during the 5th month of intrauterine life.

APPLIED ANATOMY

1. Inferior nasal concha is at great risk in cases of mid-facial injuries.
2. Inferior concha receives adequate blood supply from periosteal arteries and therefore all the fragments of the fractured bone retain a periosteal blood supply.
3. Inferior concha is clothed in nasal mucosa over large areas of its surfaces and therefore the fractures usually open to the nasal cavity with potential risk of infection.
4. Infracture of the inferior concha is some times needed during management of congenital lacrimal defects (Fig. 34.3).

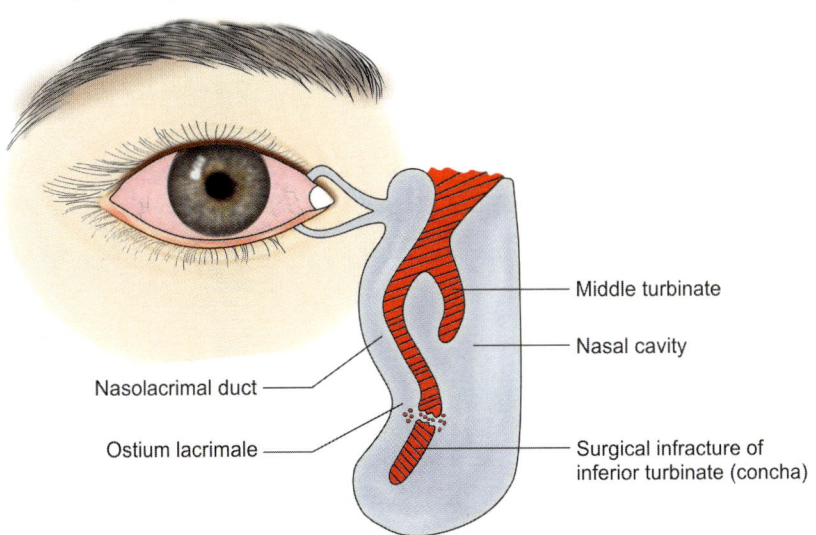

Fig. 34.3: Infracture of inferior concha (turbinate)

CHAPTER 35

The Vomer

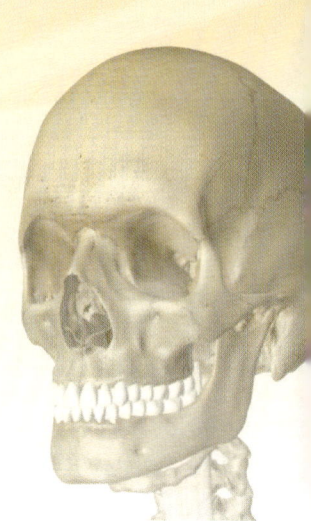

TERMINOLOGY

'Vomer' is a Latin word. The term is used for the thin plate of bone between the nostrils.

LOCATION

Vomer forms the posteroinferior part of the septum of nose (Fig. 35.1).

FEATURES AND ATTACHMENTS

Vomer has got two surfaces (right and left) and four borders (superior, inferior, anterior and posterior).

I. Surfaces

1. It has small grooves for vessels.
2. A large groove runs downwards and forwards. This is meant for *nasopalatine nerve and vessels*.

II. Borders

A. Superior border

1. It is thick.
2. Two lateral projections (*alae*) enclose a deep furrow which fits over the rostrum of sphenoid.

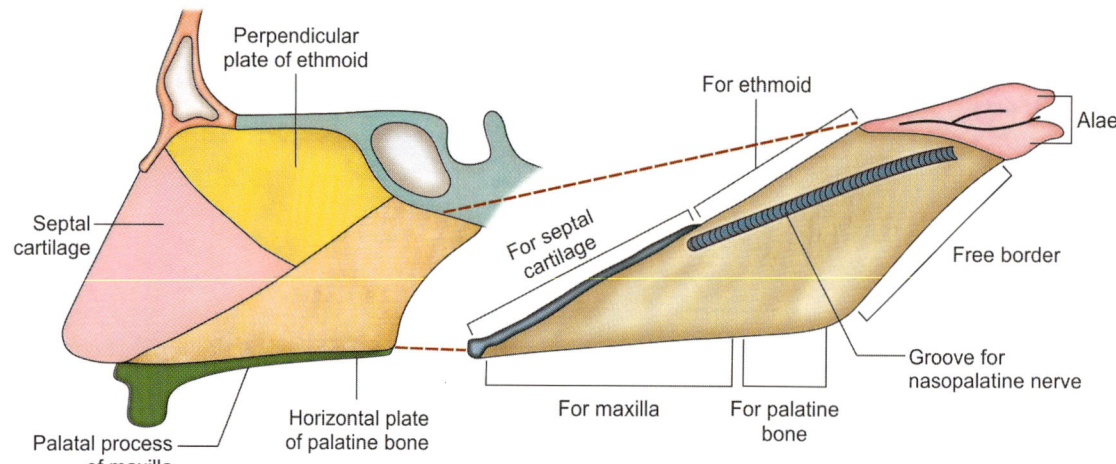

Fig. 35.1: Vomer. Left view

3. The margin of ala intervenes between body of sphenoid and vaginal process of medial pterygoid plate. Under surface of the ala forms *vomerovaginal canal* with vaginal process (Fig. 35.2).

B. Inferior border

It articulates with nasal crest formed by the maxillae and palatine bones.

C. Anterior border

1. It is the longest border.
2. Its upper half articulates with the posterior border of the perpendicular plate of ethmoid bone.
3. Its lower half is attached to septal cartilage.

D. Posterior border

1. It is free.
2. It is situated between two posterior nasal apertures (*choanae*).

OSSIFICATION

1. Vomer develops by ossification of membrane covering the median septal part of the cartilaginous nasal capsule.
2. One centre of ossification appears on each side of the cartilage at about 8th week of intrauterine life. giving rise to two bony plates separated by a cartilage.
3. Two bony plates fuse with each other in the lower part at about 12th week of intrauterine life.
4. The cartilaginous plate is gradually absorbed allowing the fusion of two bony plates which proceeds upwards from below. Fusion is completed at puberty.

APPLIED ANATOMY

1. Vomer is paper thin and does not resist much to forces responsible for fracture.
2. Vomer is involved in all three types of Le Fort fractures of mid-facial skeleton (Fig. 35.3).

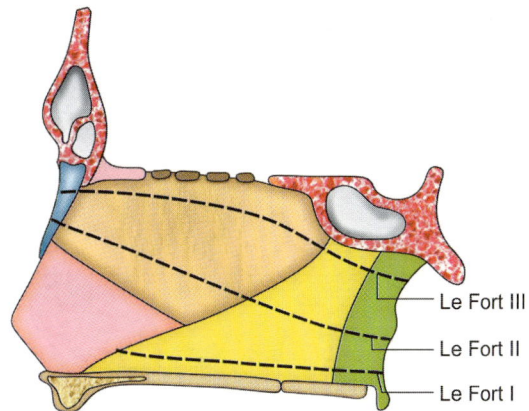

Fig. 35.3: Le Fort fractures

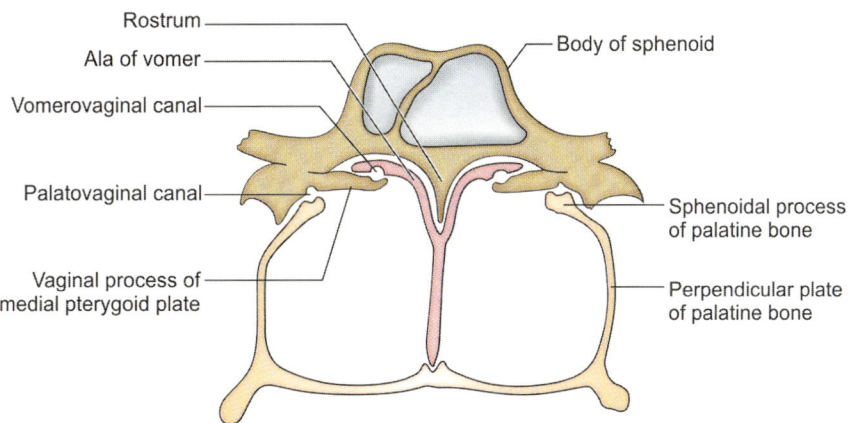

Fig. 35.2: Vomerovaginal and palatovaginal canals

3. Vomer receives adequate blood supply from periosteal arteries and therefore all the fragments of fractured bone retain a periosteal blood supply.

4. A transverse fracture of vomer due to direct blow on the nose, can lead to *deviation of nasal septum (D.N.S.)*.

5. Vomer is clothed in mucosa over large areas of its surfaces and therefore its fracture opens into nasal cavity with potential risk of infection.

6. Vomer may be deviated from the median plane as a result of birth injury or a congenital malformation.

7. In case of severe deviation, nasal septum comes into contact with the lateral wall of the nasal cavity. Surgical repair *(submucosal resection—S.M.R.)* is usually necessary to correct the deviation.

CHAPTER
36

The Sphenoid Bone

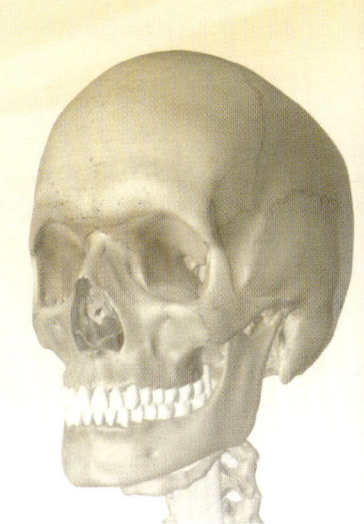

TERMINOLOGY

'Sphenoid' is derived from Greek word 'sphen' which means 'a wedge'. The bone is so named because it is wedged between the frontal bone in front and occipital bone behind.

ANATOMICAL POSITION

1. Hypophyseal fossa faces upwards.
2. Pterygoid processes descend vertically downwards.
3. Openings of sphenoidal sinuses are directed forwards.

ARTICULATIONS

Sphenoid is a key bone in the cranial skeleton as it articulates with following eight bones:

1. Frontal
2. Parietal
3. Temporal
4. Occipital
5. Vomer
6. Zygomatic
7. Palatine
8. Ethmoid

SHAPE

Sphenoid resembles a 'bat' with its wings stretched out.

FEATURES AND ATTACHMENTS

Sphenoid consists of a central body, four wings (2 greater and 2 lesser) and two pterygoid processes (right and left).

I. Body

It has six surfaces (superior, inferior, anterior, posterior and 2 lateral) and a pair of air filled cavities (sphenoidal sinuses).

A. Surfaces

a. Superior (cerebral) surface (Fig. 36.1)

It shows of following features from anterior to posterior.

   i. *Jugum sphenoidale*
      1. It is smooth.
      2. It articulates with posterior margin of cribriform plate.
      3. It is related on each side to gyrus rectus of cerebral hemisphere and olfactory tract.
   ii. *Sulcus chiasmatis*
      1. It is a transverse groove behind the jugum sphenoidale.

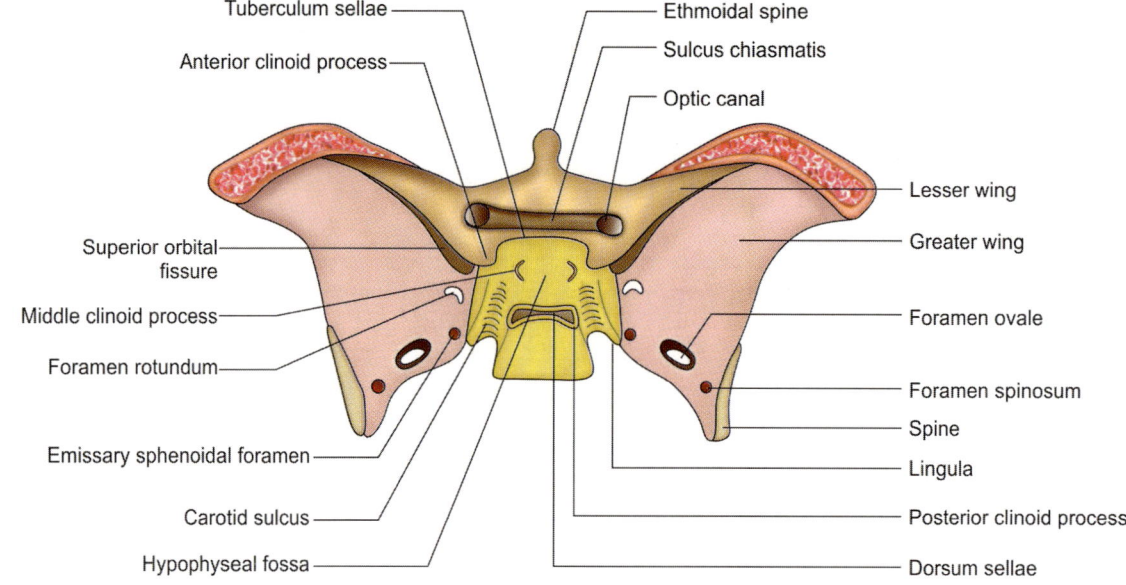

Fig. 36.1: Sphenoid bone : Superior aspect

    2. *Optic chiasma* lies just above it.

    3. It leads laterally into *optic canal*.

iii. *Tuberculum sellae*

It is an elevation just behind the sulcus chiasmatis.

iv. *Sella turcica*

    1. It is a depressed area behind the tuberculum sellae.

    2. *Hypophyseal fossa* is the deepest part of the sella turcica. It lodges *pituitary gland*.

    3. Anterior part of sella turcica is bounded on each side by an elevation called *middle clinoid process*.

v. *Dorsum sellae*

It is a square plate of bone behind the sella turcica.

vi. *Posterior clinoid process*

    1. Superior angles of dorsum sellae project laterally into *posterior clinoid processes*.

    2. Attached margin of *tentorium cerebelli* is attached to this process on each side.

vii. *Upper part of clivus*

    1. It is sloping behind the dorsum sellae.

    2. It is formed by the posterior parts of body and dorsum sellae.

    3. It supports the pons.

b. *Posterior surface* (Fig. 36.2)

    1. It is rough.

    2. It articulates with the basilar part of occipital bone.

c. *Anterior and inferior surfaces* (Fig. 36.3)

    1. Midline of the anterior surface is marked by a triangular crest called *sphenoidal crest*.

    2. Sphenoidal crest articulates with the upper part of the posterior border of perpendicular plate of ethmoid.

    3. The midline of the inferior surface is marked by a triangular spine called *sphenoidal rostrum*. It fits into the groove between the alae of vomer.

    4. Both anterior and inferior surfaces of the body on either side of midline, are

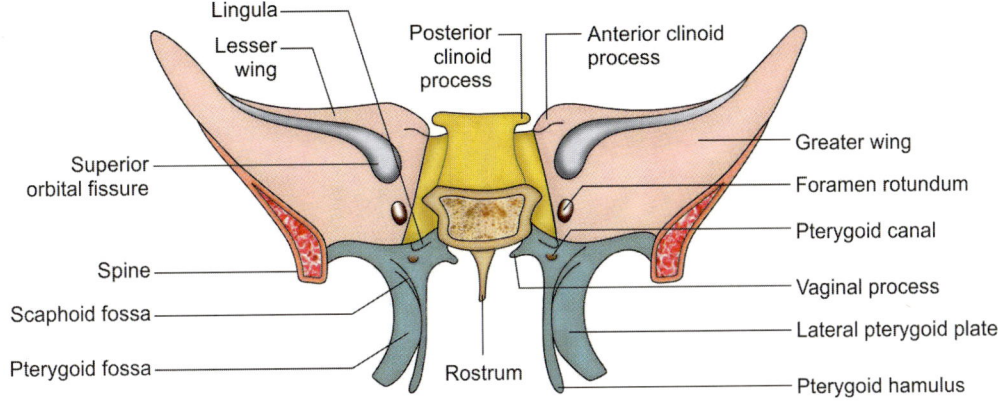

Fig. 36.2: Sphenoid bone : Posterior aspect

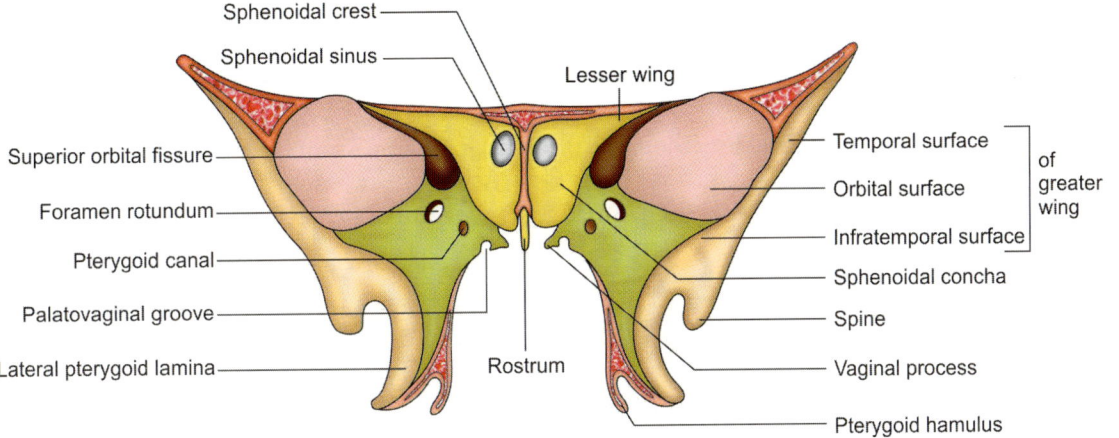

Fig. 36.3: Sphenoid bone : Anterior aspect

occupied by a thin plate of bone called *sphenoidal concha*.

5. Each sphenoidal concha consists of an anterior part which is vertical and quadrangular and a posterior part which is horizontal and triangular.

i. *Anterior part*

It consists of an upper and lateral depressed area which completes the posterior ethmoidal sinus and articulates below with the orbital process of palatine bone. Its lower and medial part forms part of the roof of the nasal cavity and is perforated above by the round opening through which sphenoidal sinus communicates with sphenoethmoidal recess of nasal cavity.

ii. *Posterior part*

It forms part of the roof of nasal cavity and completes the *sphenopalatine foramen*.

d. *Lateral surface*

1. Its lower part unites with the greater wing and medial pterygoid plate.
2. Its upper part is marked by *carotid sulcus* which lodges internal caroid artery and cavernous sinus.

3. The lateral margin of the carotid sulcus at its posterior end, projects backwards into tongue shaped *lingula*.
4. Lingula lies just above the posterior opening of *pterygoid canal*.

B. Sphenoidal sinuses

1. These are two large air spaces present in the body of sphenoid.
2. The two sinuses are separated by a septum and are rarely symmetrical.
3. *Relations*

   Superiorly – Optic chiasma.
   – Pituitary gland.
   Laterally – Internal carotid artery.
   – Cavernous sinus.
4. *Size*

   Vertical height – 2 cm (little less then 2 cm)
   Transverse breadth – 1.8 cm
   Anteroposterior depth – 2.1 cm (little more than 2 cm).

Note: *For simplification students may consider all the measurements approximately as 2 cm.*

5. Each sinus communicates with the spheno-ethmoidal recess.
6. *Development*
   i. Sphenoidal sinus starts developing as nasal mucosal evagination during intrauterine life.
   ii. These are in the form of minute cavities at birth.
   iii. It develops to its adult size in adolescence.

II. Wings

A. Greater wings

There are two greater wings, a right and a left. Each has three surfaces (cerebral, lateral and orbital) and several margins.

a. Surfaces
   i. Cerebral surface

   It is concave. It forms part of middle cranial fossa. It is related to temporal lobe of cerebrum. It possesses following foramina.

   1. *Foramen rotundum*

      It is situated in the anteromedial part. *Maxillary nerve* passes through it.
   2. *Foramen ovale*

      It is situated posterolateral to foramen rotundum. It transmits:
      – Mandibular nerve.
      – Accessory meningeal artery.
      – Lesser petrosal nerve.
      – Emissary vein.

Note: *Remember, it is the MALE which passes through foramen ovale in which M = Mandibular nerve, A = Accessory meningeal artery, L = Lesser petrosal nerve E = Emissary vein.*

   3. *Emissary sphenoidal foramen*

      It is an inconstant foramen present medial to foramen ovale. It transmits emissary vein.
   4. *Foramen spinosum*

      It is lateral to foramen ovale. It transmits:
      – Middle meningeal artery.
      – Nervus spinosus.
   5. *Canaliculus innominatus*

      It is occasionally present between foramen ovale and foramen spinosum. If present, it transmits *lesser petrosal nerve*.

   ii. Lateral surface
   1. It is convex from above downwards.
   2. *Infratemporal crest* is an anteroposterior ridge which divides the lateral surface into an upper *temporal* and a lower *infratemporal* parts.

3. *Temporal surface* forms part of temporal fossa and gives origin to *temporalis muscle*.
4. *Infratemporal surface* forms roof of infratemporal fossa and gives origin to *upper head of lateral pterygoid muscle*. This surface possesses openings of *foramen ovale* and *foramen spinosum*.
5. *Spine of sphenoid* is a projection at the posterior end of lateral surface. It shows following relations and attachments:
   - Tip gives attachment to *sphenomandibular ligament*.
   - Medially it is related to *chorda tympani nerve* and *auditory tube*.
   - Laterally it is related to *auriculotemporal nerve*.

iii. Orbital surface

1. It is quadrilateral in shape.
2. It forms posterior part of the lateral wall of orbit.
3. Its upper serrated edge articulates with orbital plate of frontal bone.
4. Its lateral serrated margin articulates with zygomatic bone.
5. Its inferior smooth border forms the posterolateral boundary of *inferior orbital fissure*.
6. Its medial sharp margin constitutes lower boundary of *superior orbital fissure*. A projection from this border provides attachment to *common tendinous ring*.
7. Below the medial end of superior orbital fissure is a depressed area pierced by *foramen rotundum*.

b. Margins

1. The tip of the greater wing is called *parietal margin*. It articulates with sphenoidal angle of parietal bone at pterion.
2. *Posterior margin* of the greater wing extends from body of sphenoid to its spine. Its medial half forms the anterior boundary of foramen lacerum and receives the opening of pterygoid canal. Its lateral half articulates with the petrous temporal.
3. *Lateral margin* extends forwards from spine to the tip of greater wing. This is also called *squasmosal margin* because it articulates with the squamous part of temporal bone.
4. Medial to the tip there is a *triangular rough area* for the frontal bone.
5. Anterior angle of the triangular area continues with a serrated margin (lateral margin of orbital surface) which articulates with zygomatic bone.

B. Lesser wings

It is a triangular bone extending laterally from the anterosuperior part of the body. It consists of a tip, two roots (anterior and posterior), two surfaces (superior and inferior) and two borders (anterior and posterior).

a. Tip

1. It is the lateral end of lesser wing.
2. It is situated near the lateral end of superior orbital fissure.

b. Roots

1. Lesser wing is connected to body by anterior and posterior roots.
2. The two roots enclose the *optic canal* which transmits *optic nerve* and *ophthalmic artery*.

c. Surfaces

i. Superior surface

It forms posterior part of the floor of anterior cranial fossa.

ii. Inferior surface

It forms superior boundary of superior orbital fissure and posterior part of the orbital roof.

d. Borders
i. Anterior border
It articulates with the posterior border of the orbital plate of the frontal bone.
ii. Posterior border
1. It is free.
2. Its medial end forms the *anterior clinoid process* to which is attached the free margin of tentorium cerebelli.

C. Superior orbital fissure
1. It is a triangular slit like communication between the orbit and middle cranial fossa.
2. **Boundaries**:
   Medial - *Body of sphenoid*
   Apex - *Frontal bone*
   Superior - *Lesser wing of sphenoid.*
   Inferior - *Greater wing of sphenoid.*
3. It transmits the following structures:
   ### a. Structures which enter the orbit
   i. Upper and lower divisions of oculomotor nerve.
   ii. Trochlear nerve.
   iii. Three branches (lacrimal, frontal and nasociliary) of ophthalmic division of trigeminal nerve.
   iv. Abducent nerve.
   v. Orbital branch of middle meningeal artery.
   vi. Sympathetic filaments.
   ### b. Structures which appear from the orbit
   i. Superior and inferior ophthalmic veins.
   ii. Recurrent meningeal branch of lacrimal artery.

III. Pterygoid processes
1. Pterygoid process on each side descends vertically downwards from the junction of body and greater wing of sphenoid.
2. Each consists of *a lateral and a medial pterygoid plate*.
3. The plates unite anteriorly in the upper part to enclose a fossa called *pterygoid fossa*.
4. The plates are not united in the lower portion to form *pterygoid fissure* which is filled by the pyramidal process of palatine bone.
5. Anterior surface of the pterygoid process forms posterior boundary of *pterygopalatine fossa*. Anterior opening of pterygoid canal is located in this region.

Some details of the two pterygoid plates are as follows:

A. Lateral pterygoid plate
It has two surfaces (lateral and medial) and two borders (anterior and posterior).

a. Surfaces
i. Lateral surface
It forms medial wall of infratemporal fossa and gives origin to *lower head of lateral pterygoid muscle*.
ii. Medial surface
It forms lateral wall of pterygoid fossa which gives origin to *deep head of medial pterygoid muscle*.

b. Borders
i. Anterior border
It forms posterior boundary of *pterygomaxillary fissure*.
ii. Posterior border
It is free.

B. Medial pterygoid plate
It has two surfaces (lateral and medial) and two borders (anterior and posterior).

a. Surfaces
i. Lateral surface
It forms medial wall of pterygoid fossa and is related to *tensor palati muscle*.
ii. Medial surface
1. It forms the lateral wall of corresponding posterior nasal aperture.
2. *Vaginal process* is a thin lamina projecting medially from its upper

part under the body of sphenoid. A groove on its anterior part of undersurface completes the *palatovaginal canal* with sphenoidal process of palatine bone. This canal transmits pharyngeal branch of maxillary artery and pharyngeal branch of pterygopalatine ganglion.
3. Vaginal process articulates medially with ala of vomer and forms *vomerovaginal canal* between the two. This canal transmits branches of pharyngeal nerve and vessels.

b. Borders

i. Anterior border
It articulates with the posterior border of perpendicular plate of palatine bone.

ii. Posterior border
1. At its upper end it splits to enclose *scaphoid fossa* which gives origin to *tensor palati muscle*.
2. Its upper end shows a small projection called *pterygoid tubercle* which lies immediately below the posterior end of pterygoid canal.
3. *Pharyngobasilar fascia* is attached to its whole extent while *superior constrictor* arises from its lower part only.
4. A hook like process at its lower end is called *pterygoid hamulus*. Tondon of tensor palati winds round this process. *Superior constrictor and pterygomandibular raphe* are also attached to it.
5. An angular process projecting from the middle of this margin is called *processus tubarius*. Posterior border above this process is called *notch of auditory tube*. This process and notch support the medial end of auditory tube.

OSSIFICATION

1. Sphenoid ossifies partly in membrane and partly in cartilage.
2. Parts ossifying in membrane are as follows:
   i. Greater wings except their roots.
   ii. Pterygoid processes except pterygoid hamuli.
3. Parts ossifying in cartilage are as follows:
   i. Body of sphenoid.
   ii. Lesser wings.
   iii. Sphenoidal conchae.
   iv. Roots of greater wings.
   v. Pterygoid hamuli.
4. From ossification point of view, the sphenoid is divided into presphenoidal and postsphenoidal parts.
   A. Presphenoidal part is comprised of parts lying in front of tuberculum sellae, i.e. anterior part of body, lesser wings and sphenoidal conchae. Two centres appear for each of these components as follows:
   Anterior body - 9th wk of intrauterine life.
   Lesser wings - 9th wk of intrauterine life.
   Conchae - 5th month of intrauterine life.
   B. Rest of the sphenoid is included in postsphenoidal part. Two centres appear for each of the following components of the postsphenoidal part.
   Sella turcica - 4th month of intrauterine life.
   Lingulae - 4th month of intrauterine life.
   Greater wings (including lateral pterygoid plates) – 8th wk of intrauterine life.
   Medial pterygoid plates – 9th wk of intrauterine life.
   Hamuli – 3rd month of intrauterine life.
5. Fusions of different components of sphenoid take place as follows:
   i. Medial and lateral pterygoid plates fuse with each other at about 6th month of intrauterine life.
   ii. Presphenoidal part of the body fuses with the postsphenoidal part of the body at about 8th month of intrauterine life.
   iii. At birth sphenoid is in three parts, a central part consisting of the body and

lesser wings and two lateral parts, each consisting of the greater wing and the pterygoid process.

iv. Greater wing fuses with the body at about 1st year.
v. Concha fuses with the ethmoidal labyrinth at about 4th year.
vi. Concha fuses with the body of sphenoid before puberty.
vii. Body of sphenoid fuses with the basilar part of occipital bone at about 25th year.

APPLIED ANATOMY

1. In the anterior part of hypophyseal fossa there is occasionally a vascular foramen termed as *craniopharyngeal* canal. The canal sometimes extends inferiorly to the exterior of the skull and is said to mark the original position of Rathke's pouch.
2. Premature ossification of sutures between pre- and post-sphenoidal parts and sphenoid and occipital bones is often observed in *achondroplasia*.
3. Anomalous development of the presphenoidal elements may lead to excessive separation of the two orbits (*hypertelorism*).
4. Observation of the sella turcica and the hypophyseal fossa in radiographs is important clinically because they may reflect pathological changes such as *pituitary tumor* or *aneurysm of internal carotid artery*.
5. Decalcification of the dorsum sellae is one of the signs of a generalized *increase in intracranial pressure*.
6. The lateral wall of optic canal is infractured during *optic nerve decompression* in the optic canal.
7. A *fracture of sphenoid bone* may lacerate the optic nerve resulting into blindness.
8. Basilar fracture of skull through the sphenoid bone may lacerate the internal carotid artery resulting into *carotid-cavernous fistula*. This leads to *pulsating exophthalmos*.
9. Collection of air in the cranial cavity (*aerocele*) may occur if the basilar fracture of the skull involves sphenoidal sinus.
10. Involvement of the pterygoid processes of sphenoid is a constant feature in cases of Le Fort fractures of mid-facial skeleton but the location of fracture depends upon its type. In Le Fort I fracture, the lower 3rd of the pterygoid plates is involved while in *Le Fort III fracture* the roots of pterygoid plates are fractured.
11. Large areas of the body and medial pterygoid plates are clothed in mucosa and therefore fractures of these parts of sphenoid may open into nasal cavity or sphenoidal sinus with *potential risk of infection*.

CHAPTER 37

The Palatine Bones

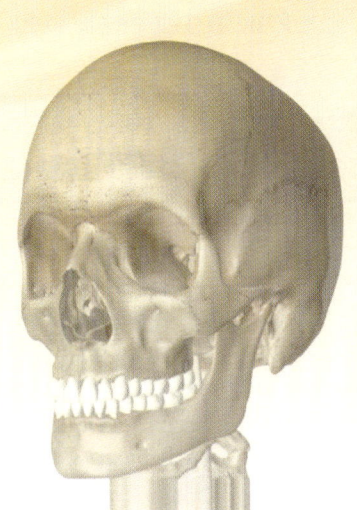

TERMINOLOGY

'Palatine' bone is so named because of its contribution to the 'hard palate'. The word 'palate' is derived from 'plate' because it forms 'plate-like' partition between nasal and oral cavities.

LOCATION

Each palatine bone is located between the maxilla and pterygoid process of sphenoid in the posterior part of nasal cavity.

FEATURES AND ATTACHMENTS

Each palatine bone is 'L' shaped in appearance and consists of two plates (horizontal and perpendicular) and three processes (pyramidal, orbital and sphenoidal).

I. Plates

A. Horizontal plate

It projects medially from the lower end of perpendicular plate. It has two surfaces (nasal and palatine) and four borders (anterior, posterior, lateral and medial).

a. Surfaces

i. Nasal surface
1. It faces superiorly.
2. It is concave from side to side.
3. It forms posterior part of the floor of nasal cavity.

ii. Palatine surface
1. It faces inferiorly.
2. With the corresponding surface of the opposite side, it forms posterior 1/4th of the hard palate.
3. Near its posterior border, this surface presents a curved ridge called *palatine crest*. This crest and the area behind it gives attachment to *palatine aponeurosis*.

b. Borders

i. Anterior border
It articulates with the posterior border of palatine process of maxilla to form *palatomaxillary suture*.

ii. Posterior border
1. It is concave.
2. It is free.
3. This gives attachment to *palatine aponeurosis* (the aponeurosis is also attached to palatine crest and the area behind it).
4. Its medial end projects backwards and with that of opposite side forms *posterior nasal spine*. To this spine is attached the *musculus uvulae*.

iii. Lateral border
1. It is attached to the lower border of perpendicular plate.
2. Its lower end is marked by greater palatine groove.

iv. Medial border
1. It articulates with that of opposite bone to form *interpalatine suture*.
2. Articulating medial borders of horizontal plates of two palatine bones project upwards to form *nasal crest*.
3. Nasal crest articulates with the posterior part of lower border of vomer and is continuous anteriorly with the nasal crests of maxillae.

B. Perpendicular plate

It has two surfaces (maxillary and nasal) and four borders (anterior, posterior, superior and inferior).

a. Surfaces

i. Maxillary surface (Fig. 37.1)
1. It faces laterally.
2. Its major part is rough to articulate with the nasal surface of maxilla.

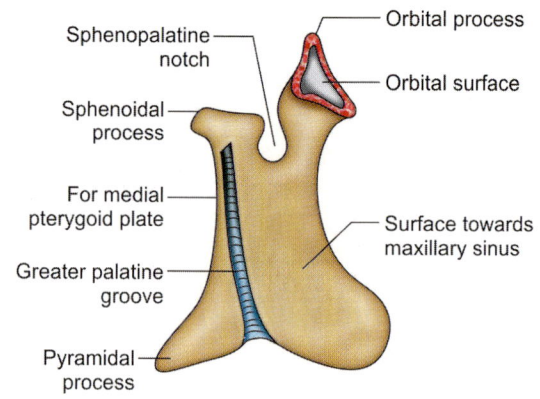

Fig. 37.1: Right palatine bone : Lateral aspect

3. Its upper and posterior part is smooth and forms medial wall of *pterygopalatine fossa*.
4. Its anterior part is also smooth and forms posterior part of medial wall of *maxillary sinus*.
5. Its posterior part shows a vertical groove (*greater palatine groove*) which is converted into *greater palatine canal* by maxilla in articulated skull. *Greater palatine vessels and nerve* pass through greater palatine canal.

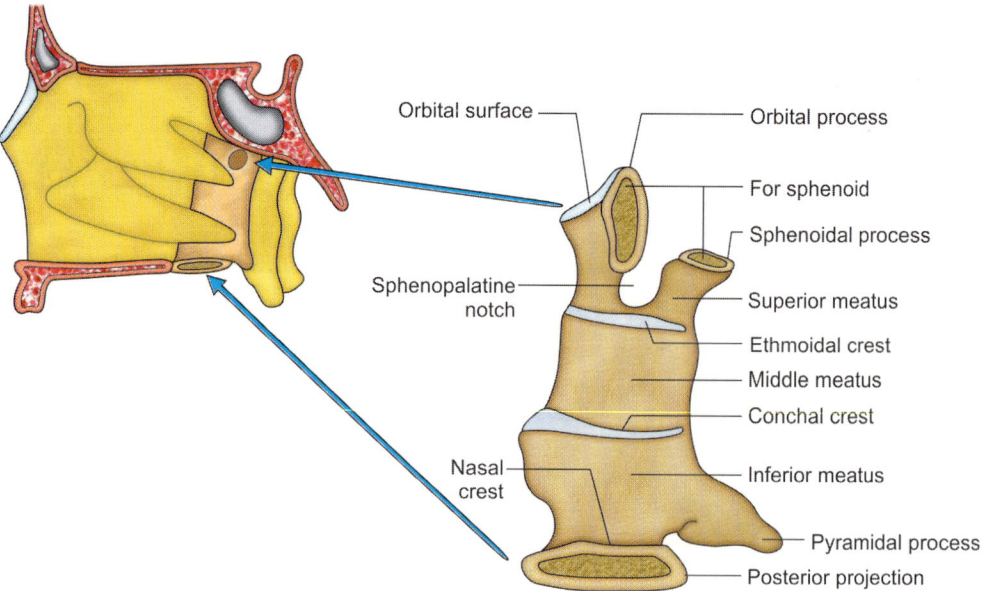

Fig. 37.2: Right palatine bone: Medial aspect

ii. Nasal surface (Fig. 37.2)
1. It faces medially.
2. It has two horizontal crests. The lower crest is called the *conchal crest* because it articulates with the inferior concha. The upper one is named as the *ethmoidal crest* because of its articulation with the middle concha of ethmoid.
3. The area below the conchal crest forms *inferior meatus* of nose.
4. The area between the two crests contributes to *middle meatus* of nose.
5. The area above the ethmoidal crest takes part in the formation of *superior meatus* of nose.

b. Borders
i. Anterior border
1. Its lower part articulates with the maxillary process of inferior concha and assists in the formation of medial wall of maxillary sinus.
2. Its upper part forms the posterior boundary of maxillary hiatus.

ii. Posterior border
It articulates with the anterior border of medial pterygoid plate of sphenoid.

iii. Superior border
1. It supports the *orbital process* in front and *sphenoidal process* behind.
2. Between the orbital and sphenoidal processes is the *sphenopalatine notch* which is converted into *sphenopalatine foramen* by the inferior surface of the body of sphenoid.
3. Sphenopalatine foramen is the communication between pterygopalatine fossa and the posterior part of superior meatus of nose.
4. Sphenopalatine foramen transmits *sphenopalatine vessels* and *posterior superior nasal nerves*.

iv. Inferior border
1. It is continuous with the lateral border of horizontal plate.
2. In front of pyramidal process it is marked by lower end of greater palatine groove.

II. Processes (Figs 37.1 to 37.3)
A. Pyramidal process
1. It projects downwards, backwards and laterally from the junction of two plates of palatine bone.
2. It fits into pterygoid fissure of pterygoid process of sphenoid.
3. Its posterior surface completes the lower part of pterygoid fossa.
4. Its lateral surface is rough anteriorly and smooth posteriorly. The rough part articulates with maxillary tuberosity. Smooth part forms the lower part of infratemporal fossa.
5. Its inferior surface presents *lesser palatine foramina* for *lesser palatine nerves and vessels*.

B. Orbital process
It projects upwards and laterally from the anterior part of upper border of perpendicular plate. A constricted neck connects it with the

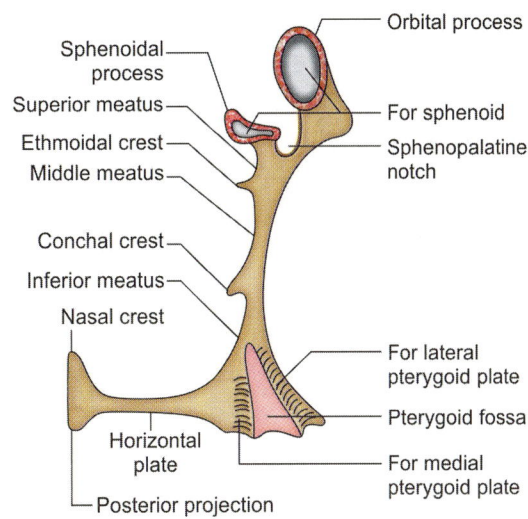

Fig. 37.3: Right palatine bone: Posterior aspect

perpendicular plate. It has three articular surfaces (anterior, posterior and medial) and two non-articular surfaces (superior and lateral)

a. *Articular surfaces*

   i. **Anterior surface**

   It articulates with maxilla.

   ii. **Posterior surface**

   It articulates with sphenoidal body.

   iii. **Medial surface**

   It articulates with ethmoidal bulla.

b. *Non-articular surfaces*

   i. **Superior surface**

   It forms posterior part of the floor of orbit.

   ii. **Lateral surface**

   It forms part of the medial wall of pterygopalatine fossa.

   The border between lateral and posterior surfaces is prolonged downwards as anterior boundary of *sphenopalatine notch*.

C. *Sphenoidal process*

It is directed upwards and medially from the posterior part of upper border of perpendicular plate. It has three surfaces (superior, inferomedial and lateral) and three borders (posterior, anterior and medial).

a. *Surfaces*

   i. **Superior surface**

   1. It articulates with under surface of sphenoidal concha and root of medial pterygoid plate.
   2. It is grooved to complete the *palatovaginal canal*.

   ii. **Inferomedial surface**

   It contributes to the roof and lateral wall of nasal cavity.

   iii. **Lateral surface**

   1. Its posterior part articulates with medial pterygoid plate.

   2. Its anterior part contributes to the medial wall of pterygopalatine fossa.

b. *Borders*

   i. **Posterior border**

   It articulates with the vaginal process of medial pterygoid plate.

   ii. **Anterior border**

   It forms posterior boundary of *sphenopalatine notch*.

   iii. **Medial border**

   It articulates with ala of vomer.

OSSIFICATION

1. Palatine bone ossifies in membrane.
2. Single centre appears in the perpendicular plate during 8th week of intrauterine life.
3. The ossification spreads into the processes and horizontal plate.
4. At birth the height of perpendicular plate is equal to the transverse width of horizontal plate.
5. Length of perpendicular plate becomes double the transverse width of horizontal plate at puberty.

APPLIED ANATOMY

1. Palatine bone may be involved in fracture of mid-facial skeleton.
2. Palatine bone receives adequate blood supply from periosteal arteries and therefore all the fragments of fractured bone retain a periosteal blood supply.
3. Palatine bone is clothed in mucosa over large areas of its surfaces. Its fracture may open into the nasal or oral cavities or maxillary sinus with potential risk of infection.
4. Le Fort fractures of midfacial skeleton always involve the perpendicular plates of palatine bones. Guerin's fracture (Le Fort I

fracture) involves lower 1/3rd of the perpendicular plates of palatine bones. In cases of Le Fort II and III fractures, upper parts of the perpendicular plates are affected.

5. Horizontal plate of palatine bone may be fractured in uncommon central split of the palate. It is actually paramedian in nature because median sutures (intermaxillary and interpalatine) are relatively strong (Fig. 37.4).

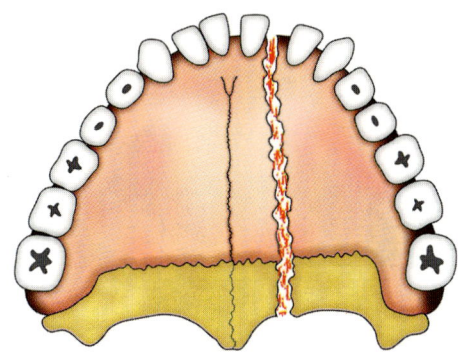

Fig. 37.4: Central split of palate

CHAPTER

38 | The Skull (General Features)

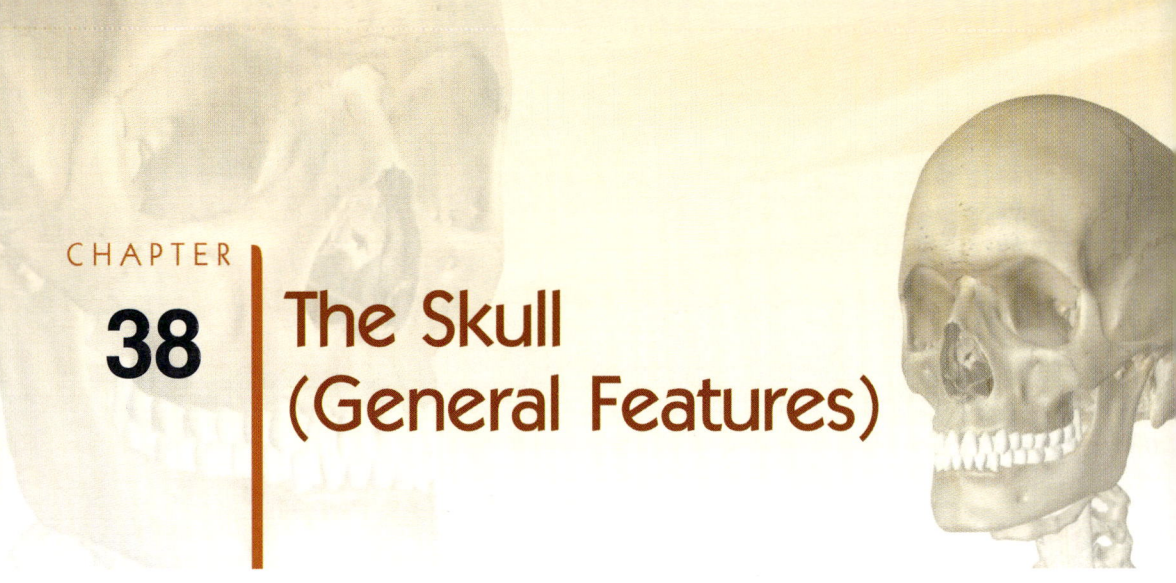

INTRODUCTION (Fig. 38.1)

1. Skull is the skeleton of the head.
2. Cranium means skull minus the mandible.
3. Neurocranium is upper part of skull which encloses the brain
4. Calvaria is the upper part of the cranium. It is also called as the skull cap.
5. Facial skeleton (viscerocranium) is skull minus the calvaria.
6. Facial skeleton is further divided into upper facial skeleton and lower facial skeleton (mandible).

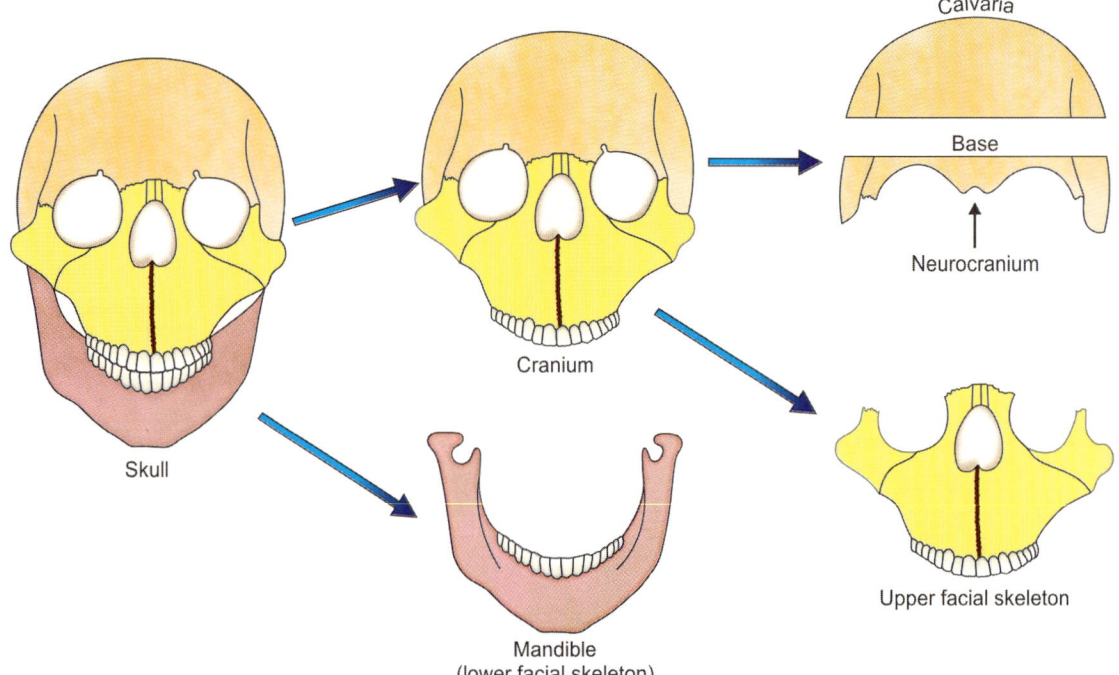

Fig. 38.1: Subdivisions of skull

NEUROCRANIUM

The bones which constitute the neurocranium can be classified as:

A. Paired bones
These include:
  a. Parietal bones.
  b. Temporal bones.

B. Unpaired bones
These include:
  a. Frontal bone.
  b. Occipital bone.
  c. Sphenoid.
  d. Ethmoid.

FACIAL SKELETON (VISCEROCRANIUM OR SPLANCHNOCRANIUM)

It is composed of following bones:

A. Paired bones
These include:
  a. Maxillae.
  b. Zygomatic bones.
  c. Nasal bones.
  d. Lacrimal bones.
  e. Palatine bones.
  f. Inferior conchae.

B. Unpaired bones
These include:
  a. Mandible.
  b. Vomer.

ANATOMICAL POSITION OF SKULL (Fig. 38.2)

Skull can be kept in normal anatomical position by Reid's baseline or Frankfurt's horizontal plane.

A. Reid's baseline
It is a horizontal line formed by the joining of infraorbital margin with the centre of the external acoustic meatus.

B. Frankfurt's horizontal plane
It is marked by the horizontal line joining the infraorbital margin with the upper margin of the external acoustic meatus.

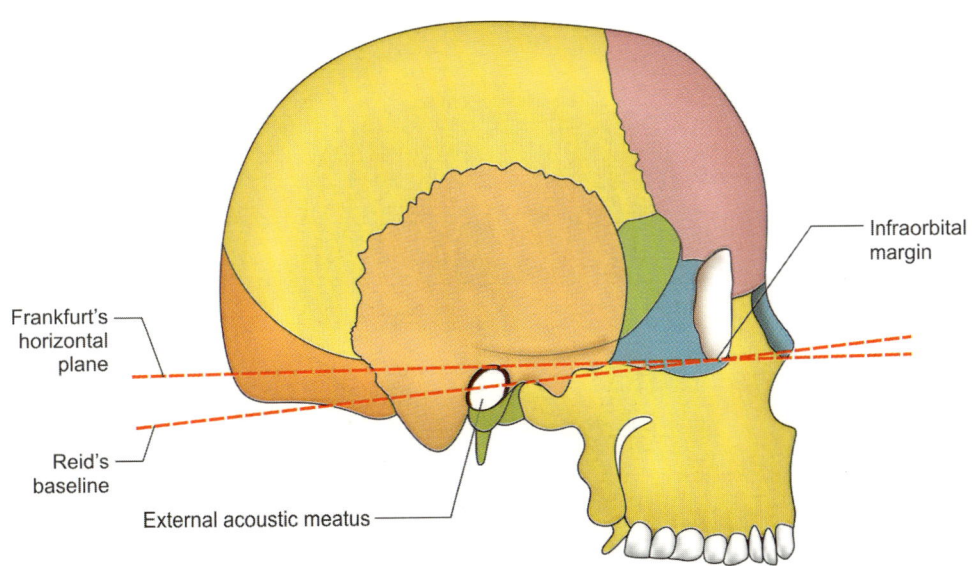

Fig. 38.2: Skull in relation to horizontal planes

> **Note:** Remember that Reid's starts with 'R' which also stands for 'Round' opening of external acoustic meatus, thus Reid's baseline passes through the rounded external acoustic meatus. On the other hand 'Frankfurt' starts with 'F' which also stands for 'Fly' and anything that has to fly has to be above, therefore, Frankfurt's horizontal plane passes above the external acoustic meatus.

APPLIED ANATOMY

Clinically the entire front of skull is considered to be facial skeleton. It is further divided into following three parts (Fig. 38.3):

I. Upper facial skeleton
1. It forms the skeleton of forehead.
2. It is comprised of frontal bone.

II. Lower facial skeleton
1. It forms the skeleton of the lower jaw.
2. It is comprised of mandible.

III. Middle facial skeleton

It is the complex middle 3rd of the facial skeleton. The region is of great clinical importance because the multiple bones constituting it are frequently involved in fractures.

A. Boundaries
a. *Upper*: Transverse line passing through fronto-zygomatic, frontomaxillary and frontonasal sutures.
b. *Lower*: Incisal edge and occlusal plane.
c. *Posterior*: Spheno-ethmoidal junction.

B. Bones involved in the fractures of middle 3rd of the facial skeleton are as follows:
1. Maxillae.
2. Palatine bones.
3. Zygomatic bones.
4. Zygomatic processes of temporal bones.
5. Nasal bones.
6. Lacrimal bones.
7. Vomer.
8. Ethmoid.
9. Pterygoid processes of sphenoid.

C. Subdivisions (Fig. 38.4)
The middle 3rd facial skeleton can be divided into:

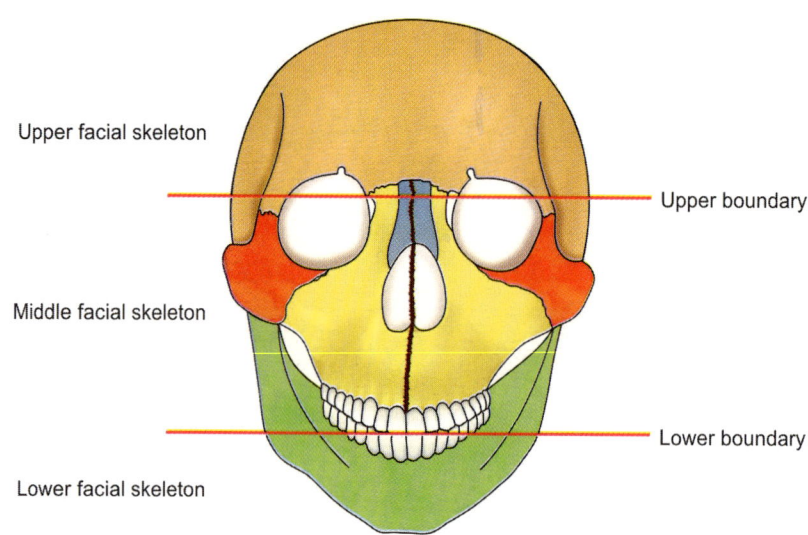

Fig. 38.3: Subdivisions of facial skeleton

The Skull (General Features)

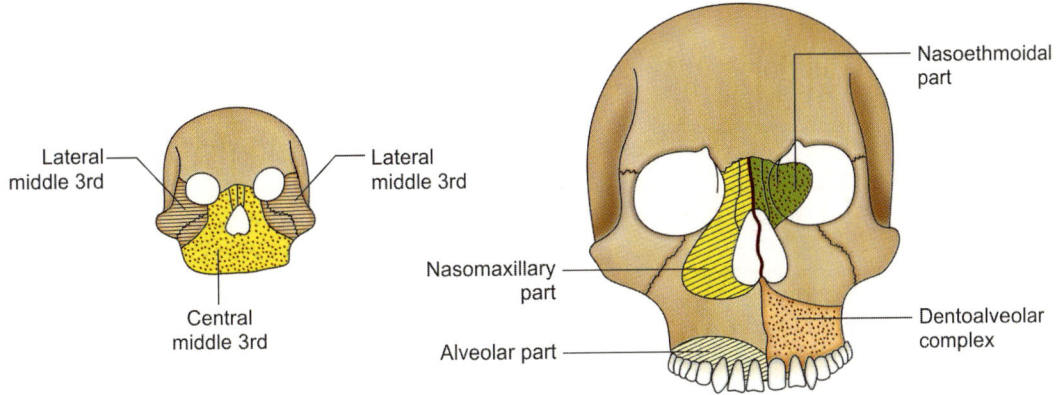

Fig. 38.4: Clinical subdivisions of middle 3rd of facial skeleton

a. **Lateral middle 3rd** also called zygomatico-maxillary part.
b. **Central middle 3rd,** which can be further subdivided into:

i. Alveolar part.
ii. Dento-alveolar complex.
iii. Naso-maxillary part.
iv. Naso-ethmoidal part.

CHAPTER 39
The Exterior of the Skull

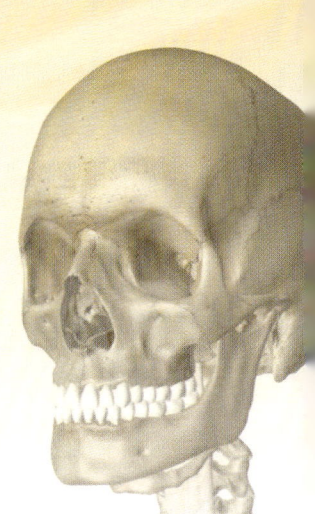

Different views of skull are considered from the description point of view. These are as follows:
- I. **Norma verticalis** – This is superior view.
- II. **Norma occipitalis** – This is posterior view.
- III. **Norma frontalis** – This is anterior view.
- IV. **Norma lateralis** – This is lateral (side) view.
- V. **Norma basalis** – This is inferior view.

I. NORMA VERTICALIS

Definition
Observation of skull from superior aspect is called norma verticalis.

Shape
Norma verticalis view of skull appears ovoid in shape. It is relatively wider posteriorly.

Bones
The following bones contribute to the norma verticalis:
1. *Frontal bone (frontal squama)* – It lies anteriorly.
2. *Occipital bone (squamous part)* – It lies posteriorly.
3. *Parietal bones (paired)* – These lie on each side of midline.

Junctions of Bones (sutures)
1. Sutures are the immovable joints of skull which are fibrous in nature.
2. In norma verticalis following sutures can be seen:
   i. *Coronal suture*: It is between frontal and parietal bones.
   ii. *Sagittal suture:* It is between the two parietal bones.
   iii. *Lambdoid suture:* It is between occipital and two parietal bones.

Features (Fig. 39.1)
a. Vertex
It is the highest point on sagittal suture.

b. Vault
It is the arched roof of skull.

c. Bregma
1. It is situated at the intersection between coronal and sagittal sutures.
2. Bregma is the site of a membranous gap in the foetal skull. This gap is known as *anterior fontanelle*.
3. Anterior fontanelle closes by 18 months.

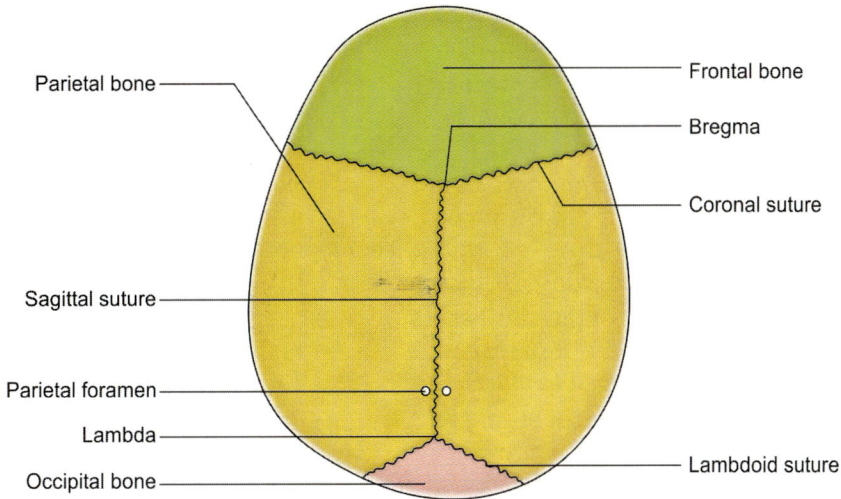

Fig. 39.1: The skull : Norma verticalis

d. Lambda
1. It is situated at the intersection of sagittal and lambdoid sutures.
2. In foetal skull there is a membranous gap at the site of lambda. This gap is known as *posterior fontanelle*.
3. Posterior fontanelle closes by 2–3 months.

e. Parietal foramen
It pierces the parietal bone on each side of midline about 3.5 cm in front of lambda. *Emissary vein* passes through it.

f. Obelion
It is the region on the sagittal suture between two parietal foramina.

g. Parietal eminence
It is the area of maximum convexity of the parietal bone.

h. Temporal lines
1. There are two temporal lines on each side:
   i. *Superior temporal line.*
   ii. *Inferior temporal line.*
2. Both the temporal lines start as single line from the zygomatic process of frontal bone.
3. The two lines arch backwards and upwards and cross the frontal bone, coronal suture and parietal bone.
4. Superior temporal line fades out in the posterior part of parietal bone.
5. *Epicranial aponeourosis* and temporal fascia are attached to superior temporal line.
6. Inferior temporal line marks the upper limit of the origin of *temporalis muscle*.

Applied anatomy
1. Fontanelles serve two important purposes:
   i. They allow moulding during birth.
   ii. They allow the brain to grow.
2. The presence of *anterior fontanelle* is both clinically and therapeutically very significant.
   i. A buldge indicates increased intracranial tension (*e.g. in case of brain tumour*).
   ii. An abnormal depression indicates excessive loss of fluid (*e.g. in case of bleeding and dehydration*).
   iii. Diagnostic and therapeutic punctures could be carried out through anterior fontanelle.

iv. Ultrasonography of brain in infants is performed through anterior fontanelle.
3. The osseous closure of the anterior fontanelle is an important milestone in the normal development of a child.
4. Soft and pliable bones of neonate can withstand considerable amount of compression and moulding, a fact clinically important during child birth.
5. In neonates the flat bones of the vault are very soft and therefore a depressed fracture is like a dimple (*pond fracture*).
6. In adult there is some amount of elasticity in flat vault bones which often prevents fractures in cases of minor trauma. But if the trauma force exceeds the minimal elasticity, fractures are bound to occur.
7. In adult a *depressed fracture* always shows an irregular line of fracture at the periphery of depressed area.
8. Almost invariably all fractures of the vault of skull in children are associated with the rupture of the dura mater.
9. When skull is compressed between two hard surfaces an axial shortening takes place along the line of the force and an axial lengthening takes place at right angle to it. This results in fracture of distant poles of the skull far from the actual site of application of force (Fig. 39.2).
10. *Fracture* of the skull is usually due to direct blow. A forceful hit on the forehead may cause linear fracture of vertex (Fig. 39.3).
11. Cranium is clinically important because it reflects the size of the brain. *Macrocephaly* (enlargement of head) can be due to hydrocephalus. *Microcephaly* may be hereditary or due to maldevelopment of brain.
12. Because of the lack of regenerating capacity of the flat bones of the vault, a gap in it should be filled with *tantalum* or *titanium*.

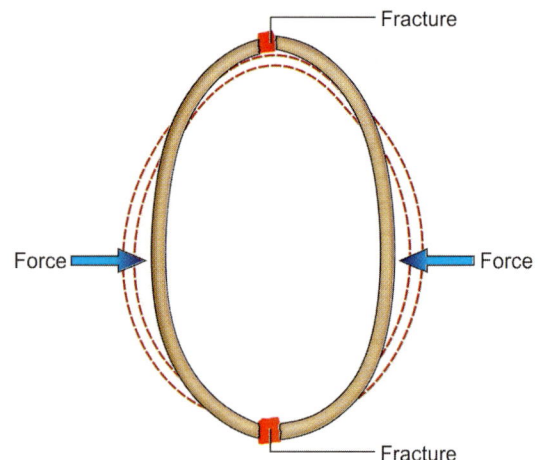

Fig. 39.2: Axial deformity of skull due to compression

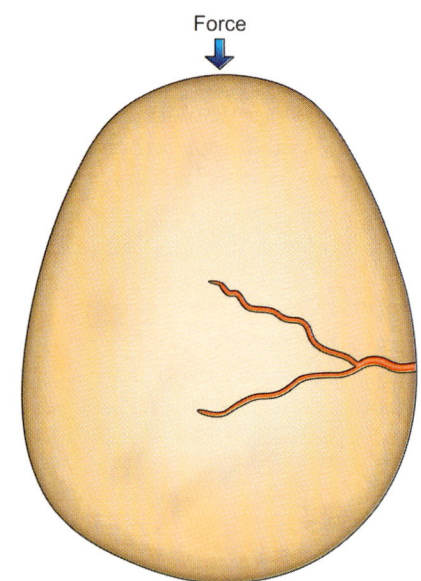

Fig. 39.3: Linear fracture of vertex

II. NORMA OCCIPITALIS

Definition

When the skull is observed from posterior aspect, it is known as norma occipitalis.

Shape
Norma occipitalis is convex upwards and flat below.

Bones
Following bones contribute to the norma occipitalis.
1. Parietal bones (paired).
2. Squamous part of occipital bone (unpaired).
3. Mastoid parts of temporal bones (paired).

Sutures
a. Posterior part of sagittal suture
b. Lambdoid suture
1. It is between the two parietal bones and the occipital bone.
2. The lower end of lambdoid suture meets with the mastoid portion of temporal bone at a point which forms the junction of *occipitomastoid* and *parietomastoid sutures*.

c. Occipitomastoid suture
It is situated between the occipital bone and the mastoid part of the temporal bone.

d. Parietomastoid suture
It is situated between the parietal bone and the mastoid part of the temporal bone.

Features (Fig. 39.4)
a. External occipital protuberance
1. It is a midline protuberance on the lower part of norma occipitalis.
2. It marks the junction of head and neck posteriorly.
3. *Inion* is the most prominent point of external occipital protuberance.
4. *Trapezius* originates from the upper part of external occipital protuberance.
5. *Ligamentum nuchae* is attached to the lower part of this protuberance.

b. Superior nuchal lines
1. These are curved ridges passing laterally from the external occipital protuberance.

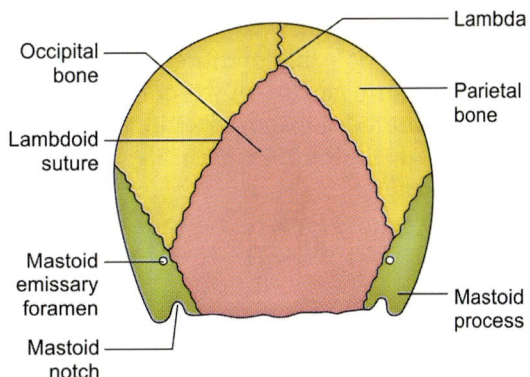

Fig. 39.4: The skull : Norma occipitalis

2. These form junction of head and neck posteriorly.
3. *Trapezius* originates from the medial 1/3rd of superior nuchal line.
4. *Sternomastoid* is inserted on the lateral part of superior nuchal line.
5. *Splenius capitis* is also inserted on the lateral part of this line below the attachment of sternomastoid.

c. Highest nuchal lines
1. These are situated about a 'cm' above the superior nuchal lines.
2. *Epicranial aponeurosis* is attached to their medial parts.
3. *Occipital belly of occipitofrontalis* originates on each side from its lateral 2/3rd.

d. Mastoid foramen
1. It is located near the occipitomastoid suture.
2. It opens internally into the sigmoid sulcus.
3. Following structures transverse through it:
   i. Meningeal branch of occipital artery.
   ii. Emissary vein.

e. Occipital point
1. It is situated in the midline a little above the inion.
2. It is farthest from glabella.

Applied anatomy

1. *Craniostenosis* is the condition in which there is premature closure of the cranial sutures. When lambdoid and coronal sutures are involved, skull grows vertically leading to *tower skull*.
2. The squamous part of the occipital bone is prone to both *fissured and depressed fractures*.
3. A cack in the inner table of squamous part of occipital bone may damage the large diploeic vein and produce small *epidural haematoma*.
4. Almost invariably fractures of the occipital squama in children are associated with *rupture of the dura mater*.
5. A gap in the occipital squama is usually filled with *tantalum or titanium* due to lack of regeneration in this part whose periosteum is devoid of cambium layer.
6. Inner table of cranial vault bones (including squamous part of occipital bone) is more brittle than the outer table, therefore, fractures are more extensive in the inner table.

III. NORMA FRONTALIS

Definition

When the skull is observed from the anterior aspect it is known as norma frontalis.

Shape

It is oval in shape being wider above than below.

Bones

Major bones contributing to the surface features of norma frontalis (excluding bones contributing to deeper orbits, nasal cavity and oral cavity) are as follows:
1. Frontal bone (unpaired).
2. Maxillae (paired).
3. Nasal bones (paired).
4. Zygomatic bones (paired).
5. Mandible (unpaired).

Junctions of Bones (Sutures)

a. Junction between zygomatic process of frontal bone and frontal process of zygomatic bone is called *frontozygomatic suture*. It is observed along the lateral margin of orbital opening.
b. Junction between nasal part of frontal bone and frontal process of maxilla (*frontomaxillary suture*) is observed along the medial margin of orbital opening in its upper part.
c. Junction between nasal part of frontal bone and nasal bones are called *fronto-nasal sutures*.
d. Junction between two nasal bones is a midline suture just above the anterior nasal aperture. This is called *internasal suture*.
e. Junction between maxilla and zygomatic bone (*zygomaticomaxillary suture*) is an oblique suture extending downwards and laterally from the lower border of each orbital opening.
f. Junction between two maxillae is called *intermaxillary suture*. It is a midline suture just below the anterior nasal aperture.

Note: *Intermaxillary suture is also observed in hard palate between palatine processes of two maxillae.*

Features (Fig. 39.5)

A. Three large apertures

One anterior nasal aperture and two orbital openings form the most striking feature of the norma frontalis.

a. Anterior nasal aperture

1. It is a midline aperture.
2. It is piriform in shape and wider below than above.
3. Its upper boundary is formed by lower borders of nasal bones.
4. Its lateral and inferior boundaries are contributed by nasal notches of two maxillae.

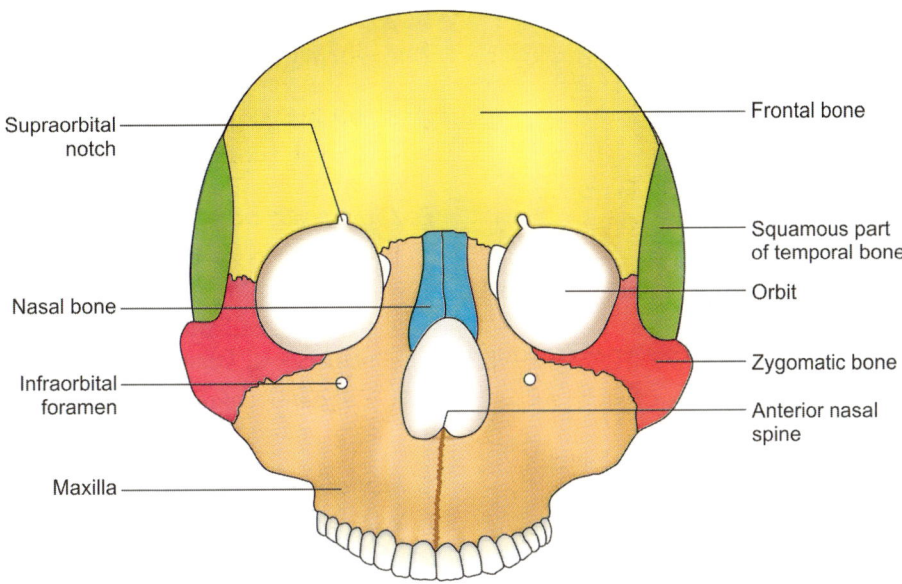

Fig. 39.5: The skull : Norma frontalis

5. *Anterior nasal spine* is a sharp projection at the lower margin of nasal aperture, in the midline.
6. *Rhinion* is the lower end of internasal suture.
7. A notch at the inferior border of nasal bone is meant for passage of *external nasal nerve*.
8. Margins of aperture give attachments to the *nasal cartilages*.

b. Orbital openings

Each is present above and lateral to the anterior nasal aperture. It is quadrangular in shape and possesses four margins (supraorbital, infraorbital, lateral and medial).

  i. *Supraorbital margin*
  1. It is formed by frontal bone.
  2. *Supraorbital notch (or foramen)* is situated at the junction of medial 1/3rd (rounded) and lateral 2/3rd (sharp) of supraorbital margin.
  3. Supraorbital notch transmits *supraorbital nerve and artery and a communicating vein between angular and superior ophthalmic veins*.

  ii. *Infraorbital margin*
  It is formed by *maxilla* medially and *zygomatic bone* laterally.

  iii. *Lateral orbital margin*
  It is formed by the *frontal process* of zygomatic bone below and the *zygomatic process of frontal bone* above.

  iv. *Medial orbital margin*
  It is formed by the *frontal bone* above and the *lacrimal crest of frontal process of maxilla* below.

B. Frontal region

a. Superciliary arch

It is curved elevation above the medial part of the supraorbital margin.

b. Glabella

It is median elevation between two superciliary arches.

c. Nasion

It is the junction of internasal and frontonasal sutures.

d. Frontal eminence (frontal tuber)
It is rounded elevation above each superciliary arch.

C. Maxillae
Each maxilla shows following features:

a. Infraorbital foramen
1. It is situated about 1 cm below the infraorbital margin.
2. *Infraorbital nerve and vessels* pass through infraorbital foramen.

b. Incisive fossa
It is situated above the incisor teeth.

c. Canine eminence
It is produced by the root of canine tooth.

d. Canine fossa
It is situated just lateral to canine eminence.

e. Frontal process
It is sandwiched between nasal bone and lacrimal bone.

f. Zygomatic process
It articulates with the zygomatic bone.

g. Alveolar process
It bears the sockets for the upper teeth.

D. Zygomatic bones
1. Each bone is situated below and lateral to the orbital opening.
2. It is marked by a foramen called *zygomaticofacial foramen*.
3. *Zygomaticofacial nerve* traverses the zygomaticofacial foramen.

E. Mandible
It forms the lower facial skeleton. For details of the features please consult the description of individual bone.

Attachments (Fig. 39.6)
A. Nasal bone – *Procerus*
B. Superciliary arch – *Corrugator supercilii*
C. Frontal process of maxilla.

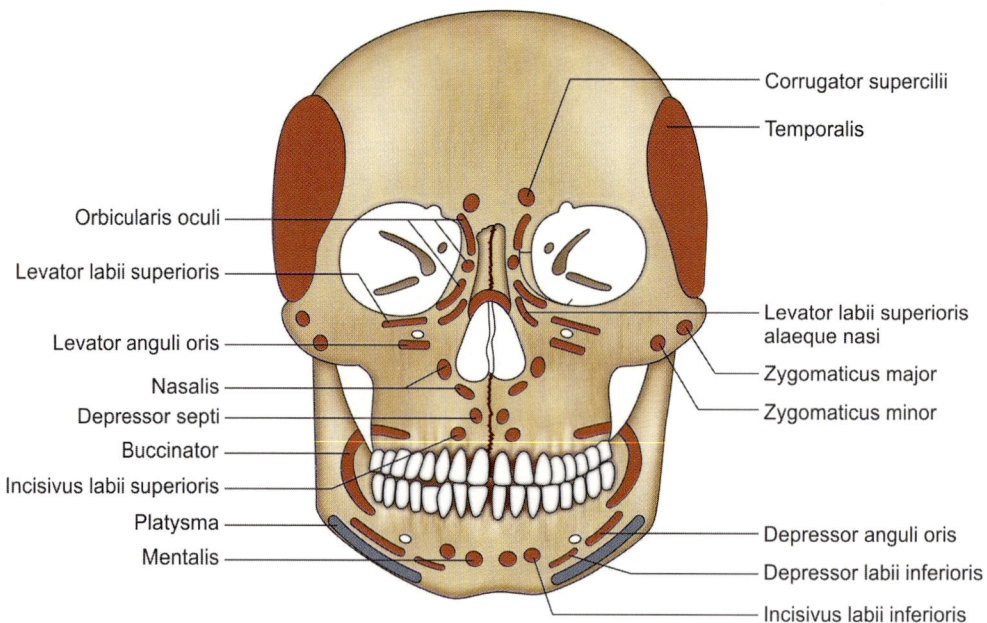

Fig. 39.6: Attachments on skull – Norma frontalis

1. *Orbital part of orbicularis oculi* (it is also attached to nasal part of frontal bone).
2. *Medial palpebral ligament.*
3. *Levator babii superioris alaeque nasi.*
D. Between infraorbital margin and infraorbital foramen-*Levator labii superioris.*
E. Below the infraorbital foramen (to canine fossa) – *Levator anguli oris.*
F. Zygomatic bone just below the zygomaticofacial foramen –*Zygomaticus minor.*
G. Lateral to zygomaticus minor – *Zygomaticus major.*
H. Adjacent to nasal notch – *Nasalis* (transverse part above and alar part below).
I. Incisive fossa.
   Medially – *Depressor septi*
   Laterally – *Incisivus labii superioris.*
J. Alveolar process of maxilla opposite to molar teeth – *Buccinator.*
K. Mandible – Please consult the description of individual bone.

Applied anatomy

1. In about 8% of adult skulls a remnant of lower part of the suture between two halves of frontal bone (*metopic suture*) may persist. This suture is some times confused for a fracture in radiograph.
2. Superciliary arches are elevated ridges from the surface of bone and any injury in this region will cause laceration of skin and severe bleeding.
3. Compression of supraorbital nerves causes nerve pain. This fact may be used by anaesthetists to determine the depth of anesthesia.
4. If the fracture of the frontal bone involves inner table forming the roof of the frontal sinus, then the air may enter the cranial cavity (*aerocele*) causing meningitis or brain abscess.
5. An impact on the nose directed in the anteroposterior plane will cause a depression of the nasal bridge due to fracture of nasal bones, frontal processes of maxillae and septal cartilage.
6. A force on the nasal bridge directed from the lateral aspect will result in a deviation of the nasal bridge to opposite side.
7. Traumatic alteration in the shape of nose because of fractures of nasal bones is of great clinical importance due to cosmetic reasons specially in young females.
8. A severe impact on the nasal bridge may involve frontal processes of maxillae.
9. Mid-facial skeleton is commonly involved in facial injuries. It includes maxillae, zygomatic bones, nasal bones and most of the bones which form nasal cavity.
10. Mid-facial skeleton receives adequate blood supply from periosteal arteries and therefore all the fragments of fractured bone retain a periosteal blood supply.
11. Fractures of maxillae and zygomatic bones show a constant pattern. Le Fort has classified such fractures into three types (Fig. 39.7):

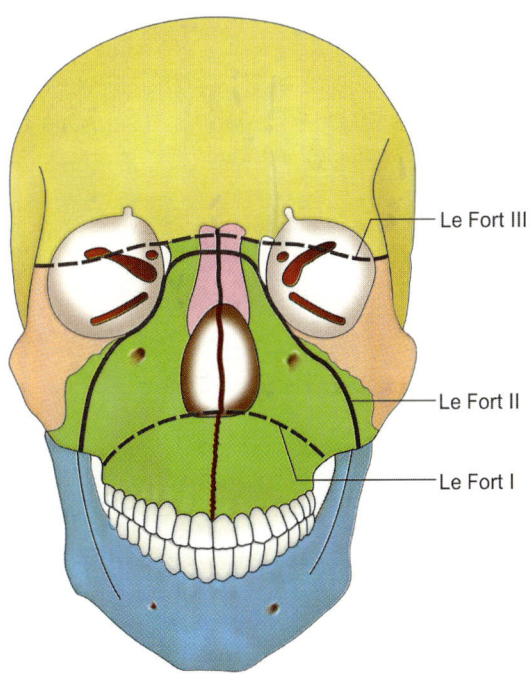

Fig. 39.7: Common fractures of maxillae and other bones of skull

i. *Le Fort I fracture (Guerin's fracture)*
   It shows fractures of lower 3rd of nasal septum, maxillae and lower 3rd of pterygoid plates.
ii. Le Fort II fracture
   It includes fractures of nasal bones, frontal processes of maxillae, lacrimal bones, ethmoid, vomer and pterygoid plates.
iii. Le Fort III fracture
   In this fracture facial skeleton is separated from skull base. It involves upper parts of nasal bones, frontal processes of maxillae, ethmoid, lesser wings of sphenoid and roots of pterygoid plates.
12. Zygomatic bone is very commonly involved in cases of fractures of middle 3rd of face. Fracture of the frontal process of the zygomatic bone may occur in conjunction with a comminuted fracture of the orbital rim and frontal bone.
13. Any of the four margins of the orbit may fracture as isolated fracture or in combination.

Note: *For applied anatomy of mandible and other bones of norma frontalis, discussion on individual bone may be consulted.*

IV. NORMA LATERALIS

Definition
When skull is observed from side, it constitutes norma lateralis.

Bones
Following bones can be visualized in this view:
1. Frontal.
2. Parietal.
3. Occipital.
4. Nasal.
5. Zygomatic.
6. Temporal.
7. Sphenoid.
8. Maxilla.

Features and attachments (Fig. 39.8)
A. Temporal lines
There are two temporal lines, superior and inferior.

a. Superior temporal line
1. It commences at frontal process of zygomatic bone.
2. It arches upwards and backwards across parietal bone.

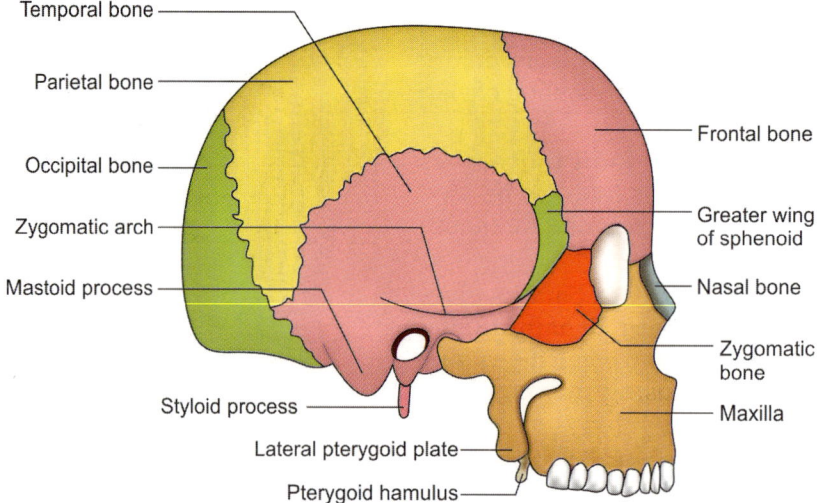

Fig. 39.8: The skull : Norma lateralis

3. It fades away on temporal bone.
4. *Temporal fasia* is attached to it.

b. Inferior temporal line
1. It commences at the same point.
2. It runs inferior and parallel to the superior temporal line.
3. Posteriorly it curves downwards and forwards on the temporal bone to continue with supramastoid crest.
4. It limits the attachment of *temporalis muscle*.

B. Temporal fossa
i. Boundaries
1. Anteriorly – *Zygomatic bone.*
2. Superiorly – *Superior temporal line.*
3. Posteriorly – *Superior temporal line.*
   – *Supramastoid crest.*
4. Inferiorly – *Zygomatic arch.*

ii. Anterior wall of the fossa is formed by:
1. *Temporal surface of zygomatic bone.*
2. *Greater wing of sphenoid.*
3. *Frontal bone.*

iii. Its floor is formed by following bones:
1. *Frontal.*
2. *Parietal.*
3. *Temporal.*
4. *Greater wing of sphenoid.*

iv. Temporalis muscle is attached to the floor and inferior temporal line.

v. Other contents of fossa are:
1. *Middle temporal artery* (a branch of superficial temporal artery).
2. *Deep temporal arteries* arising from maxillary artery.
3. *Zygomaticotemporal nerve and a minute artery* appears from the zygomaticotemporal foramen located on the temporal surface of zygomatic bone.
4. *Deep temporal nerves* arising from mandibular nerve.

C. Pterion
1. It is a circular area in the anterior part of temporal fossa which encloses four bones, frontal, parietal, sphenoid and temporal. These four bones form an 'H' shaped suture.
2. It is located 4 cm above the zygomatic arch and 3.5 cm behind the fronto-zygomatic suture.
3. *Middle meningeal vein, anterior branch of middle meningeal artery* and *stem of the lateral sulcus of brain* lie deep to pterion.

D. Zygomatic arch
1. It is formed by the *temporal process of zygomatic bone* and *zygomatic process of temporal bone.*
2. It has two surfaces (outer and inner) and two borders (upper and lower).
3. Its outer surface is subcutaneous and crossed by following structures from posterior to anterior:
   i. *Auriculotemporal nerve.*
   ii. *Superficial temporal vein.*
   iii. *Superficial temporal artery.*
4. *Masseter* originates from its inner surface and lower border.
5. *Temporal fascia* is attached to its upper border.
6. Posterior end of lower border is marked by *tubercle of root of zygoma.* To this is attached *lateral ligament of temporomandibular joint.*
7. Roots of zygomatic arch diverge from tubercle. Anterior root (*articular tubercle*) passes medially in front of mandibular fossa. Posterior root continues with *supramastoid crest.*

E. External acoustic meatus
1. It is located behind the mandibular fossa below the posterior root of zygoma.
2. Its anterior wall, floor and lower part of posterior wall is formed by the tympanic part while its roof and upper part of posterior wall is contributed by squamous part of temporal bone.

3. Margins of the meatus give attachment to *cartilaginous part of external acoustic meatus*.

f. Macewen's triangle (suprameatal triangle)
1. It is situated posterosuperior to external acoustic meatus.
2. *Spine of Henle (suprameatal spine)* may be present at the anteroinferior part of triangle.
3. Mastoid antrum is situated about 12.5 mm deep to suprameatal triangle.

g. Mastoid process
1. It is a downward projection from the mastoid part of temporal bone.
2. It is present below and behind the external acoustic meatus.
3. The muscles attached to it from anterior to posterior are:
   i. *Sternocleidomastoid.*
   ii. *Splenius capitis.*
   iii. *Longissimus capitis.*
4. *Posterior belly of digastric* originates from its medial aspect (*digastric notch*).

H. Styloid process
1. It is a slender, elongated projection below the external acoustic meatus and in front of mastoid process.
2. It provides attachments to following five structures:
   i. Anteriorly – *Styloglossus muscle.*
   ii. Posteriorly – *Stylohyoid muscle.*
   iii. Medially – *Stylopharyngeus muscle.*
   iv. Laterally – *Stylomandibular ligament.*
   v. On the tip – *Stylohyoid ligament.*

I. Infratemporal fossa
It is an irregular space below the zygomatic arch.

a. Boundaries
Anterior – Posterior surface of body of maxilla.

Medial – Lateral pterygoid plate and pyramidal process of palatine bone.
Lateral – Ramus of mandible
Roof – Infratemporal surface of greater wing of sphenoid.

b. Contents
i. Muscles
  1. *Lateral and medial pterygoids.*
  2. *Temporalis.*
ii. Arteries
  1. *Maxillary artery* (Ist and 2nd parts) with its branches.
  2. *Posterior superior alveolar branch* of 3rd part of maxillary artery.
iii. Veins
  1. *Maxillary vein.*
  2. *Pterygoid venous plexus.*
  3. *Posterior superior alveolar vein.*
iv. Nerves
  1. *Mandibular nerve and its branches.*
  2. *Chorda tympani.*
  3. *Maxillary nerve.*
  4. *Posterior superior alveolar nerve.*

c. **Anterior wall** of the fossa shows two to three perforations for the *posterior superior alveolar nerve and vessels.*

d. Junction of anterior and medial walls is marked by a fissure (***pterygomaxillary fissure***) through which it communicates with pterygopalatine fossa.

e. The junction of roof and anterior wall is marked by **lateral part of inferior orbital fissure.**

f. *Foramen ovale* and *foramen supinosum* are present in the **roof of the fossa.**

g. **Lateral part of fossa** communicates with temporal fossa through a gap between zygomatic arch and side of skull.

J. Pterygomaxillary fissure
1. It is a gap which leads into pterygopalatine fossa.

2. **Boundaries**
   Anterior – Maxilla.
   Posterior – Pterygoid process.
3. *Maxillary artery* enters the pterygopalatine fossa through pterygomaxillary fissure.
4. *Maxillary nerve* courses forwards through it from pterygopalatine fossa to enter the orbit through inferior orbital fissure.

K. Pterygopalatine fossa

a. Boundaries

Anterior – Posterior surface of *maxilla*.
Posterior – 1. *Pterygoid process.*
          2. *Greater wing of sphenoid.*
Medial – Perpendicular plate of *palatine bone.*
Floor – Fusion of anterior and posterior walls.

b. Communications

The pterygopalatine fossa communicates with,
1. The orbit, through the inferior orbital fissure.
2. The middle cranial fossa, through foramen rotundum.
3. The infratemporal fossa, through pterygomaxillary fissure.
4. The nasal cavity, through palatovaginal canal and sphenopalatine foramen.
5. The foramen lacerum, through pterygoid canal.

c. Contents

1. *Third part of maxillary artery and its branches.*
2. *Maxillary nerve with its branches.*
3. *Pterygopalatine ganglion and its branches.*

Applied anatomy

1. *Spine of Henle* is an important surgical landmark for surgery on mastoid antrum.
2. *Pterion* is very important clinically because the anterior branch of middle meningeal artery and accompanying vein lie on its internal aspect and are vulnerable to tearing if there are fractures of bone forming this region.
3. If the meningeal vessels in the region of pterion are damaged, an *extradural haematoma* is formed. Such haematoma may exert pressure on the cerebral cortex.
4. Decompression of brain in cases of extradural haematoma in the region of pterion can be done by the method of *trephining* (burr hole) at this site.
5. Temporal fascia is commonly used for making *tympanic membrane graft* during surgery for repair of ear drum.
6. Deep temporal vessels and nerves along with the tendon of temporalis muscle, transverse the gap deep to zygomatic arch whose fracture can involve these structures.
7. An *elongated styloid process* usually needs surgical correction because it leads to multiple complications in the neck.
8. An *oblique line drawn from the frontozygomatic suture to the pterion* corresponds with inferior surface of frontal lobe. This surface landmark is of great neurosurgical importance.
9. In radiographs of skull, the *diploic canals* containing the diploic veins may be mistaken for the fractures of skull.
10. *Calvaria* is very thin in the region of temporal fossa and therefore is likely to get fractured because of hard blows to the head.
11. In *depressed fractures*, the inner table of calvaria is often more extensively fractured than the outer table.
12. *Zygomatic fracture* is very common in facial injuries due to its prominent position.
13. *Fracture of skull* is usually due to direct blows. A forceful hit on the forehead causes linear fractures of both vertex and base (Fig. 39.9).

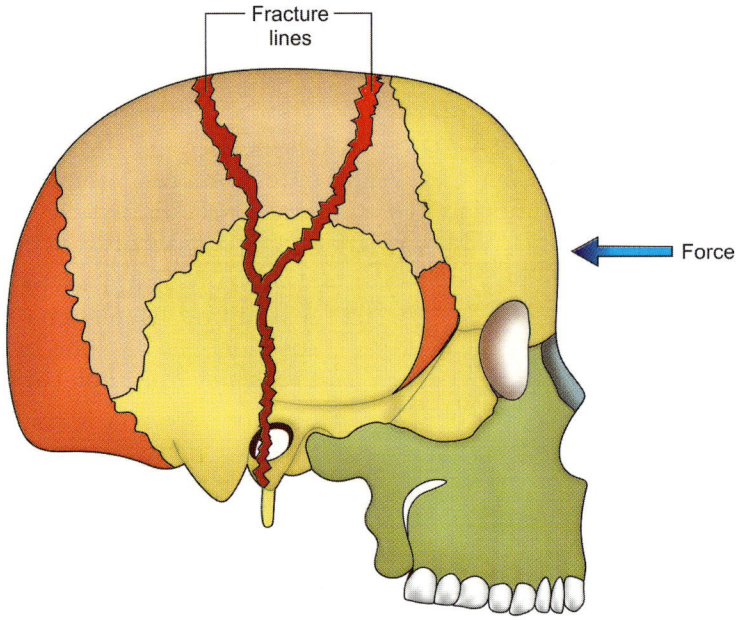

Fig. 39.9: Fracture of skull due to blow on the forehead

14. Junctions of frontal and temporal processes of zygomatic bone form surgically important landmark in the treatment of *maxillofacial injuries*.
15. The periosteum and attachment of strong temporal fascia limit the *displacement of zygomatic bone* following injuries.
16. In *depressed fracture* of zygomatico-maxillary complex the maxilla is greatly damaged and there is displacement of zygomatic bone without its fracture (Fig. 39.10).
17. If *fracture of zygomatic arch* is associated with separation from temporal fascia, then there occurs a downward displacement of arch.
18. The weakest point of zygomatic arch is its middle, just behind the temporo-zygomatic suture. This point is the commonest to fracture in cases of injuries to the arch.
19. *Frontozygomatic suture*, the *zygomatic prominence, the zygomatic buttress* and *1st molar tooth lie in the same vertical line*. In majority of zygomatic-complex (zygomatic bone + adjacent bones like maxilla and zygomatic process of temporal) fracture, the zygomatic bone rotates along this axis (Fig. 39.11).

V. NORMA BASALIS

Definition

Observation of cranium (skull without mandible) from inferior aspect is called norma basalis.

Boundaries

Anterior – *Incisor teeth.*
Posterior – *Superior nuchal line.*
Lateral (side)-
    1. *Rest of teeth.*
    2. *Zygomatic arch.*
    3. *Posterior root of zygoma.*
    4. *Mastoid process.*

Subdivisions

For the sake of convenience, norma basalis is divided into anterior, middle and posterior

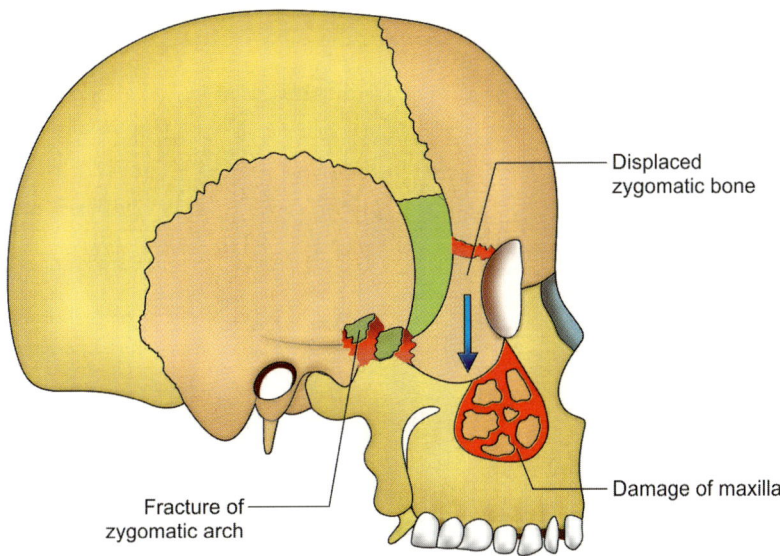

Fig. 39.10: Depressed fracture of zygomatico-maxillary complex

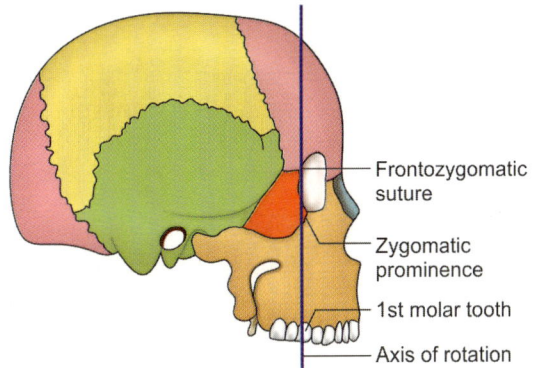

Fig. 39.11: Axis of rotation of zygomatic bone in zygomatic complex fracture

parts. Hard palate and alveolar arch are included in the anterior part. An imaginary horizontal line passing through the anterior margin of foramen magnum separates the posterior part from the middle part of norma basalis.

Features and attachments
(Figs 39.12 and 39.13)

A. Anterior part of norma basalis

a. Posterior border of hard palate

1. It forms the junction of anterior and middle parts of norma basalis.
2. *Posterior nasal spine* is a spinous projection from its middle in the median plane.
3. *Musculus uvulae* is attached to posterior nasal spine.

b. Alveolar arch

1. It possesses *sockets for the roots of upper teeth*.
2. Number of sockets depends upon number of roots. There is single socket for each of the incisors, canines and premolars. There are three sockets for each of the upper molars.

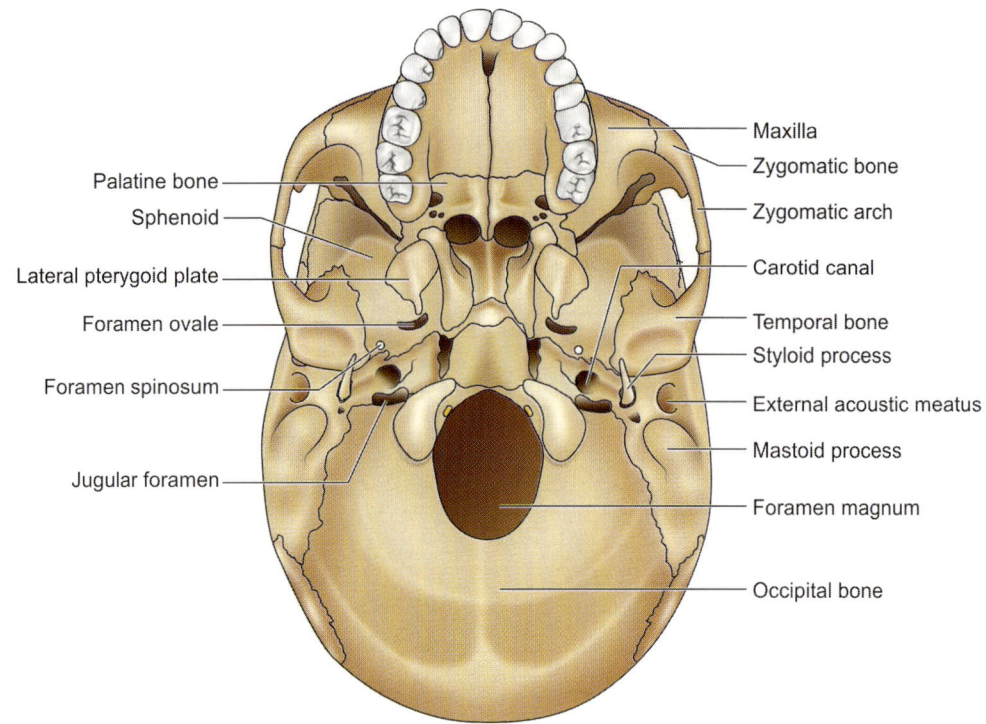

Fig. 39.12: The skull : Norma basalis

c. **Bones contributing to hard palate**
  1. *Palatine processes* of *two maxillae* contribute to the anterior 2/3rd of the hard palate.
  2. Posterior 1/3rd of the hard palate is formed by the *horizontal plates* of *palatine bones*.
  3. Bony palate is marked by several depressions produced by *palatine glands*.

d. **Cruciform suture**
  It is formed by the following three sutures.
  i. *Intermaxillary suture.*
  ii. *Interpalatine suture.*
  iii. *Palatomaxillary sutures.*

e. **Incisive fossa**
  1. It is present anteriorly in the median plane of hard palate.
  2. *Incisive foramen* (right and left) pierces its corresponding side.
  3. Each incisive foramen is transvered by *nasopalatine nerve* and *greater palatine vessels*.

f. **Greater palatine foramen**
  1. It is present behind the lateral part of palatomaxillary suture.
  2. *Greater palatine vessels and nerve* pass through it.
  3. A groove observed between greater palatine foramen and incisive fossa is meant for greater palatine vessels.

g. **Lesser palatine foramina**
  1. These are 1–3 foramina in the pyramidal process of palatine bone and located just behind the greater palatine foramen on each side.
  2. *Lesser palatine nerves and vessels* pass through these foramina.

h. **Palatine crest**
  1. It is a curved ridge observed in the hard palate near its posterior border.

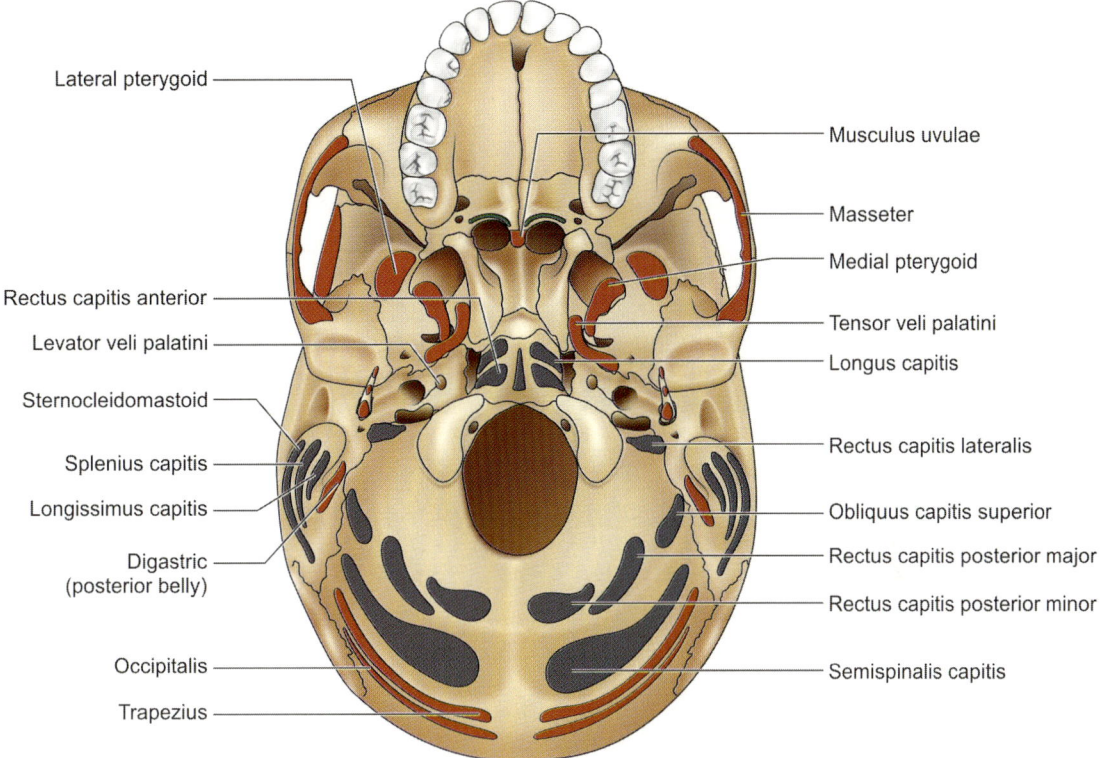

Fig. 39.13: The skull: Norma basalis showing muscular attachments

2. *Palatine aponeurosis* is attached to the palatine crest, posterior border of hard palate and the area between the two.

i. Premaxilla

1. It is a triangular piece of maxilla holding four incisor teeth.
2. It is a separate bone in most vertebrates.

B. Middle part of norma basalis

For the sake of convenience it is divided into a median area and two lateral areas (right and left).

a. Median area

i. *Posterior nasal apertures*

These are also known as *choanae*.

ii. *Posterior border of vomer*

It separates two choanae.

iii. *Alae of vomer*

1. These are two bony plates formed by the splitting of vomer superiorly.
2. It articulates with the rostrum of sphenoid.

iv. *Vomerovaginal canal*

1. It is formed between the lateral border of each ala of vomer and the vaginal process of the medial pterygoid plate.
2. It transmits *branches of pharyngeal nerve and vessels*.

v. *Palatovaginal canal*

1. It is a canal between *vaginal process of medial pterygoid plate* and *sphenoidal process of the palatine bone*.
2. This canal leads anteriorly into posterior wall of pterygopalatine fossa.
3. It transmits *pharyngeal branches of pterygopalatine ganglion* and *pharyngeal branches of 3rd part of maxillary artery*.

> **Note:** *Students are invariably confused as to which is the palatovaginal canal and which one is vomerovaginal canal. To differentiate keep in mind that vaginal process of medial pterygoid plate is common to both but as the palatine bone is anterior to medial pterygoid plate the palatovaginal canal is relatively anterior to vomerovaginal canal.*

    vi. *Broad bar of bone behind the alae*
1. It is formed by the continuation of inferior surface of body of sphenoid and that of basilar part of occipital bone.
2. It extends upto *foramen magnum.*
3. *Pharyngeal tubercle* is a median elevation just in front of foramen magnum. It is better felt than seen.
4. Pharyngeal tubercle gives attachments to:
   - Highest fibres of superior constrictor.
   - Pharyngeal raphe.
5. *Longus capitis* is inserted on the basilar part of occipital bone just lateral to pharyngeal tubercle.
6. *Rectus capitis anterior* is inserted on each side just in front of occipital condyle.

b. **Lateral area**
    i. *Pterygoid processes*
1. Pterygoid processes are located just behind the posterior ends of alveolar arch.
2. Each pterygoid process descends vertically downwards from the junction of body and greater wing of sphenoid.
3. Pterygoid process consists of a lateral and a medial plate.
4. Ptergoid plates unite anteriorly in the upper part to enclose a fossa called *pterygoid fossa*.
5. The lower ununited portions form *pterygoid fissure* which is filled by the pyramidal process of palatine bone.
6. Anterior surface of pterygoid process forms posterior boundary of *pterygopalatine fossa*.
7. Lateral surface of lateral pterygoid plate forms medial wall of *infratemporal fossa* and gives origin to lower head of *lateral pterygoid muscle*.
8. Medial surface of lateral pterygoid plate forms lateral wall of *pterygoid fossa* and gives origin to *deep head of medial pterygoid muscle*.
9. Lateral surface of medial pterygoid plate forms medial wall of pterygoid fossa and is related to *tensor palati* muscle.
10. Medial surface of the medial pterygoid plate forms the lateral wall of corresponding posterior nasal aperture.
11. Posterior border of the medial pterygoid plate shows following features:
    - At its upper end it splits to enclose *scaphoid fossa* which gives origin to *tensor palati* muscle.
    - Its upper end shows a small projection called *pterygoid tubercle* which lies immediately below the posterior end of *pterygoid canal*.
    - *Pharyngobasilar fascia* is attached to its whole extent while *superior constrictor* arises from its lower part only.
    - A hook like process at its lower end is called *pterygoid hamulus*. Tendon of *tensor palati* winds round this process. *Superior constrictor* and *pterygomandibular raphe* are also attached to it.
    - An angular process projecting from the middle of this margin is called *processus tubarius*. Posterior border above this process is called *notch of auditory tube*. This process and notch support the medial end of *auditory tube*.

ii. *Infratemporal surface of greater wing of sphenoid*
   1. It is pentagonal in shape.
   2. It forms roof of *infratemporal fossa*.
   3. It gives origin to the *upper head of lateral pterygoid muscle*.
   4. It is crossed by *deep temporal* and *masseteric nerves*.
   5. *Spine of sphenoid* is a projection from posteriormost part of infratemporal surface.
   6. *Infratemporal crest* is the lateral limit of infratemporal surface.
   7. From scaphoid fossa to spine of sphenoid, four foramina can be noticed i.e. *foramen of Vesalius, foramen ovale, canaliculus innominatus* and *foramen spinosum*.

iii. *Foramen ovale*
   1. It is an oval foramen.
   2. It transmits the *mandibular nerve, accessory meningeal artery, lesser petrosal nerve and emissary vein*.

Note: *For remembering the structures passing through foramen ovale remember MALE, in which M = Mandibular nerve, A = Accessory meningeal artery, L = Lesser petrosal nerve and E = Emissary vein.*

iv. *Foramen spinosum*
   1. It is situated near the spine of sphenoid, posterolateral to foramen ovale.
   2. It transmits *middle meningeal artery, nervus spinosus* (meningeal branch of mandibular nerve) and *parietal trunk of middle meningeal vein*.

v. *Foramen of Vesalius (sphenoidal emissary foramen)*
   1. It is an infrequently seen foramen between scaphoid fossa and foramen ovale.
   2. It transmits an emissary vein connecting cavernous sinus with pterygoid venous plexus.

vi. *Canaliculus innominatus (foramen innominatum)*
   1. This is also an infrequently seen foramen between foramen ovale and foramen spinosum.
   2. It transmits *lesser petrosal nerve*.

vii. *Spine of sphenoid*
   1. It is related laterally to *auriculotemporal nerve* and medially to *chorda tympani nerve* and *Eustachian tube*.
   2. *Sphenomandibular ligament* is attached to its tip.
   3. Most posterior fibres of *tensor palati* originate from its anterior surface.

viii. *Sulcus tubae*
   1. It is a groove between posteromedial margin of infratemporal surface of greater wing of sphenoid and inferor surcace the petrous part of temporal bone.
   2. *Cartilaginous part of Eustachian tube* (also called auditory tube or pharyngotympanic tube) occupies this sulcus.

ix. *Inferior surface of petrous part of temporal bone*
   1. It is located just behind the infratemporal surface of greater wing of sphenoid.
   2. Its anteromedial serrated end marks the apex of petrous part.
   3. The quadrilateral area near the apex provides attachment to *levator palati muscle*.
   4. Lower opening of *carotid canal* is located just behind the quadrilateral area. It *transmits internal carotid artery with its sympathetic and venous plexuses*.
   5. Carotid canal runs forwards and medially in petrous part and perforates its apex as upper opening of carotid canal.

x. *Foramen lacerum*
   1. It is located between sphenoid and apex of petrous temporal.

2. It is named *'lacerum'* because of irregular margins.
3. *Carotid canal* and *pterygoid canal* open into it.
4. Only two structures pass through it, i.e. *meningeal branch of ascending pharyngeal artery* and *emissary vein*.
5. *Internal carotid artery* traverses its upper part *with its sympathetic and venous plexuses*.
6. *Nerve of pterygoid canal (Vidian nerve)* is formed in its upper part by the union of *greater superficial petrosal and deep petrosal nerves*.

xi. *Tympanic part of temporal bone*
  1. It is a triangular bone which occupies the angle between the petrous and squamous parts of temporal bone.
  2. Its anterior surface is related to *parotid gland*.

xii. *Squamous part of temporal bone*
  Only a small part of squamous part of temporal bone is seen in norma basalis and shows following features from posterior to anterior:
  1. Anterior (articular) part of *mandibular fossa*.
  2. Articular tubercle.
  3. Part of the roof of infratemporal fossa.

xiii. *Squamotympanic fissure*
  1. It marks the junction of squamous and tympanic parts of temporal bone.
  2. Downward edge of tegmen tympani (a part of petrous part of temporal bone) divides the squamotympanic fissure into *petrotympanic* (posterior) and *pterosquamous* (anterior) *fissures*.
  3. *Chorda tympani nerve, anterior tympanic artery* and *anterior ligament of malleus* pass through petrotympanic fissure.

C. Posterior part of norma basalis

For the sake of convenience this part can be divided into a median area and two lateral areas (right and left).

a. **Median area**

It consists of foramen magnum, external occipital crest and external occipital protuberance from anterior to posterior.

  i. *Foramen magnum*
  1. It is the largest foramen in skull.
  2. It is single foramen located in the lowest part of posterior cranial fossa.
  3. It is oval in shape.
  4. It is the communication between cranial cavity and vertebral canal.
  5. *Anterior atlanto-occipital membrane* is attached to its anterior margin.
  6. *Posterior atlanto-occipital membrane* is attached to its posterior margin.
  7. Lateral margins provide attachments to *alar ligaments*.
  8. Following structures pass through its anterior part:
     • Apical ligament of dens.
     • Superior longitudinal band of cruciform ligament.
     • Membrana tectoria.
  9. Following structures pass through its posterior part:
     • Medulla oblongata.
     • Meninges.
     • Spinal roots of accessory nerves.
     • Meningeal branches of upper cervical nerves (C_{1-3}).
     • Vertebral arteries.
     • Sympathetic plexuses around vertebral arteries.
     • Anterior and posterior spinal arteries.

  ii. *External occipital crest*
  1. It extends from posterior margin of foramen magnum to external occipital protuberance.

2. Upper margin of *ligamentum nuchae* is attached to it.
   iii. *External occipital protuberance*
   Trapezius is attached to it superiorly and ligamentum nuchae inferiorly.

b. **Lateral area**
   i. *Occipital condyles*
      1. These are located lateral to anterior half of foramen magnum.
      2. Each is oval and convex to articulate with concave superior articular process of atlas.
   ii. *Condylar fossa*
      1. It is present just behind the occipital condyle.
      2. It may have *condylar canal for emissary vein* from sigmoid sinus.
   iii. *Hypoglossal canal*
      1. Lateral to anterior part of condyle is the outer opening of hypoglossal canal.
      2. It transmits:
         - Hypoglossal nerve.
         - Meningeal branch of ascending pharyngeal artery.
         - Emissary vein from basilar venous plexus.
   iv. *Squamous part of occipital bone*
      1. Superior nuchal line is a well defined ridge which extends laterally from external occipital protuberance on each side. Its medial 1/3rd provides origin to *trapezius* while lateral 1/3rd receives insertions of *sternomastoid* (above) and *splenius capitis* (below).
      2. Running laterally on each side from the middle of external occipital crest is another ridge called *inferior nuchal line*.
      3. A vertical line on each side along with inferior nuchal line divides the region below the superior nuchal line into four areas, each meant for the attachment of a muscle as follows:
         - Upper medial area for *semispinalis capitis*.
         - Upper lateral area for *obliquus capitis superior*.
         - Lower medial area for *rectus capitis posterior minor*.
         - Lower lateral area for *rectus capitis posterior major*.
   v. *Jugular foramen*
      1. It is an interosseous foramen situated between anterior margin of jugular process of occipital bone and posterior margin of petrous part of temporal bone at the petro-occipital suture.
      2. It is divided into anterior, middle and posterior parts.
      3. *9th, 10th and 11th cranial nerves* pass through its middle part.
      4. *Inferior petrosal sinus* and *meningeal branch of ascending pharyngeal artery* pass through its anterior part.
      5. *Sigmoid sinus* and *meningeal branch of occipital artery* traverse through its posterior part.
      6. At its posterior end the anterior wall (petrous temporal) is hollowed out to form the *jugular fossa* which lodges the superior bulb of internal jugular vein.
      7. *Mastoid canaliculus* is a minute canal in the lateral wall of jugular fossa which transmits the *auricular branch of vagus*.
      8. *Glossopharyngeal notch* is on the posterior border of petrous temporal bone near the medial end of jugular foramen.
      9. *Cochlear canaliculus* is located at the apex of glossopharyngeal notch. The *aqueduct of cochlea* opens into the cochlear canaliculus.
      10. *Tympanic canaliculus* is present in the ridge between jugular fossa and lower opening of carotid canal. It transmits the *tympanic branch of glossopharyngeal nerve* to middle ear.
   vi. *Inferior surface of jugular process of occipital bone*
      1. It is the area just lateral to occipital condyle behind the jugular foramen.

2. It provides attachment to *rectus capitis lateralis*.

vii. *Styloid process*
   1. It is a conical projection just below the tympanic part of temporal bone.
   2. It is directed downwards, forwards and slightly medially.
   3. It sprovides attachments to 3 muscles and 2 ligaments. Three muscles attached to it are *styloglossus* (anteriorly), *stylohyoid* (posteriorly) and *stylopharyngeus* (medially). Two ligaments attached to it are *stylomandibular* (laterally) and *stylohyoid* (on the tip).
   4. It is interposed between *parotid gland* (laterally) and *internal jugular vein* (medially).
   5. Two structures cross it superficially i.e. *facial nerve* (near the base) and *external carotid artery* (near the tip).

viii. *Mastoid process*
   1. It is a prominent projection from the temporal bone posterolateral to styloid process.
   2. The medial aspect of this process shows a deep groove (*digastric notch*) which provides attachment to *posterior belly of digastric*.
   3. Medial to digastric notch, there can be another *groove for occipital artery*.

ix. *Stylomastoid foramen*
   1. It is present between styloid and mastoid processes.
   2. *Facial nerve* and *stylomastoid artery* pass through this foramen.

APPLIED ANATOMY

1. A forceful hit on the forehead causes linear fracture of both vertex and base (Fig. 39.14).
2. Due to the presence of natural thick bony buttresses at the base of skull, the fracture lines often converge towards the foramen magnum or sella turcica.
3. In case of basal fractures, loceration of structures passing through the basal foramina may complicate the issue.
4. A fracture line passing through the foramen lacerum may tear the internal carotid artery with a resultant *caroticocavernous fistula*.
5. If the fissure lines involve grooves having meningeal vessels and dural sinuses, then *epidural haematoma* might result.
6. Fractures of skull base are often zig-zag in appearance because the fracture lines avoid

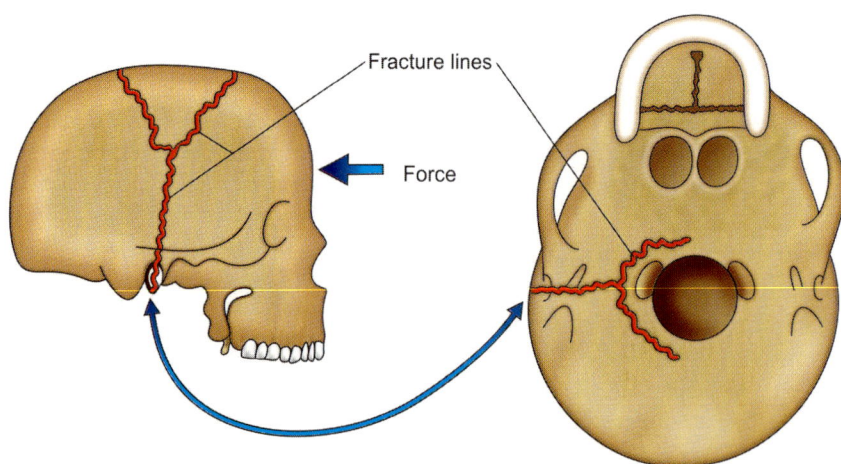

Fig. 39.14: Fracture of skull base due to hit on forehead

the thickenings and pass through the lines of least resistance.

7. Tumours of the base of skull
    A. *Transitional cell carcinoma* arising from mucous membrane of paranasal sinuses or fossa of Rosenmuller of nasopharynx usually erodes the skull base.
    B. Some of the very rare tumours which may arise from the base of skull or adjacent tissue, are as follows:
        i. *Osteomas.*
        ii. *Chondromas.*
        iii. *Giant cell tumours of bone.*
    C. Many malignant tumours metastasize to the base of skull bones from distant organs, e.g. prostate, lung and breast.
8. Bony palate may be fractured in uncommon central split of palate. It is actually paramedian in nature because median sutures (intermaxillary and interpalatine) are relatively strong (Fig. 39.15).
9. Clinical signs and symptoms which support the involvement of base of skull, are as follows:
    i. Discharge of C.S.F. through external acoustic meatus (C.S.F. otorhea)
    ii. Tear of tympanic membrane.

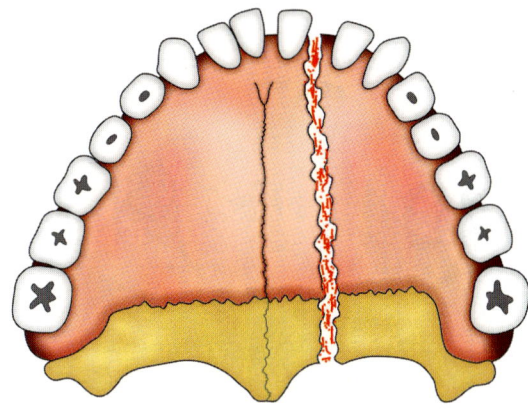

Fig. 39.15: Central split of palate

    iii. Collection of blood in the middle ear.
    iv. Facial paralysis due to damage of 7th cranial nerve.
    v. Loss of hearing, vertigo and nystagmus due to involvement of 8th cranial nerve. Aforementioned signs are indicative of fracture of petrous part of temporal bone.
    vi. Discolouration and edema of tissue over mastoid process is indication of sigmoid sinus damage.
10. Cranial nerve damage is due to involvement of foramina in the skull base by the fracture lines.

CHAPTER

40 | The Orbital Cavity

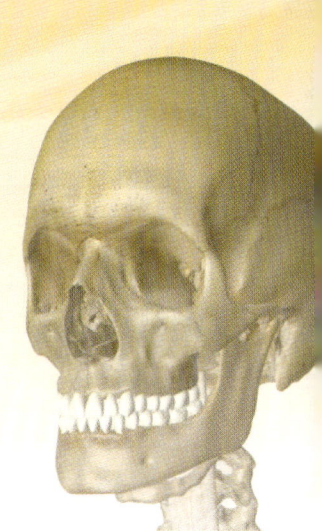

DEFINITION

Orbits are two bony sockets which lodge the eye balls and the associated structures.

SHAPE AND PARTS (Fig. 40.1)

Each orbit is pyramidal in shape having an anterior base (orbital opening), posterior apex and four walls (medial, lateral, roof and floor).

BONY CONTRIBUTIONS (Fig. 40.2)

A. Orbital opening (base)

It consists of four margins (supraorbital, infraorbital, lateral and medial).

a. Supraorbital margin
  1. It is formed by the frontal bone.
  2. *Supraorbital notch (or foramen)* is situated at the junction of its medial 1/3rd (rounded) and lateral 2/3rd (sharp) parts.
  3. Supraorbital notch transmits:
     i. *Supraorbital nerve.*
     ii. *Supraorbital artery.*
     iii. *Communicating vein between angular and superior ophthalmic veins.*

b. Infraorbital margin
  It is formed by maxilla medially and zygomatic bone laterally.

c. Lateral orbital margin
  It is formed by the frontal process of zygomatic bone below and the zygomatic process of frontal bone above.

d. Medial orbital margin
  It is formed by the frontal bone above and the lacrimal crest of frontal process of maxilla below.

B. Apex

1. It forms the posterior end of orbit.
2. It is contributed by sphenoid.
3. Usually the medial end of superior orbital fissure is said to mark the apex.

C. Medial wall

It is formed by the following bones from anterior to posterior:

a. Posterior part of the frontal process of *maxilla.*
b. *Lacrimal bone.*
c. The orbital plate of *ethmoid.*
d. Body of *sphenoid.*

D. Lateral wall

It is contributed by:

a. *Greater wing of sphenoid bone* posteriorly.
b. *Orbital surface of zygomatic bone* and *medial aspect of its frontal process* anteriorly.

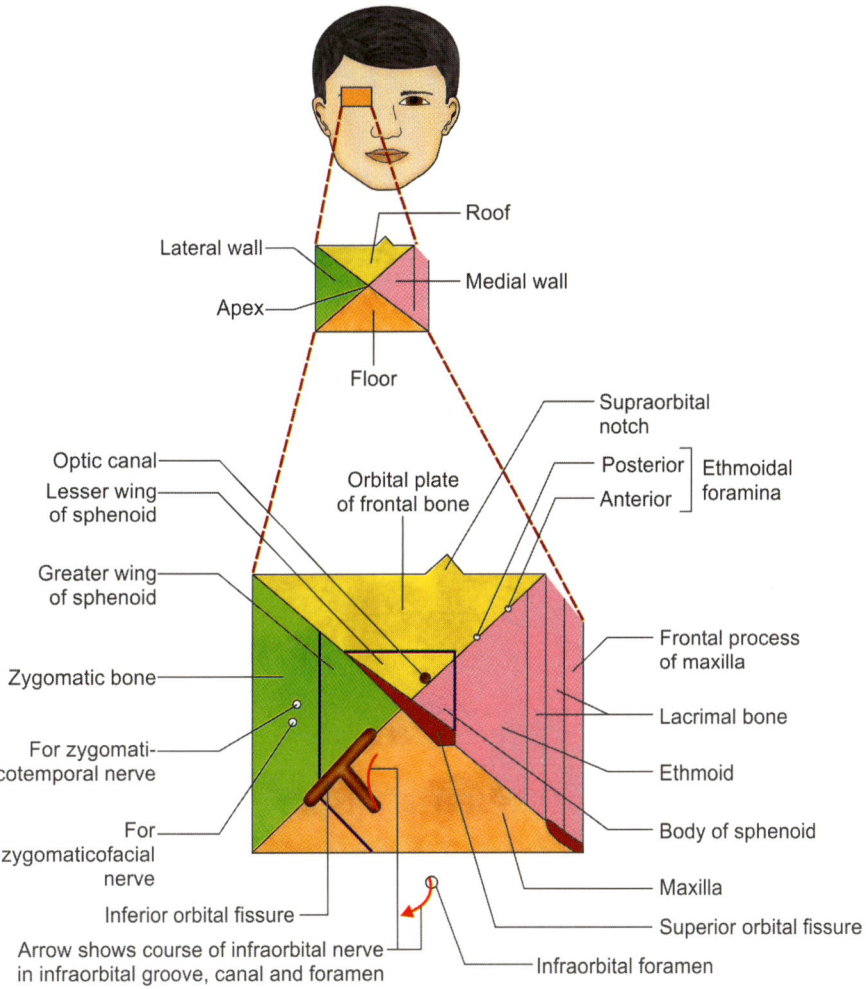

Fig. 40.1: Right orbit : Anterior view

E. Roof

It is formed by :
a. *Orbital plate of frontal bone* anteriorly.
b. *Lesser wing of sphenoid* posteriorly.

F. Floor

It is formed by :
a. *Orbital surface of maxilla* medially. It is the major contribution.
b. *Orbital surface of zygomatic bone.*
c. *Orbital process of palatine bone.* It is an insignificant contribution near the posterior end at the junction of medial wall and floor.

COMMUNICATIONS (Fig. 40.3)

The orbit communicates through several passages with adjacent regions as shown below:

Passages	Adjacent regions
1. Orbital opening	Face
2. Infraorbital canal	Face
3. Optic canal	Middle cranial fossa
4. Superior orbital fissure	Middle cranial fossa
5. Inferior orbital fissure	
a. Medially	Pterygopalatine fossa
b. Laterally	Infratemporal fossa

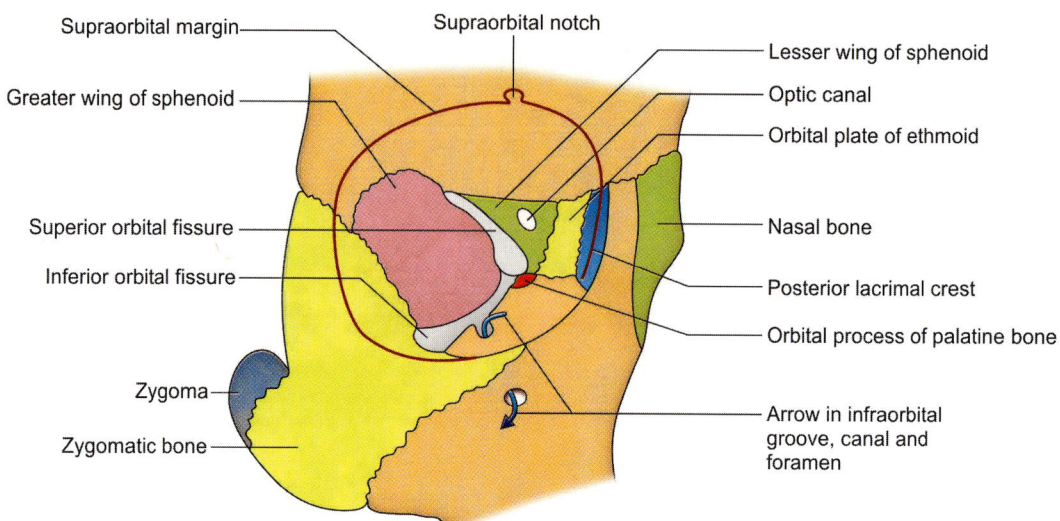

Fig. 40.2: Right orbit : Anterior view

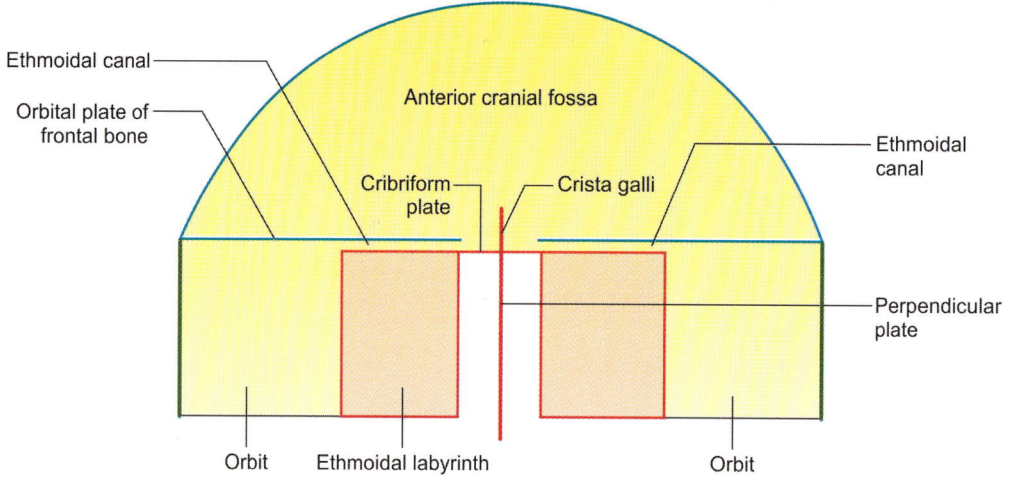

Fig. 40.3: Diagramatic representation of ethmoidal canal in coronal sectional view

6. Zygomatico-orbital foramina	Face and temporal fossa
7. Anterior and posterior ethmoidal canals	Anterior cranial fossa
8. Nasolacrimal canal	Nasal cavity

MEASUREMENTS (Fig. 40.4)

1. Length of medial wall – 50 mm.
2. Length of lateral wall – 50 mm.
3. Width of orbital opening, i.e. distance between medial and lateral orbital margins – 40 mm.
4. Distance between two lateral orbital margins – 100 mm.
5. Distance between two medial orbital margins – 25 mm.
6. Angle between two lateral walls – 90°.
7. Angle between lateral and medial walls of each orbit – 45°.

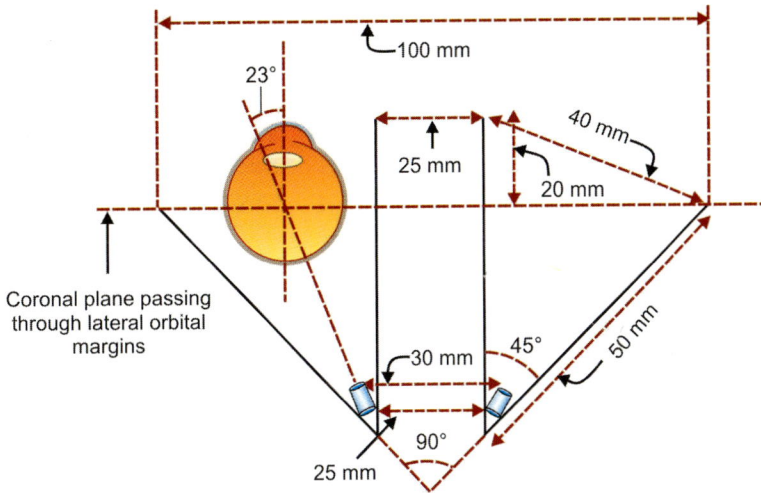

Fig. 40.4: Horizontal sectional view of orbits showing measurements

8. Angle between long axis of orbit and anteroposterior axis of eye ball – 23°.
9. Distance between medial orbital margin and coronal plane passing through lateral orbital margins – 20 mm.
10. Measurements of optic canal:
    i. Length – 3-9 mm.
    ii. Diameter – 5 mm.
    iii. Distance between orbital openings of optic canals – 30 mm.
    iv. Distance between cranial openings of optic canals – 25 mm.

FEATURES

1. Anterolateral part of roof is slightly hollowed out to form *fossa for lacrimal gland*.
2. The anteromedial part of roof near the orbital opening is marked by the *trochlear fovea* or *spine* for the attachment of fibrocartilaginous pulley meant for the tendon of superior oblique muscle.
3. *Optic canal* is present at the posterior end of junction of roof and medial wall. *Optic nerve* and *ophthalmic artery* pass through optic canal.
4. The posterior part of the junction of lateral wall and floor is marked by **inferior orbital fissure**. It transmits the following structures:
    i. *Maxillary nerve.*
    ii. *Infraorbital vessels.*
    iii. *Zygomatic nerve.*
    iv. *A branch from inferior ophthalmic vein.*
    v. *Some twigs (orbital branches) from pterygopalatine ganglion.*

    Boundaries of inferior orbital fissure are as follows:
    a. Superiorly – *Greater wing of sphenoid.*
    b. Inferiorly – *Body of maxilla* and *orbital process of palatine bone*
    c. Laterally – *Zygomatic bone.*
5. Maxillary part of the floor is marked by a groove (*infraorbital groove*) in the posterior part. This groove is directed forwards and continues with the *infraorbital canal* in the anterior part of floor and ultimately opens on the face as *infraorbital foramen*. Infraorbital groove, canal and foramen are meant for the passage of infraorbital nerve and vessels.

6. In the anterior part of medial wall, the posterior part of frontal process of maxilla (behind the anterior lacrimal crest) and anterior part of lacrimal bone (anterior to posterior lacrimal crest) form a vertical fossa called *lacrimal fossa*. This fossa continues down with the beginning of *nasolacrimal canal*. The fossa and canal are meant for *lacrimal sac* and *nasolacrimal duct* respectively.
7. *Anterior lacrimal crest* provides attachments to:
   i. *Lacrimal fascia.*
   ii. *Medial palpebral ligament.*
   iii. *Orbicularis oculi.*
8. *Posterior lacrimal crest* gives attachments to:
   i. *Lacrimal fascia.*
   ii. *Lacrimal part of orbicularis occuli.*
9. The junction of orbital plate of frontal bone (roof) and orbital plate of ethmoid (medial wall) shows two openings which lead into *anterior and posterior ethmoidal canals*. These transmit corresponding ethmoidal nerves and vessels.
10. Orbital surface of zygomatic bone in the lateral wall possesses *zygomatico-orbital foramina* meant for the passage of zygomaticotemporal and zygomaticofacial nerves and zygomatic branches of lacrimal artery.
11. **Superior orbital fissure**
    A. *Location*
       It is located at the junction of roof and lateral wall of orbit.
    B. *Shape*
       It is triangular in shape with base medially and apex laterally.
    C. *Communication*
       It connects orbit with middle cranial fossa.
    D. *Boundaries*
       i. Medial – Body of sphenoid bone.
       ii. Apex – Frontal bone.
       iii. Superior – Lesser wing of sphenoid.
       iv. Inferior – Greater wing of sphenoid.
    E. *Common annular tendon*
       The lower margin of fissure presents a bony projection for the attachment of common tendinous ring (common annular tendon) for the attachment of recti of eye ball.
    F. *Structures passing through*
       Common annular tendon divides the fissure into three compartments for the passage of number of structures as shown below:
       a. Lateral part
          i. *Lacrimal nerve.*
          ii. *Frontal nerve.*
          iii. *Trochlear nerve.*
          iv. *Superior ophthalmic vein.*
          v. *Meningeal branch of lacrimal artery.*
          vi. *Orbital branch of middle meningeal artery.*
       b. Part within tendinous ring
          i. *Upper and lower divisions of the oculomotor nerve.*
          ii. *Nasociliary nerve.*
          iii. *Abducent nerve.*
       c. Part below the tendinous ring
          i. *Inferior ophthalmic vein*
          ii. *Sympathetic twigs.*
12. The lateral wall of orbit near the lateral orbital margin presents an ill defined *Whitnall's tubercle*. It is located on the orbital surface of frontal process of zygomatic bone about 1 cm below the frontozygomatic suture. Following structures are attached to this tubercle:
    i. *Lateral palapebral ligament.*
    ii. *Lateral check ligament.*
    iii. *Suspensory ligament of eye ball.*
    iv. *Aponeurosis of levator palpebrae superioris.*

APPLIED ANATOMY

1. *Maxillectomy* should be performed below the attachements of check ligaments to avoid the sagging of eye ball (Fig. 40.5).

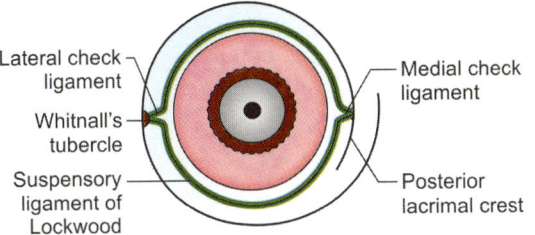

Fig. 40.5: Check ligaments located in the right orbit

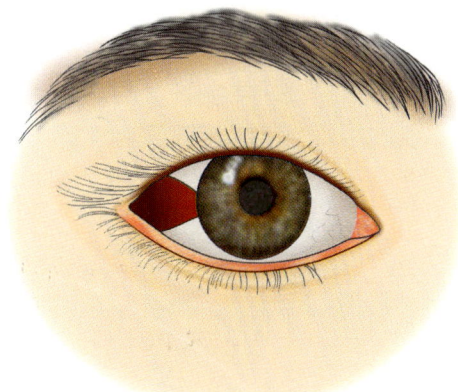

Fig. 40.6: Haemorrhage in orbit

2. Normal amount of orbital fat stabilizes the eye ball from behind. An increase in the orbital fat as observed in *hyperthyroidism*, will push the eye ball forwards leading to *exophthalmos* (bulging of eye).

3. The floor and medial wall of the orbit are relatively thin therefore *tumours* arising from ethmoidal and maxillary sinuses may push into the orbital cavity and displace the eye ball.

4. In *Graves' disease* there is hypertrophy of extraocular muscles which is responsible for increased intraorbital pressure and exophthalmos.

5. Eye ball occupies the anterior half of orbit and it is joined by the optic nerve from behind. Optic nerve runs a tortuous course to allow the movements of eye ball without being damaged. Inflammation of optic nerve is called *retrobulbar neuritis*.

6. There may be isolated fracture of single orbital margin or wall or there can be involvement of multiple margins or walls in different combinations.

7. Fracture of the orbital plate of frontal bone causes *haemorrhage* into the orbit. The haemorrhage acquires a triangular shape under the conjunctiva whose apex is towards the corneoscleral junction and base towards the orbital margin (Fig. 40.6).

8. A severe impact on the nasal bridge may involve the medial wall of orbit. Involvement of lacrimal bone will damage the lacrimal passage.

9. A fracture of sphenoid may lacerate the optic nerve in the optic canal resulting into *blindness*.

10. Frontozygomatic suture located in the leteral orbital margin forms an important landmark in the treatment of *maxillofacial injuries*.

11. Fracture of the frontal process of the zygomatic bone may occur in conjunction with a *comminuted fracture* of the orbital rim and frontal bone.

12. Orbit is an anatomical region which is of great clinical and surgical interest due to many disciplines in its surrounding relations.

13. Floor of the orbit is very thin and further weakened by the presence of infraorbital groove. A fracture which is common in this part, invariably involves infraorbital nerve and vessels.

14. *Le Fort (II and III) fractures* of mid-facial skeleton involve the walls of orbit. Fracture line in case of Le Fort II fracture crosses the lower part of frontal process of maxilla and lacrimal bone. In Le Fort III fracture both medial and lateral walls are involved near the roof (Fig. 40.7).

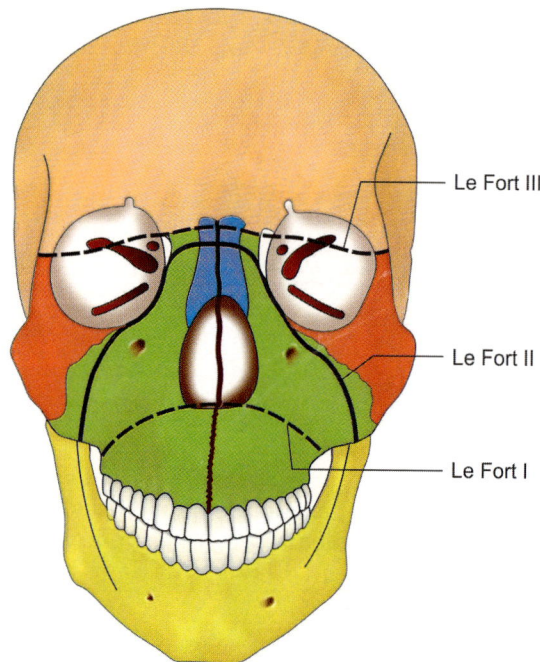

Fig. 40.7: Le Fort fractures

15. For *optic nerve decompression* in the optic canal, posterior lacrimal crest, ethmoid and sphenoid are infractured to reach the medial wall of optic canal.
16. Lacrimal bone is very fragile therefore an extra precaution should be taken to avoid trauma in cases of surgery of the lacrimal system.
17. A *penetrating object* will enter the orbit through orbital opening and damage the adjacent regions depending upon its directions e.g.,
    a. Directed upwards and medially – It will enter the frontal sinus in the anterior part and anterior cranial fossa more posteriorly.
    b. Directed towards the floor – It will enter the maxillary sinus.
    c. Directed backwards – It will enter the middle cranial fossa through superior orbital fissure and damage temporal lobe.
18. *Ethmoidal malignancy* may erode the optic canal and compress the optic nerve.
19. *Tumours in the adjacent regions* may enter the orbit through large communications. From middle cranial fossa it passes through superior orbital fissure while from temporal fossa it traverses the inferior orbital fissure.
20. An *orbital tumour* will push the eye ball forwards producing *exophthalmos*.
21. Since lateral orbital margin is lying relatively more posteriorly than medial orbital margin, a lateral approach is preferred for the operations on eye ball.

CHAPTER 41

The Nasal Cavity

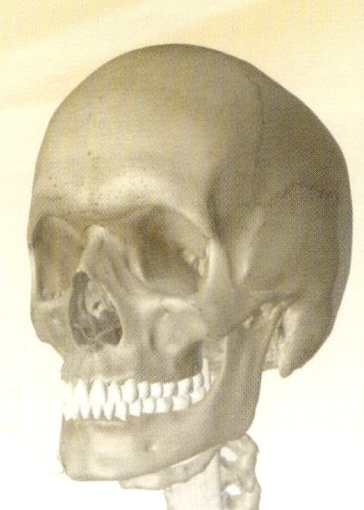

Nasal cavity is the beginning of respiratory system. It is divided into right and left halves by a midline partition called *nasal septum*. To study the cavity, a sagittal section of skull is considered in which one half of the skull shows *lateral wall of nasal cavity* and the second half shows *nasal septum*.

FEATURES

Each half of the nasal cavity consists of a roof, floor, medial wall and lateral wall.

I. Roof

It has anterior and posterior slopings and middle horizontal part.

A. Anterior sloping

It is formed by the *nasal bone* and *nasal spine* of the frontal bone.

B. Posterior sloping

1. It is formed by the following bones from anterior to posterior:
   i. Anterior surface of *body of sphenoid*.
   ii. *Ala of vomer*.
   iii. *Sphenoidal process of palatine bone*.
2. It possesses *opening of sphenoidal sinus*.

C. Middle horizontal part

1. It is formed by the *cribriform plate* of ethmoid bone.

2. Number of foramina in it provide passages for *filaments of olfactory nerve*.
3. One of these perforations in its anterior part transmits *anterior ethmoidal nerve and vessels*.

II. Floor

1. It is formed by the superior surface of bony palate, i.e. *palatine process of maxilla* and *horizontal plate of palatine bone*.
2. Anteriorly near the septum a small *infundibular opening* leads into *incisive canal*.
3. *Nasopalatine nerve* and *greater palatine* vessels traverse the incisive canal.

III. Medial wall (Fig. 41.1)

1. It is formed by bony septum in a dried skull.
2. Posteroinferior part of the bony septum is contributed by *vomer*.
3. Its anterosuperior part is formed by *perpendicular plate of ethmoid*.
4. *Nasal crest* (below), *sphenoidal crest* and *rostrum* (above and behind) provide minor contributions to bony septum.
5. A groove on each side of vomer descends downwards and forwards towards incisive canal. It lodges nasopalatine nerve.

IV. Lateral wall (Fig. 41.2)

1. This is very irregular.
2. This is marked by three bracket like projections which run anteroposteriorly

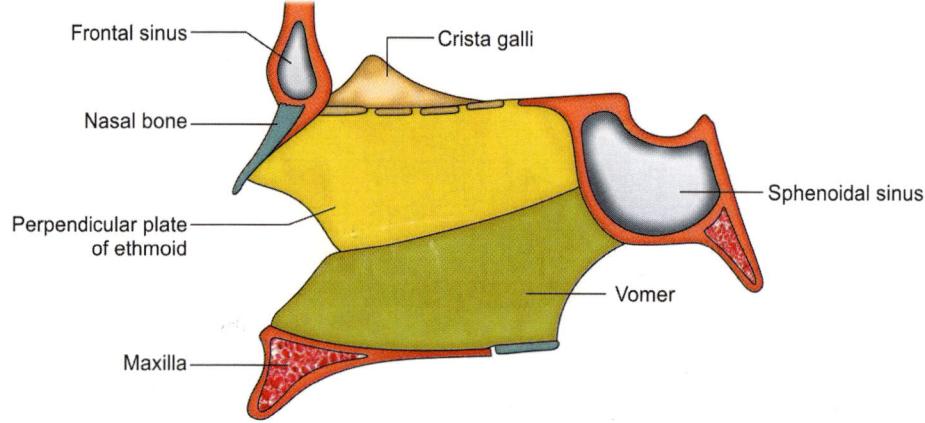

Fig. 41.1: Left surface of bony nasal septum

and lie one above the other. These projections are named from above downwards, *superior, middle and inferior conchae*.

3. Each concha forms medial wall and roof of corresponding meatus. Therefore there are three *meatuses, superior, middle and inferior*.

4. The part of the lateral wall above the superior concha is called *sphenoethmoidal recess*.

5. Main bony contributions in the lateral wall are as follows:
   i. Below and in front – *Nasal surface of maxilla*.
   ii. Behind – *Perpendicular plate of palatine bone*.
   iii. Above – *Ethmoidal labyrinth* (with superior and middle conchae).
   iv. Below – *Inferior concha* (an independent bone).

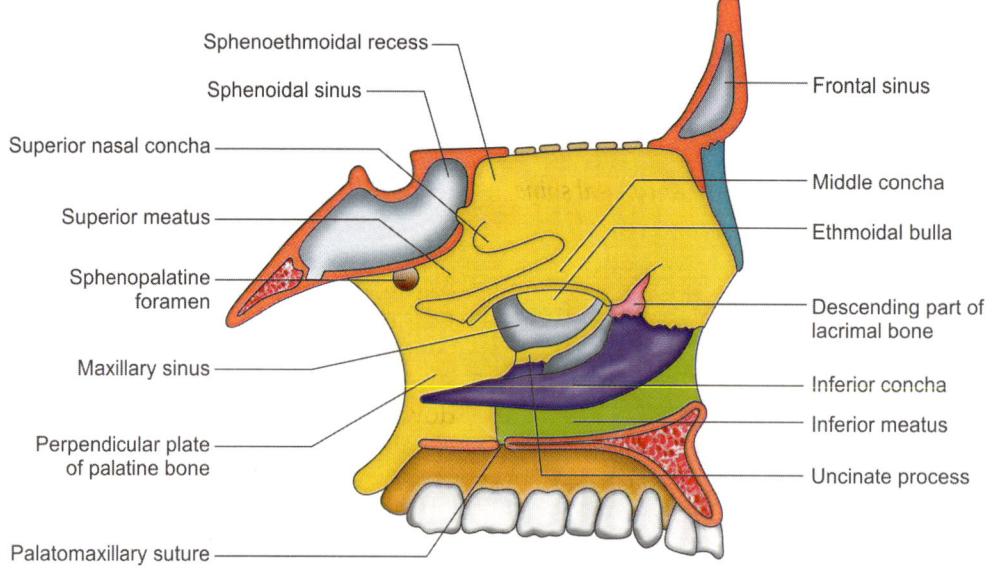

Fig. 41.2: Lateral wall of left nasal cavity

6. *Inferior meatus*
   a. It lies below and lateral to inferior concha.
   b. It receives *opening of nasolacrimal duct* in its anterior part.
7. *Middle meatus*
   i. It is situated between middle and inferior conchae.
   ii. A rounded elevation in its upper part is called *ethmoidal bulla* produced by middle ethmoidal air cells.
   iii. On the surface or just above the bulla is the *opening of middle ethmoidal sinus*.
   iv. Behind the bulla is the *opening of maxillary* sinus.
   v. Anteroinferior to bulla is a curved, thin bony projection called as *uncinate process of ethmoid*.
   vi. Uncinate process passes backwards and encloses a curved gap between it and bulla. This gap is called *hiatus semilunaris*.
   vii. Upper end of hiatus semilunaris continues with *ethmoidal infundibulum*.
   viii. Infundibulum of ethmoid receives *opening of anterior ethmoidal sinus* and itself continues up as *frontonasal duct* to reach the frontal sinus.
8. *Superior meatus*
   i. It is situated between superior and middle conchae.
   ii. *Opening of posterior ethmoidal sinus* is located in the superior meatus.
9. *Sphenoethmoidal recess*
   i. It is situated between roof and superior concha.
   ii. It receives the *opening of sphenoidal air sinus*.
10. *Sphenopalatine foramen*
    i. It is located just behind the superior concha.
    ii. It transmits *sphenopalatine artery* and *nasal branches of pterygopalatine ganglion*.

APPLIED ANATOMY

1. Fracture of base of skull involving anterior cranial fossa might lead to communication between nasal cavity and subarachnoid space resulting C.S.F. leak into the nose. This condition is called *CSF rhinorrhoea*.
2. An impact on the nasal bridge will lead to fracture and displacement of nasal septum.
3. Fracture of cribriform plate will result into *anosmia* (loss of smell sensation) due to damage of olfactory nerve filaments.
4. Fracture of cribriform plate may cause infection to enter the cranial cavity from nasal cavity resulting into *meningitis*.
5. *Le Fort fractures* of mid-facial skeleton always involve the nasal septum (Fig. 41.3).
6. All the bones of nasal cavity are clothed in mucosa therefore their fractures open to nasal cavity with potential risk of infection.
7. The bones of nasal cavity receive adequate blood supply from periosteal arteries and therefore all the fragments of fractured bone retain a periosteal blood supply.

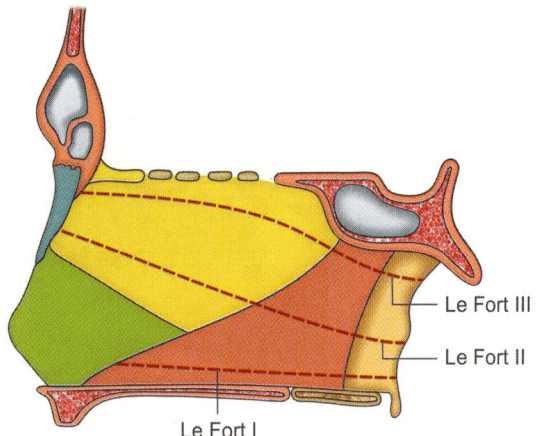

Fig. 41.3: Fracture lines of Le Fort fractures crossing the nasal septum

8. Bony septum is papery thin and does not resist much to forces responsible for fracture.
9. Floor of the nasal cavity may be fractured in uncommon central split of the palate. It is actually paramedian in nature because median sutures (intermaxillary and interpalatine) are relatively strong.
10. *Nasal ethmoidostomy* (an artificial opening to drain the ethmoidal air cell) is a common practice in several surgical procedures involving ethmoidal labyrinth.
11. Lacrimal bone is very fragile therefore an extra-precaution should be taken to avoid trauma in cases of surgery of the lacrimal system.
12. In the management of congenital lacrimal defect, *infracture of the inferior concha* is some times needed (Fig. 41.4).
13. In cases of obstruction of lacrimal sac or nasolacrimal duct, *dacryocystorhinostomy* is performed. In this operation an artificial passage is made by breaking lacrimal bone.
14. *Congenital atresia of the choanae* is an uncommon condition in which there is occlusion of the posterior naris by a bony or membranous diaphragm.
15. *Antral puncture* is a common procedure performed by ENT surgeons to wash out infected fluid in maxillary sinus (*antral lavage*). The antrum is punctured through the inferior meatus by a trocar and cannula (Fig. 41.5).

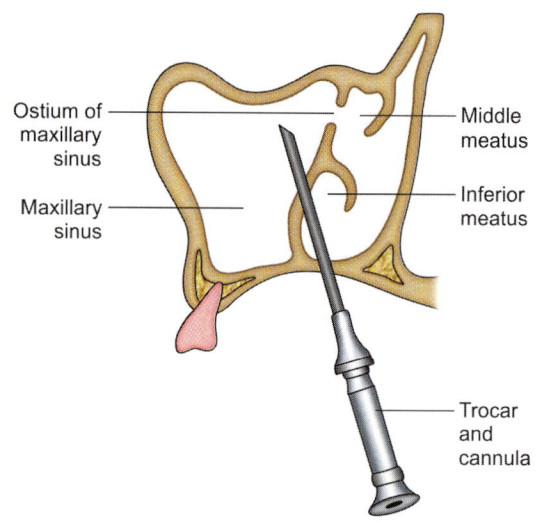

Fig. 41.5: Antral puncture

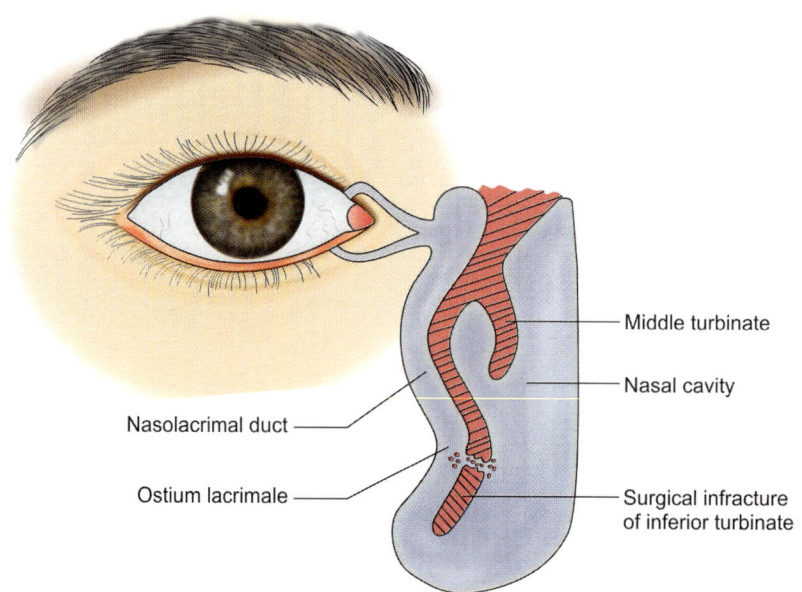

Fig. 41.4: Infracture of inferior concha

16. *Deviation of nasal septum (DNS)* is a common condition which may be developmental in origin or may arise from trauma.
17. A *perforated septum* may be due to septal surgery or syphilis or tuberculosis.
18. Some times a permanent opening is made in the inferior meatus to encourage the drainage of the pus in the maxillary sinus. This operation is called *intranasal antrostomy*.

CHAPTER 42
Interior of the Cranial Vault

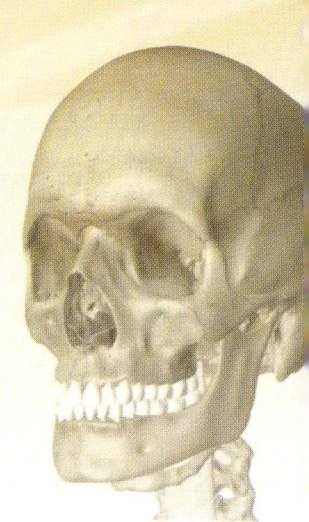

DEFINITION
It is the internal surface of the skull cap.

SHAPE
This is ovoid like norma verticalis.

BONES
Same bones contribute to this part which were observed in norma verticalis, i.e.
1. Frontal bone, anteriorly.
2. Occipital bone, posteriorly
3. Parietal bones, on each side.

SUTURES
Sutures correspond with those observed in norma verticalis which are as follows:
1. *Coronal suture*, between frontal and parietal bones.
2. *Sagittal suture*, between two parietal bones.
3. *Lambdoid suture*, between parietal and occipital bones.

FEATURES (Fig. 42.1)

A. Frontal crest
1. It is a midline crest seen at its anterior part.
2. *Falx cerebri* is attached to it.

B. Sagittal sulcus
1. It is an anteroposterior groove in the median plane.
2. It is narrow anteriorly but widens posteriorly.
3. It contains superior *sagittal sinus*.
4. *Falx cerebri* is attached to its margins.

C. Bregma and lambda
These mark the junctions of sagittal suture with coronal and lambdoid sutures respectively (see norma verticalis).

D. Parietal foramen
It pierces the parietal bone on each side of midline about 3.5 cm in front of lambda. Emissary vein passes through it.

E. Granular foveolae
1. These are irregular depressions on each side of sagittal sulcus.
2. These are produced by *arachnoid granulations*.
3. These are deep and more abundant in aged skull.

F. Grooves for meningeal vessels
1. Grooves for anterior (frontal) twigs of middle meningeal vessels are located just behind the coronal suture.
2. Grooves for parietal twigs of middle meningeal vessels are more posteriorly

Interior of the Cranial Vault

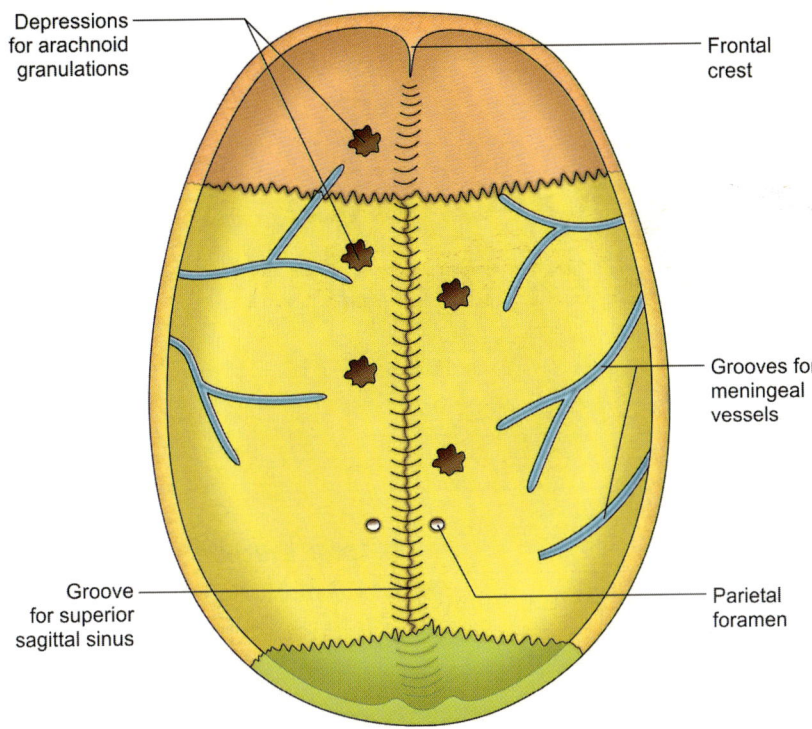

Fig. 42.1: Skull cap. Internal surface

placed. These run backwards and upwards.

G. Impressions for cerebral gyri

These are less marked in cranial vault in contrast to the interior of the base of skull where cerebral impressions are well defined.

APPLIED ANATOMY

(Please see the chapter of applied anatomy in norma verticalis).

CHAPTER 43

Interior of the Base of the Skull

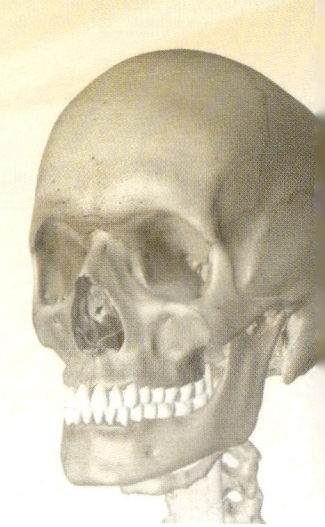

DEFINITION

It is the base of skull (neurocranium minus skull cap) observed from inside, i.e. the cavity side.

SUBDIVISIONS

Internal surface of the base of the skull is naturally demarcated into three fossae known as the anterior, middle and posterior cranial fossae.

I. ANTERIOR CRANIAL FOSSA

A. Boundaries
a. Anterior and lateral
Frontal bone.

b. Posterior
   i. *Posterior border of lesser wing of sphenoid.*
   ii. *Anterior clinoid process.*
   iii. *Anterior margin* of *sulcus chiasmatis.*

B. Floor
a. Median region
   i. Anteriorly – *Cribriform plate of ethmoid.*
   ii. Posteriorly – Anterior part of superior surface of body of sphenoid (*jugum sphenoidale*).

b. Lateral region
   i. Anteriorly – *Orbital plates of frontal bone.*
   ii. Posteriorly – *Lesser wings of sphenoid.*

C. Features and attachments (Figs 43.1 and 43.2)
a. Frontal crest
   1. It is a median crest in the anterior wall of fossa.
   2. It provides attachment to *falx cerebri*.

b. Crista galli of cribriform plate
   1. It is an upward tooth like projection in the midline of cribriform plate just behind the frontal crest.
   2. This projection receives attachment of *anterior end of falx cerebri.*

c. Foramen caecum
   1. It is situated between crista galli and crest of frontal bone.
   2. It is usually blind but some times may transmit an *emissary vein* from nasal cavity to superior sagittal sinus.

d. Cribriform plate of ethmoid on each side of crista galli
   1. It is a sieve-like (perforated) bony plate.

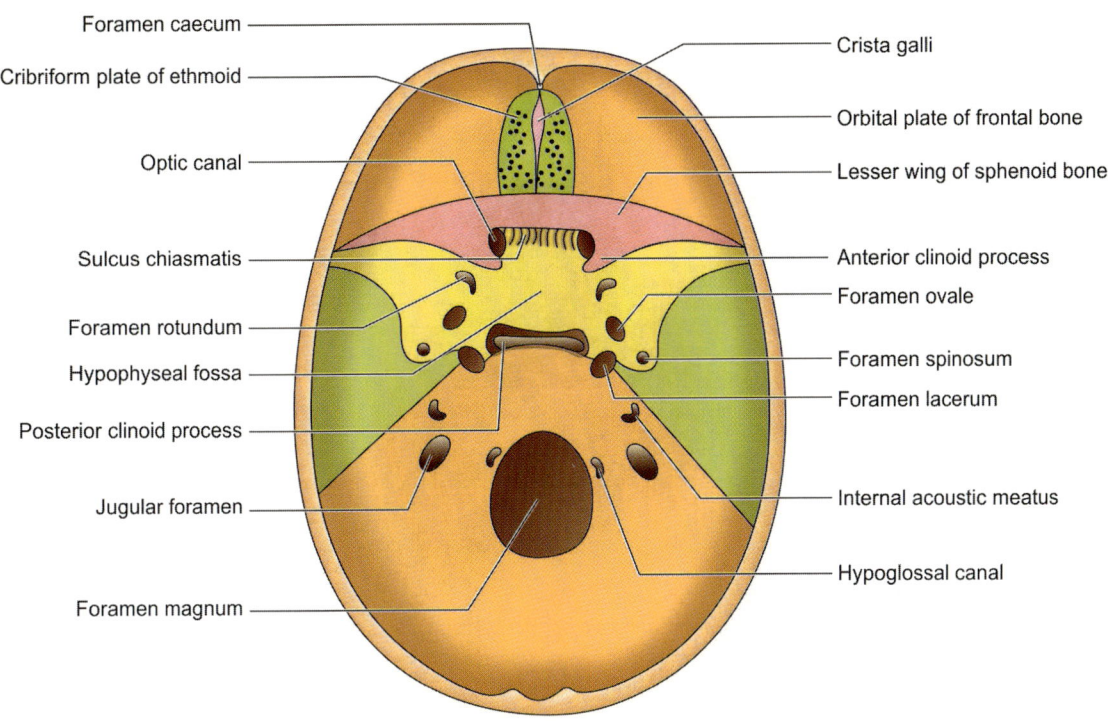

Fig. 43.1: Base of skull. Internal surface

2. 15–20 filaments of olfactory nerve pass through each perforate plate from olfactory mucosa of nose to olfactory bulb.
3. Groove just lateral to crista galli is related to:
   i. *Olfactory bulb.*
   ii. *Gyrus rectus.*
4. Anterior ethmoidal canal
   i. It opens in the *cribrofrontal suture* behind the crista galli.
   ii. *Anterior ethmoidal nerve and vessels* pass through it.
5. A *slit like aperture* by the side of anterior part of crista galli is meant for a process of dura mater.
6. A foramen just lateral to anterior end of slit.
   Through this passage, *anterior ethmoidal nerve and vessels* enter the nose from anterior cranial fossa.
7. Posterior ethmoidal canal
   i. It is present in the posterolateral corner of cribriform plate.
   ii. It transmits *posterior ethmoidal vessels.*

e. Jugum sphenoidale
1. It is most anterior part of the superior surface of body of sphenoid.
2. Its anterior margin meets the posterior margin of cribriform plate.
3. Posteriorly it is limited by sulcus chiasmatis.
4. It separates anterior cranial fossa from two sphenoidal sinuses located in the body of sphenoid.

f. Orbital plates of frontal bone
1. Each of the two orbital plates separates anterior cranial fossa from corresponding orbit just lateral to cribriform plate.

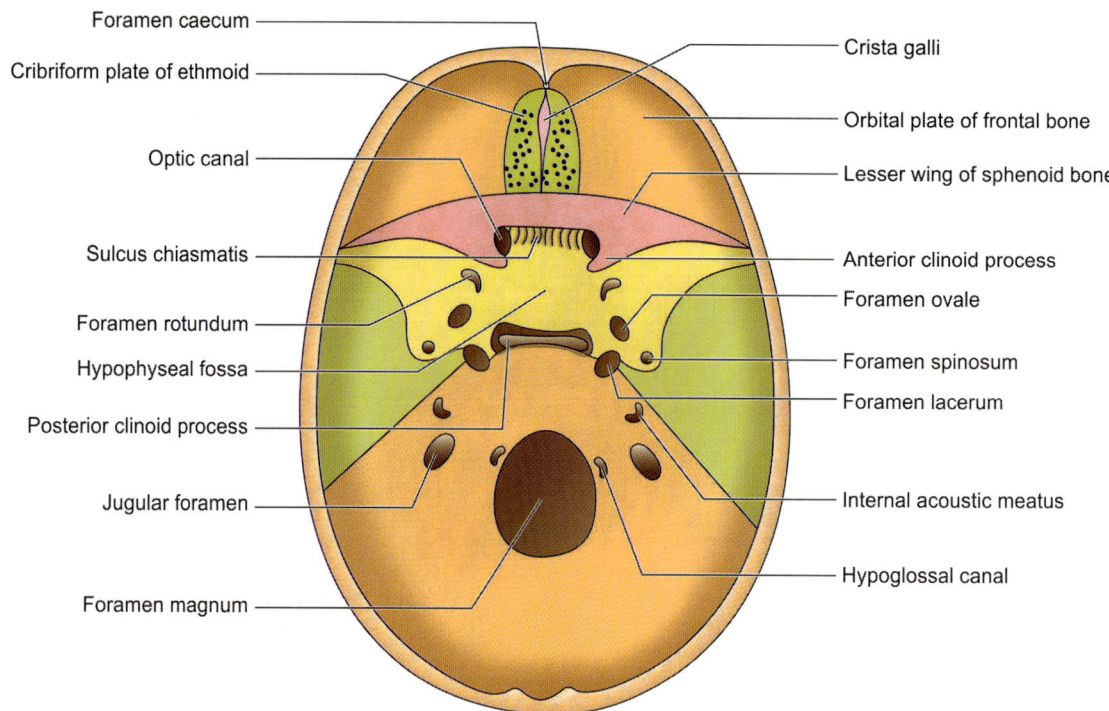

Fig. 43.2: Base of skull : Internal surface

2. It shows impressions for cerebral gyri.
3. It supports the orbital surface of frontal lobe of cerebrum.
4. Medially it covers the superior surface of ethmoidal labyrinth (anterior and posterior ethmoidal canals intervening between the two).
5. Posteriorly it meets the anterior margin of lesser wing of sphenoid.

g. Lesser wings of sphenoid

1. Jugum sphenoidale continues laterally with superior surface of lesser wing.
2. It is broad medially and tapers laterally.
3. Posterior margin of lesser wing is related to:
    i. *Sphenoparietal sinus*.
    ii. *Lateral sulcus* of cerebral hemisphere.
4. Posterior border of lesser wing ends medially into *anterior clinoid process* which receives attachment of free margin of tentorium cerebelli.

II. MIDDLE CRANIAL FOSSA

A. Boundaries

a. Anterior
  i. Posterior border of *lesser wing of sphenoid*.
  ii. *Anterior clinoid process*.
  iii. Anterior border of *sulcus chiasmatis*.

b. Posterior
  i. Superior border of *petrous part of temporal bone*.
  ii. *Posterior clinoid process*.
  iii. *Dorsum sellae*.

c. Lateral (on each side)
  i. *Greater wing of sphenoid*.
  ii. Anteroinferior angle of *parietal bone*.
  iii. Squamous part of *temporal bone*.

B. Floor

a. Central portion
Body of sphenoid.

b. Lateral portion (on each side)
 i. Greater wing of sphenoid.
 ii. Squamous part of temporal bone.
 iii. Anterior surface of petrous temporal.

C. Features and attachments

a. Sulcus chiasmatis
1. It is transversely running groove just behind the jugum sphenoidale.
2. It is named after its relation with the *optic chiasma* which never comes in contact with it but lies posterosuperior to sulcus.
3. Sulcus chiasmatis leads laterally into optic canals.

b. Optic canal
1. It connects the middle cranial fossa with the orbit.
2. It is bounded by anterior and posterior roots of lesser wing and body of sphenoid.
3. It transmits:
    i. *Optic nerve.*
    ii. *Ophthalmic artery.*
    iii. *Meninges.*

c. Tuberculum sellae
1. It forms an elevation just behind the sulcus chiasmatis.
2. *Middle clinoid processes* are the lateral prominent ends of tuberculum sellae.
3. It receives attachment of anterior margin of *diaphragma sellae*.

d. Sella turcica
1. It is the depressed area behind the tuberculum sellae.
2. It is shaped like a Turkish saddle and therefore named as sella turcica.
3. *Hypophyseal fossa* is the deepest part in it.

It lodges *pituitary gland*.
4. *Sphenoidal air sinus* is present below the floor of the hypophyseal fossa.

e. Dorsum sellae
1. It is the back of Turkish saddle.
2. It is the square plate of bone behind the sella turcica.
3. Superior angles of dorsum sellae project laterally into *posterior clinoid processes*.
4. *Diaphragma sellae* is attached to the upper margin of dorsum sellae.
5. Anterior end of attached margin of *tentorium cerebelli* is attached to posterior clinoid process.

f. Carotid sulcus
1. It is observed as a shallow groove on each side of the body of sphenoid.
2. It lodges *cavernous sinus* enclosing cavernous part of *internal carotid artery*.
3. It extends posteriorly upto foramen lacerum where it is deepened.
4. The lateral margin of carotid sulcus at its posterior end, projects backwards into tongue shaped *lingula*.
5. Lingula lies over the *posterior opening of pterygoid canal*.

g. Superior orbital fissure
1. It is a triangular fissure connecting the lateral portion of middle cranial fossa with orbit.
2. It is bounded above by the *lesser wing*, below by the *greater wing* and medially by the *body of sphenoid*.
3. Common annular tendon (tendinous ring of Zinn) is attached to a small projection seen on the lower border of fissure.
4. Common annular tendon divides the fissure into lateral, middle and medial parts through which following structures traverse:

Through lateral part
    i. *Lacrimal nerve.*

ii. *Frontal nerve.*
iii. *Trochlear nerve.*
iv. *Superior ophthalmic vein.*
v. *Meningeal branch of lacrimal artery.*
vi. *Orbital branch of middle meningeal artery.*

Through common annular tendon, i.e. middle part

  i. Upper and lower divisions of *oculomotor nerve.*
  ii. *Nasociliary nerve.*
  iii. *Abducent nerve.*

Through medial part

  i. *Inferior ophthalmic vein.*
  ii. *Sympathetic twigs* form internal carotid sympathetic plexus.

Note: *To remember structures passing through superior orbital fissure, remember 'I Slept One Night And Left For Tokyo' in which I = Inferior ophthalmic vein, S = Sympathetic twigs, Superior ophthalmic vein; O = Oculomotor nerve, N = Nasociliary nerve, A = Abducent nerve, L = Lacrimal nerve, F = Frontal nerve, T = Trochlear nerve.*

h. Foramen rotundum

1. It is present in the greater wing of sphenoid.
2. It is located just below and behind the medial end of superior orbital fissure.
3. It leads forwards into pterygopalatine fossa.
4. It transmits *maxillary nerve.*

Note: *Remember, it is not visible in norma basalis.*

i. Foramen ovale

1. It is located posterolateral to foramen rotundum.
2. It leads inferiorly into infratemporal fossa.
3. It transmits:
    i. *Mandibular nerve.*
    ii. *Accessory meningeal artery.*
    iii. *Lesser petrosal nerve.*
    iv. *Emissary vein.*

Note: *Remember Ovale = MALE, where M = Mandibular, A = Accessory, L = Lesser and E = Emissary.*

j. Foramen spinosum

1. It is situated posterolateral to foramen ovale.
2. It leads inferiorly into infratemporal fossa.
3. It transmits:
    i. *Middle meningeal artery.*
    ii. *Nervus spinosus.*
    iii. *Parietal trunk of middle meningeal vein.*

k. Foramen of Vesalius (sphenoidal emissary foramen)

1. It is inconstant.
2. It is located between foramen rotundum and foramen ovale.
3. It transmits emissary vein connecting the cavernous sinus and pterygoid venous plexus.

l. Foramen innominatum

1. This is also an inconstant foramen.
2. It is located between foramen ovale and foramen spinosum.
3. It transmits *lesser petrosal nerve.*

m. Foramen lacerum

1. It is a foramen with irregular margin between sphenoid and apex of petrous temporal.
2. *Carotid* and *pterygoid canals* open into it.
3. Only two structures pass through it, i.e. *meningeal branch of ascending pharyngeal artery* and *emissary vein.*
4. *Internal carotid artery* traverses its upper part *with its sympathetic and venous plexuses.*

5. *Nerve of pterygoid canal* (*Vidian nerve*) is formed in its upper part by the union of *greater superficial petrosal* and *deep petrosal nerves*.

n. Anterior surface of petrous temporal

1. *Trigeminal impression* is a depression for trigeminal ganglion adjacent to apex.
2. A ridge limits the trigeminal impression posteriorly.
3. *Roof of internal acoustic meatus* is a depressed area behind the ridge.
4. *Arcuate eminence* is a prominent elevation behind the second depression. It is produced by superior semicircular canal. Its posterior sloping lies over lateral and posterior semicircular canals.
5. Area anterolateral to trigeminal impression forms the *roof of anterior part of carotid canal*.
6. Area anterolateral to arcuate eminence forms *roof of vestibule and beginning of facial canal*.
7. Thin plate of bone between squamous temporal and features described above is called *tegmen tympani*. It forms roof of mastoid antrum, middle ear and canal for tensor tympani from posterior to anterior. Tegmen tympani projects downwards to form lateral walls of canal for tensor tympani and bony Eustachian tube and appears in norma basalis in the squamotympanic fissure.
8. A hiatus lateral to arcuate eminence leads into a *groove for greater superficial petrosal nerve* which runs towards foramen laerum on the tegmen tympani.
9. Lateral to aforementioned groove is present another *groove for lesser petrosal nerve* which runs towards foramen ovale.

o. Superior border of petrous temporal

1. It is gooved by the superior petrosal sinus.
2. Margins of groove provide attachment to tentorium cerebelli.

3. It is crossed by the trigeminal nerve near the apex of petrous temporal.

p. Lateral part of the fossa shows following additional features:

1. Markings for the middle meningeal vessels.
2. Depressions produced by the gyri of temporal lobe of cerebral hemisphere.

III. POSTERIOR CRANIAL FOSSA

It is largest and the deepest of all cranial fossae. It lodges cerebellum, pons and medulla.

A. Boundaries

a. Anterior
i. *Dorsum sellae*.
ii. *Posterior clinoid process*.
iii. *Superior border of petrous temporal*.

b. Posterior
Squamous part of occipital bone.

c. Lateral
i. *Mastoid part of temporal bone*.
ii. *Mastoid angle of parietal bone*.

B. Floor
1. *Basisphenoid and basiocciput*.
2. Posterior surface of petrous temporal.
3. Mastoid part of temporal bone.
4. Posteroinferior angle of the parietal bone.
5. Squamous part of occipital bone.

C. Features and attachments

a. Clivus
1. It is sloping surface in front of foramen magnum.
2. It is formed by the superior surface of basilar part of occipital bone, posterior part of superior surface of body of sphenoid and dorsum sellae.
3. It supports *pons* and *medulla*.

4. It is related to *basilar plexus of veins* and *basilar artery*.
5. Its lower part receives attachments of following structures from above downwards:
   i. *Membrana tectoria.*
   ii. *Superior longitudinal band of cruciform ligament.*
   iii. *Apical ligament of dens.*

b. Petro-occipital fissure
1. It is the junction between clivus and petrous temporal.
2. It is grooved by the *inferior petrosal sinus*.

c. Foramen magnum
1. It is largest foramen.
2. It is located in the floor of posterior cranial fossa.
3. Its margins provide attachments to following structures:
   i. *Anterior margin – Anterior atlanto-occipital membrane.*
   ii. *Posterior margin – Posterior atlanto-occipital membrane.*
   iii. *Lateral margins – Alar ligaments.*
4. Structures passing through its anterior part are:
   i. *Apical ligament of dens.*
   ii. *Superior longitudinal band of cruciform ligament.*
   iii. *Membrana tectoria.*
5. Structures passing through its posterior part are:
   i. *Medulla oblongata.*
   ii. *Meninges.*
   iii. *Spinal roots of accessory nerves.*
   iv. *Meningeal branches of upper cervical nerves.*
   v. *Vertebral arteries.*
   vi. *Sympathetic plexuses around the vertebral arteries.*
   vii. *Anterior and posterior spinal arteries.*

d. Internal occipital protuberance
1. It is situated opposite the external occipital protuberance.
2. It is related to *confluence of dural venous sinuses*.
3. On each side it is grooved by *transverse sinus*.

e. Internal occipital crest
1. It is a midline crest between internal occipital protuberance and the foramen magnum.
2. *Falx cerebelli* is attached to it.
3. *Cerebellar hemisphere* occupies the deep fossa on each side of the internal occipital crest.

f. Vermian fossa
1. It is a midline fossa at the lower end of internal occipital crest adjacent to foramen magnum.
2. It is related to *inferior vermis of the cerebellum*.

g. Transverse sulcus
1. It runs laterally on each side from the internal occipital protuberance.
2. At the mastoid angle of the parietal bone it continues as sigmoid sulcus.
3. It lodges the *transverse sinus*.
4. *Attached margin of tentorium cerebelli* is attached to its lips.
5. Right transverse sulcus is wider than the left one and is continuous posteriorly with superior sagittal sulcus.

h. Sigmoid sulcus
1. It is downward continuation of transverse sulcus at the mastoid angle of parietal bone.
2. It ends at the lateral end of jugular foramen.
3. It lodges *sigmoid sinus* which enters the jugular foramen to continue with internal jugular vein.

i. Jugular foramen
1. It is located at the posterior end of *petro-occipital fissure*.
2. It is an interosseous foramen situated between the anterior margin of jugular process of occipital bone and posterior margin of petrous part of temporal bone.
3. It is divided into anterior, middle and posterior parts.
4. *9th, 10th and 11th cranial nerves* pass through its middle part.
5. *Inferior petrosal sinus* and *meningeal branch of ascending pharyngeal artery* traverse its anterior part.
6. Sigmoid sinus and meningeal branch of occipital artery pass through its posterior part.

j. Jugular tubercle
1. Medial to the lower margin of jugular foramen there is a rounded elevation known as *jugular tubercle*.
2. It is located anterosuperior to the internal opening of hypoglossal canal.
3. It is grooved by the 9th, 10th and 11th cranial nerves.

k. Hypoglossal canal
1. Its internal opening is located just above the tubercle for alar ligament on the medial aspect of occipital condyle.
2. It transmits:
    i. *Hypoglossal nerve*.
    ii. *Meningeal branch of ascending pharyngeal artery*.
    iii. *Emissary vein from basilar venous plexus*.

l. Condylar canal
1. It is inconstant.
2. Its internal orifice is located posterolateral to that of hypoglossal canal.
3. It transmits emissary vein from sigmoid sinus.

m. Internal acoustic meatus
1. Its *porus* (inlet or medial end) is present in the centre of the posterior surface of petrous temporal.
2. It is about 1 cm in length.
3. It transmits:
    i. *Facial nerve*.
    ii. *Vestibulocochlear nerve*.
    iii. *Labyrinthine vessels*.
4. *Fundus* of internal acoustic meatus is a plate of bone at its lateral end. The plate is divided into upper and lower areas by a transverse ridge (*crista falciformis*). The upper area is further divided into anterior and posterior areas by a vertical crest called *Bill's bar*. Anterior to bar is the *facial canal* for facial nerve. Area behind the bar is called *superior vestibular area* which presents number of small openings for the nerve fibres supplying utricle and superior and lateral semicircular ducts.
Below the transverse crest, anteriorly is the *cochlear area* (which possesses number of foramina called *tractus spiralis foraminosus*) and posteriorly is the *inferior vestibular area*. Fibres of cochlear nerve enter the cochlear area while nerve fibres supplying the saccule enter the inferior vestibular area. Below and behind the inferior vestibular area is *foramen singulare* for the passage of nerve to posterior semicircular duct (Fig. 43.3).

n. Aqueduct of vestibule
1. A slit behind the porus of internal acoustic meatus leads into aqueduct of vestibule.
2. Aqueduct of vestibule contains *saccus and ductus endolymphaticus* along with the small artery and vein.

o. Subarcuate fossa
1. It is an irregular depression located above and between the openings of internal acoustic meatus and aqueduct of vestibule.
2. It lodges a process of dura mater.

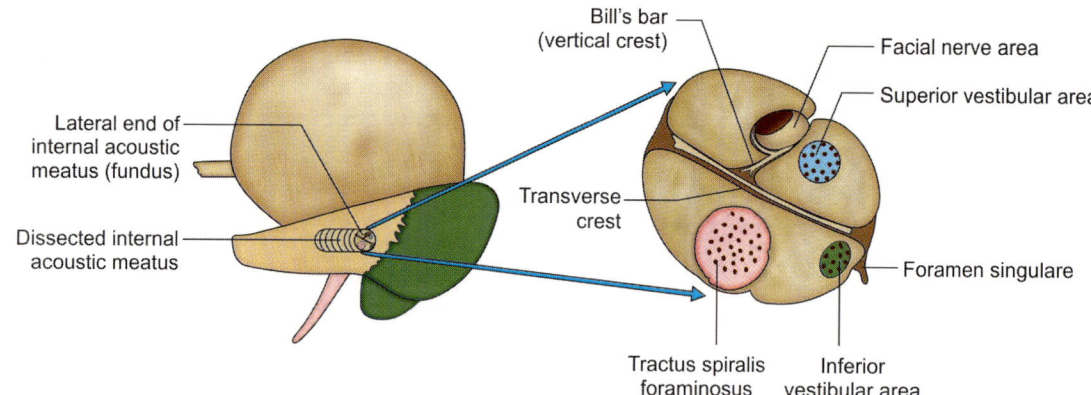

Fig. 43.3: Fundus of right internal acoustic meatus

APPLIED ANATOMY

1. Thickenings of bones in the base of skull form strengthening buttresses of the skull and exert a direct effect on the pattern of fracture. Fracture lines avoid the thickenings and pass through the line of least resistance. Therefore fractures are often zig-zag in appearance and for the same reason fracture lines often converge towards the foramen magnum or sella turcica.

2. In cases of basal fractures, laceration of structures passing through basal foramina may complicate the issue, e.g. fracture line passing through the foramen lacerum may tear the internal carotid artery with a resultant *caroticocavernous fistula* which produces *pulsating exophthalmos*.

3. If the fissure lines involve the grooves having meningeal vessels and dural sinuses, then *epidural haematoma* might result.

4. Basal fractures involving anterior cranial fossa might lead to communication between nasal cavity and subarachnoid space resulting into CSF leak into the nose. This condition is called *CSF rhinorrhea*.

5. Fracture of tegmen tympani might connect the subarachnoid space with middle ear leading to CSF leakage into the middle ear. If the tympanic membrane is also damaged then the CSF will appear as discharge through external acoustic meatus. This condition is called *CSF otorrhea*.

6. Communications between cranial cavity and nasal and middle ear cavities due to basal fractures may act as portal for sepsis of meninges and brain.

7. Fracture of orbital plate of frontal bone causes haemorrhage into the orbit. This haemorrhage acquires a triangular shape under the conjunctiva whose apex is towards the corneoscleral junction and base towards the orbital margin, but the exact peripheral limit of the base is not visible (Fig. 43.4).

8. Petrous temporal is very strong and therefore most fracture lines end here

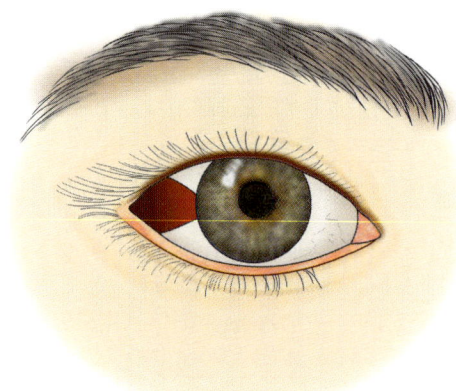

Fig. 43.4: Haemorrhage in the orbit

without making a tear in it. A bullet entering the middle cranial fossa through orbit, is prevented from entering the posterior cranial fossa due to the same reason.

9. A forceful hit on the forehead causes linear fracture of both vertex and base (Fig. 43.5).
10. Clinical signs and symptoms which support the involvement of base of skull, are as follows:
    i. *CSF otorrhea* (discharge of CSF from ear).
    ii. *Tear of tympanic membrane.*
    iii. *Collection of blood in the middle ear.*
    iv. *Discolouration and edema of tissue of mastoid process* (it is due to sigmoid sinus damage).
    v. *CSF rhinorrhea* (this is due to damage of cribriform plate).
    vi. *Cranial nerve damage* (it is due to involvement of foramina).
11. A fracture near the sella turcica may tear the stalk of pituitary gland with resulting *diabetes insipidus, impotence* and *amenorrhea*.
12. A fracture of sphenoid may lacerate the optic nerve in optic canal resulting into blindness.
13. Fracture of cribriform plate may damage the filaments of olfactory nerve and result into *anosmia* (loss of smell sensation).
14. Petrous fracture often leads to *facial paralysis* if the facial nerve is damaged and *vertigo* and *nystagmus* if the 8th cranial nerve is involved.
15. Orbital plate of frontal bone is very important clinically:
    i. A penetrating object entering the orbit might damage its roof and then involve the frontal lobe of brain.
    ii. Orbital roof may be selected by surgeons as route to approach frontal lobe of brain.
16. A tumour in the middle cranial fossa enters the orbit through superior orbital fissure.
17. Some of the tumours which might involve the skull base are as follows:
    i. *Transitional cell carcinoma* arising from mucous membrane of paranasal sinuses or fossa of Rosenmuller of nasopharynx usually erodes the skull base.
    ii. Some of the other tumours, though very rare, arising from the base of skull or adjacent tissue are as follows: *osteomas, chondromas, chordomas, giant cell tumours of bones.*
    iii. Many malignant tumours metastasize to the basal skull bones from distant organs e.g. prostate, lung and breast.

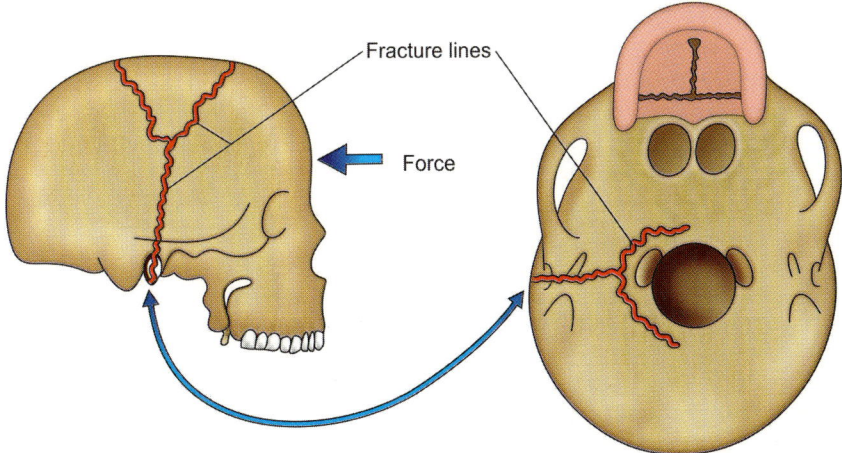

Fig. 43.5: Basal fracture due to blow on forehead

CHAPTER 44

Ossification at a Glance

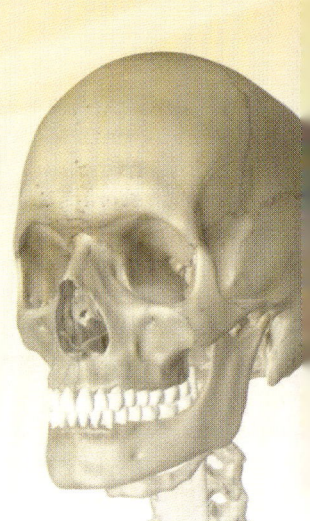

DEFINITION

Ossification is defined as deposition of calcium salts in the membranous or cartilaginous background of a bone. The former is called intramembranous while latter, endochondral ossification.

CENTRE OF OSSIFICATION

The site in the developing bone where calcium salts start depositing, is called centre of ossification. The centre of ossification is first microscopic but soon becomes macroscopic.

EXAMPLES

Bones ossifying in membrane are clavicle, most of the mandible, upper part of squamous part of occipital bone, frontal bone, parietal bones, squamous and tympanic parts of temporal bones, upper parts of greater wings and pterygoid processes of sphenoid; palatine, lacrimal and zygomatic bones; maxillae, vomer and nasal bones. Rest of the bones in the body are endochondral in origin.

PRIMARY AND SECONDARY CENTRES

Though many bones (e.g. carpal, tarsal, lacrimal, nasal, zygomatic bones; inferior nasal conchae and auditory ossicles) ossify from a single centre, majority of them ossify from several foci. One centre in these bones appears first in late embryonic and early foetal life (7th week to 4th month of intrauterine life). This is called primary centre of ossification. Remaining centres, called secondary centres appear later during period from birth to 12 years.

FUSION OF OSSIFICATION CENTRES

The secondary centres fuse with each other and then with the bone derived from primary centre. The process of fusion begins as early as 3 months of intrauterine life (e.g. fusion between 4 centres of squamous part of occipital bone) or may be observed as late as 40 years of age (e.g. fusion between body and xiphoid process of sternum).

FUSION BETWEEN ADJACENT BONES

Some adjacent bones may fuse to develop continuity, e.g. basilar parts of both sphenoid and occipital bones fuse at the age of 25 years.

EPIPHYSIS AND DIAPHYSIS

In long bones of limbs primary centres usually appear at 8th week of intrauterine life and give rise to shafts of these bones. Their ends remain cartilaginous till birth and are known as cartilaginous epiphyses (Sing., epiphysis). The long bony shaft between epiphyses is called diaphysis. Secondary centres appear in these cartilaginous ends resulting into formation of bony epiphyses. Epiphyseal plate is the cartilaginous plate between epiphysis and diaphysis, before their fusion with each other.

In miniature long bones (metacarpal and metatarsal bones) and clavicle, the epiphysis is located at one end only. Usually only one centre appears in the cartilaginous epiphysis forming single bony epiphysis. Even if multiple centres appear (e.g. at the upper end of the humerus), these fuse to form single epiphysis. But the upper end of femur and medial epicondyle of humerus are exceptions. Former has three secondary centres (one each for head, greater trochanter and lesser trochanter), each forming its own bony epiphysis which fuses separately with diaphysis. Similarly the secondary centre for medial epicondyle of humerus develops into an independent epiphysis fusing separately with diaphysis.

CLINICAL SIGNIFICANCE

Following are some examples of ossification of great clinical importance.

1. Centres of lower end of femur and cuboid appear at the time of birth (9 months of intrauterine life) and therefore of medicolegal importance. Its existence is the proof for viability of baby.
2. Eight carpal bones ossify after birth and almost all the centres appear at different periods ranging from 3rd month to 12th year. Therefore these centres very much help in determining the age of individuals before 12 years.
3. Xiphoid process fuses with body of sternum at the age of 40 years, therefore enhancing the scope of age determination at a later age.

CARTILAGINOUS NASAL CAPSULE (Fig. 44.9)

It is the cartilage which forms medial and lateral walls as well as roof of nasal cavity. It plays important role in development of nasal framework. Structures derived from this capsule are sphenoidal conchae, ethmoidal bone, inferior nasal conchae, vomer, nasal bones and septal, lateral nasal and alar cartilages.

Nasal bones and vomer develop in membrane while rest of the above bones are endochondral in origin.

APPEARANCE AND FUSION OF OSSIFICATION CENTRES (Figs 44.1 to 44.9)

The times of appearance of ossification centre (in case of single focus) or appearance as well as fusion of primary and secondary centres (in case of multiple foci) are represented diagrammatically as follows:

334 Human Osteology

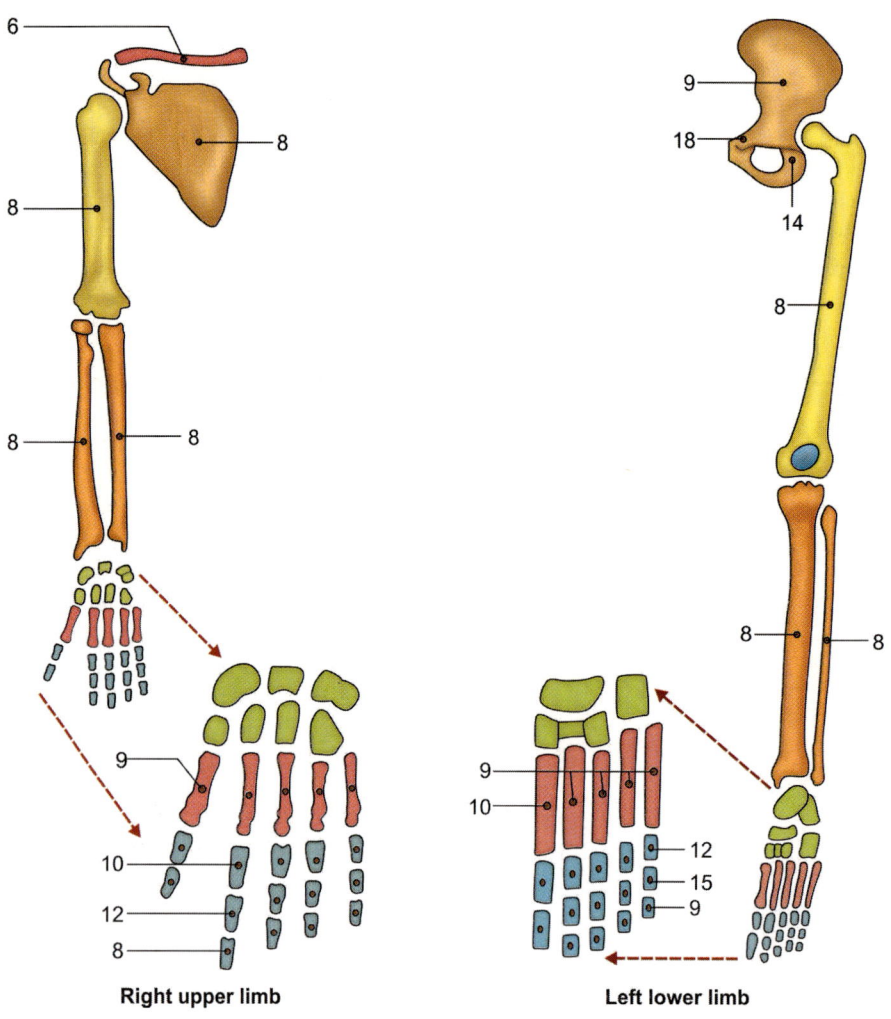

Fig. 44.1: Appearance of primary centres in appendicular skeleton (weeks of intrauterine life)

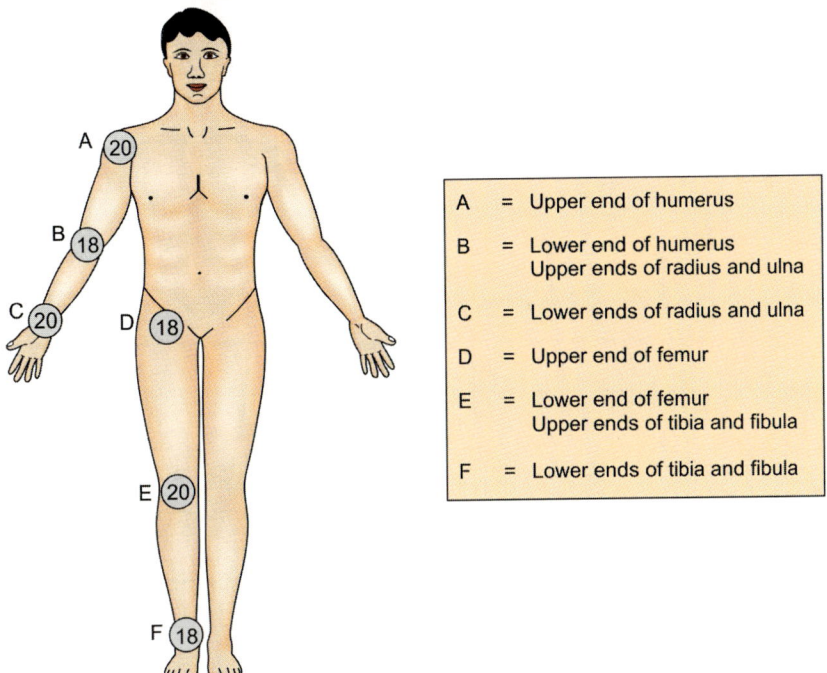

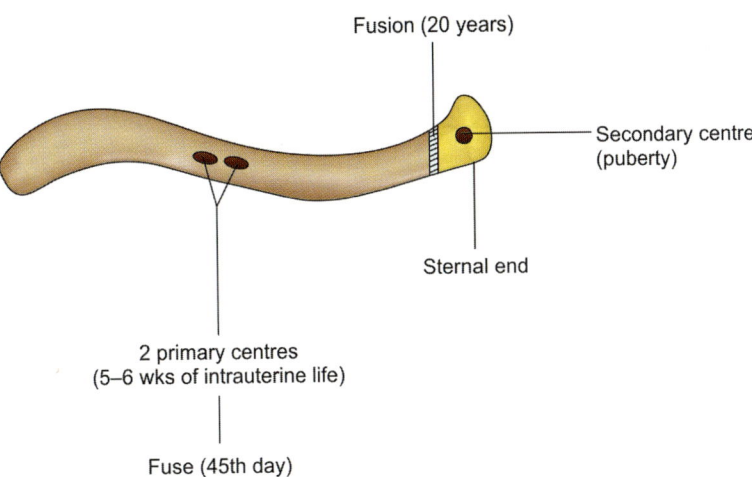

Fig. 44.2: Upper, times of the fusion of epiphyses with diaphyses in appendicular skeleton; Lower, ossification of clavicle

Human Osteology

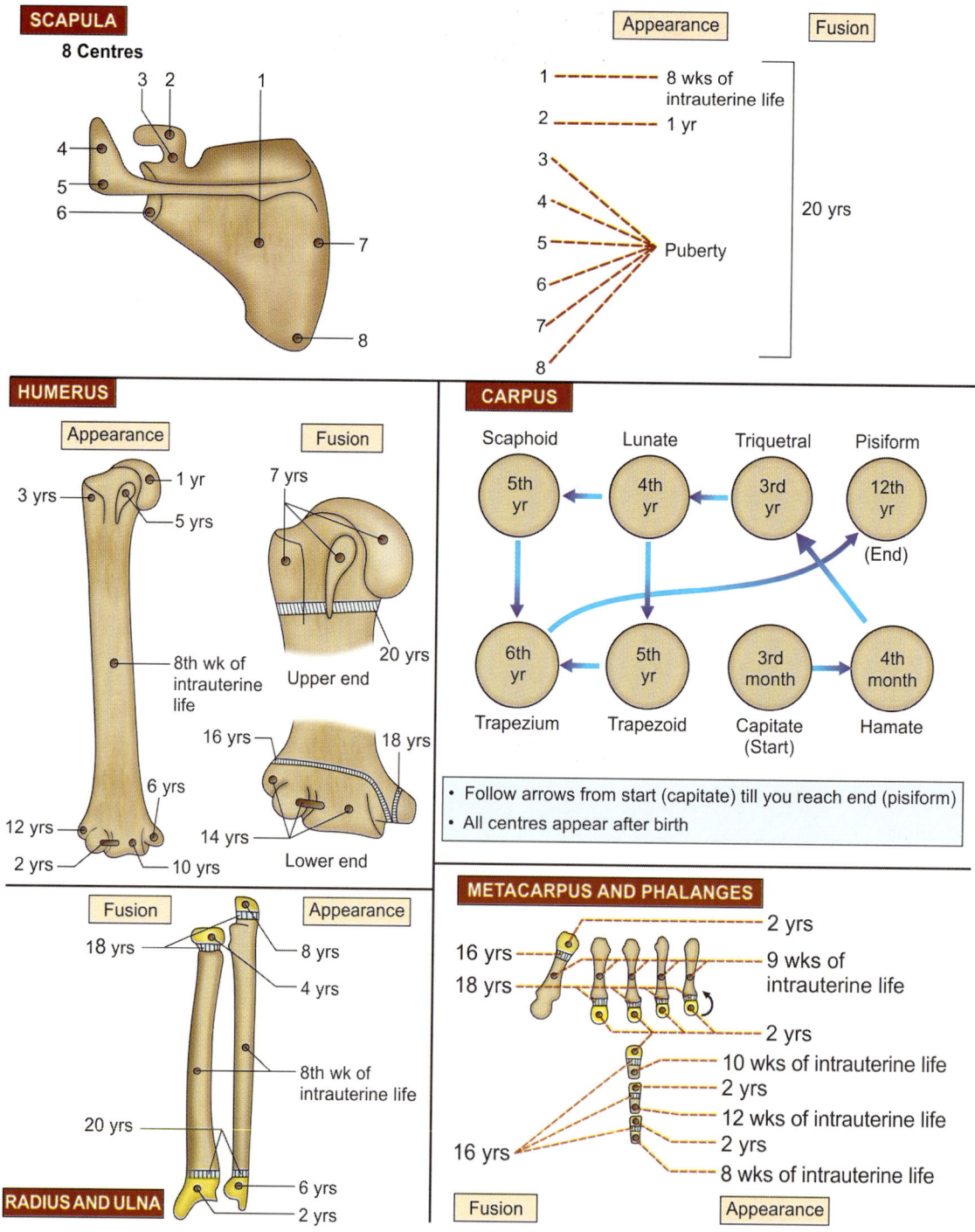

Fig. 44.3: Ossification of bones of upper limb (except clavicle)

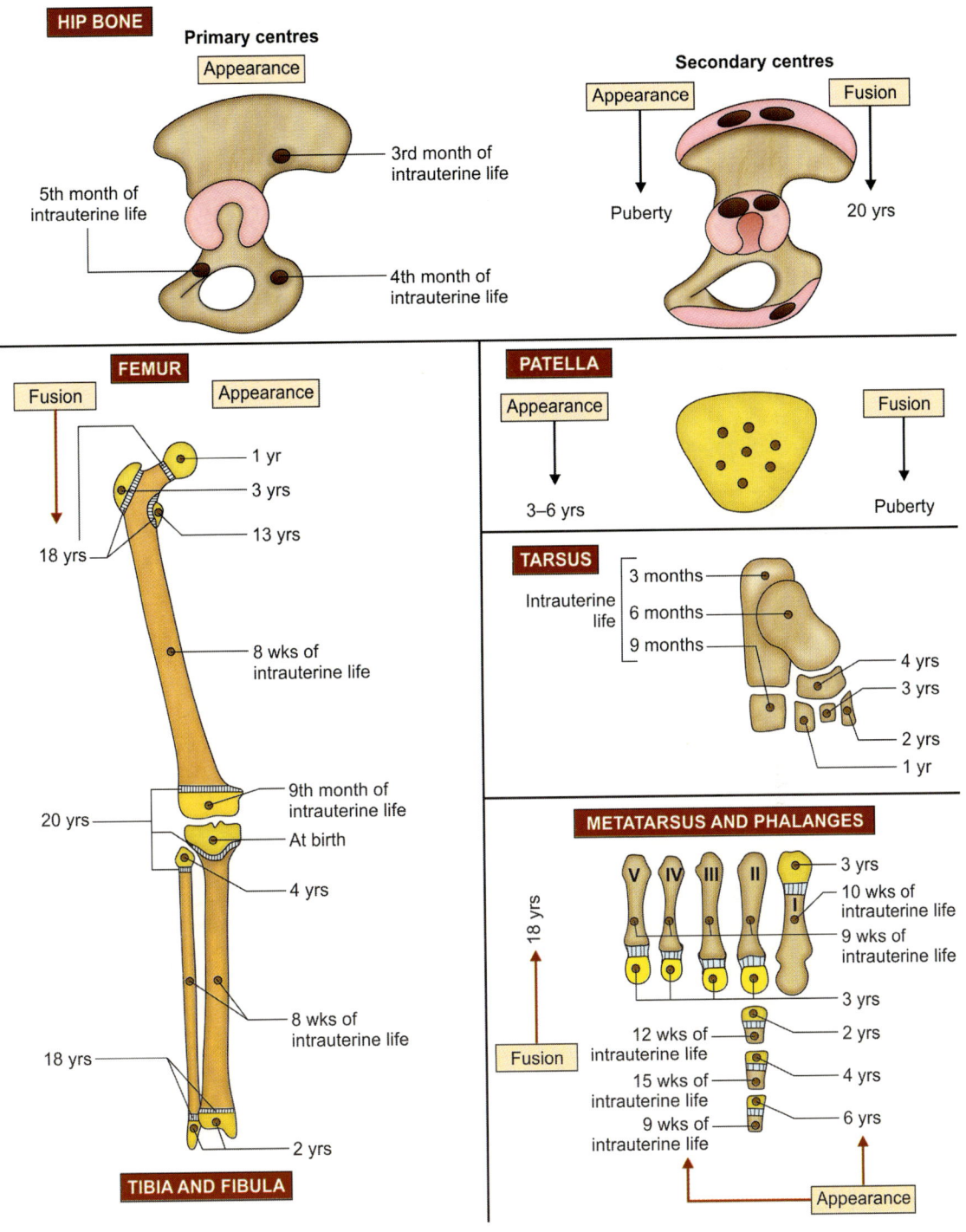

Fig. 44.4: Ossification of bones of lower limb

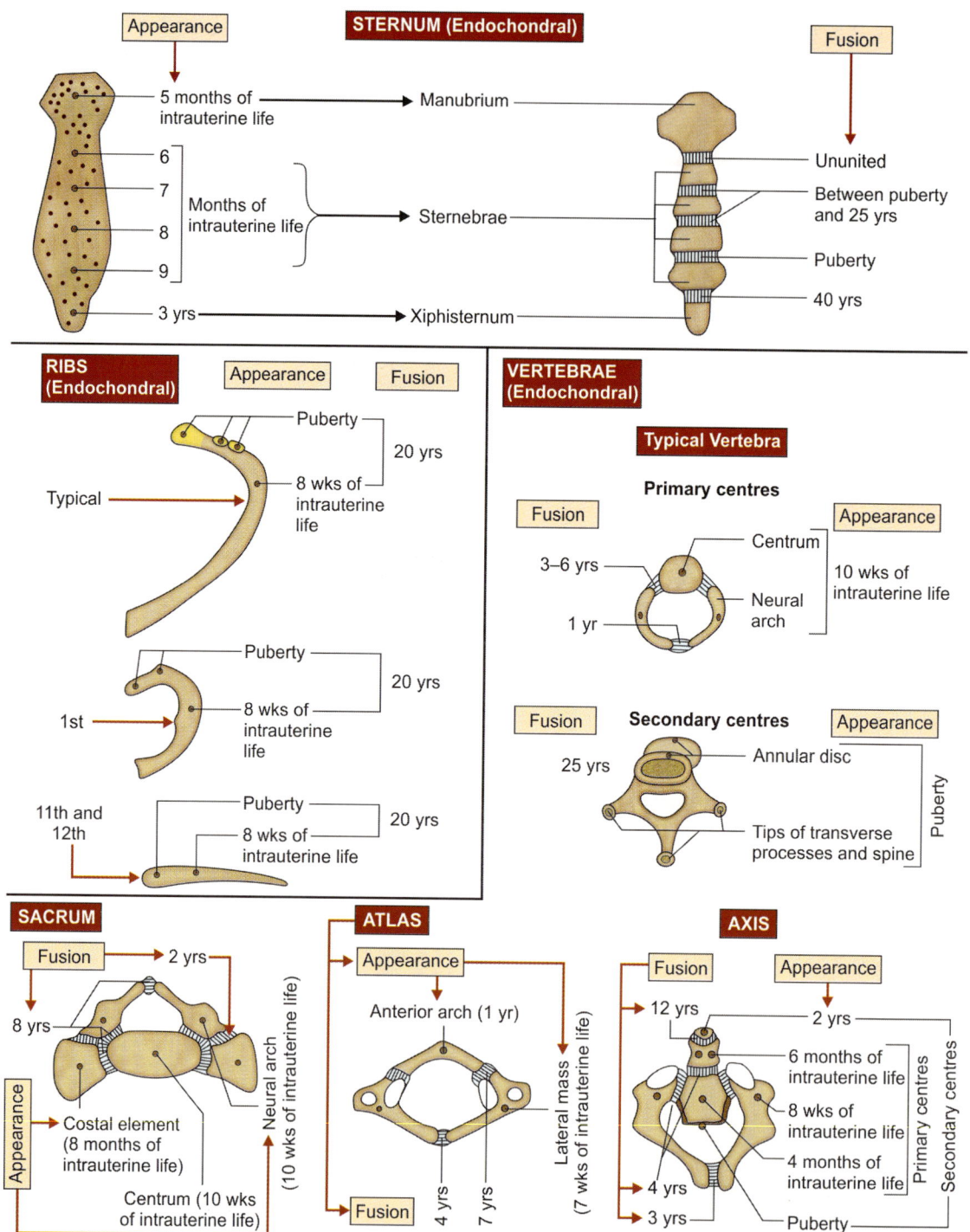

Fig. 44.5: Ossification of sternum, ribs and vertebrae

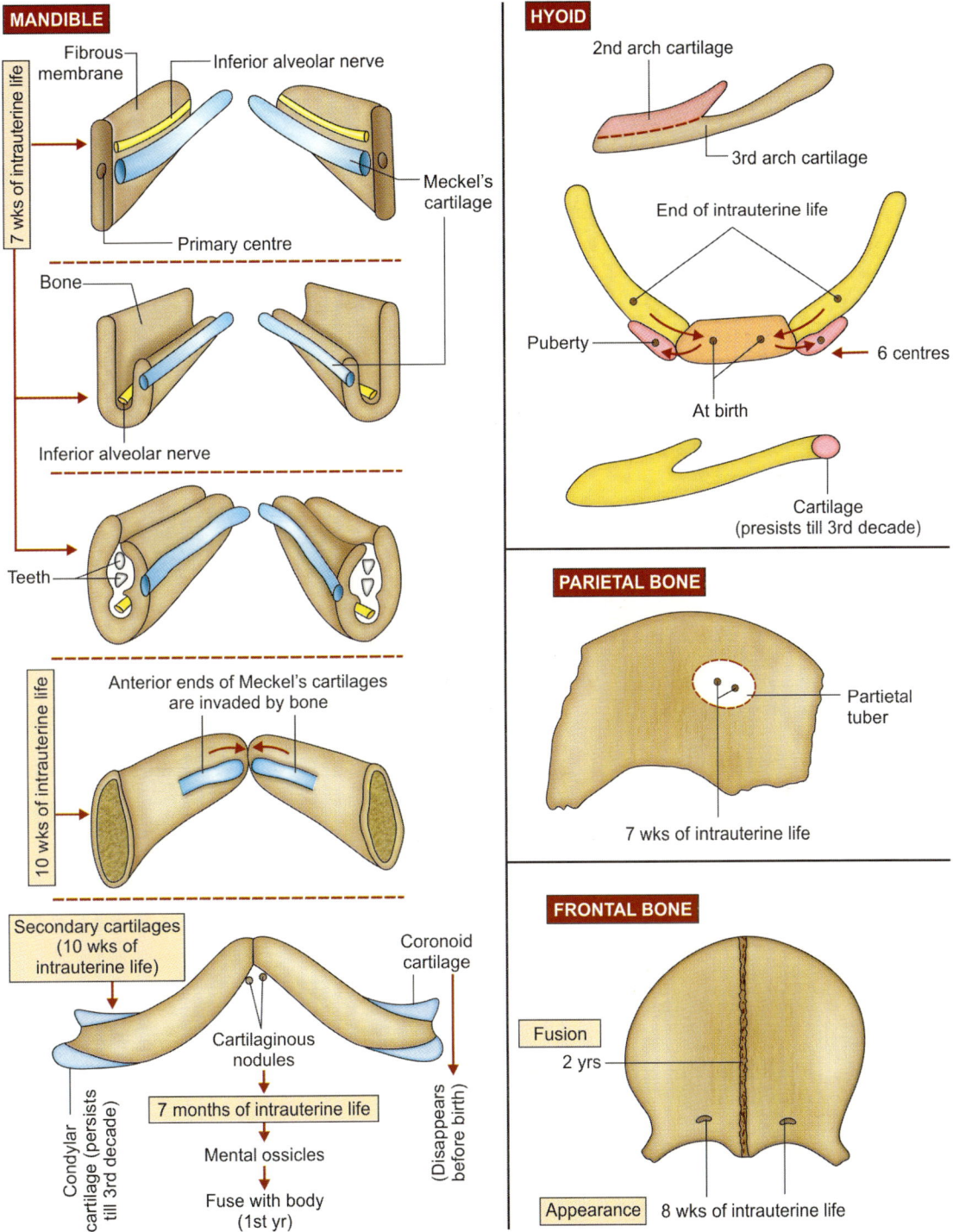

Fig. 44.6: Ossification of mandible, hyoid, parietal bone and frontal bone

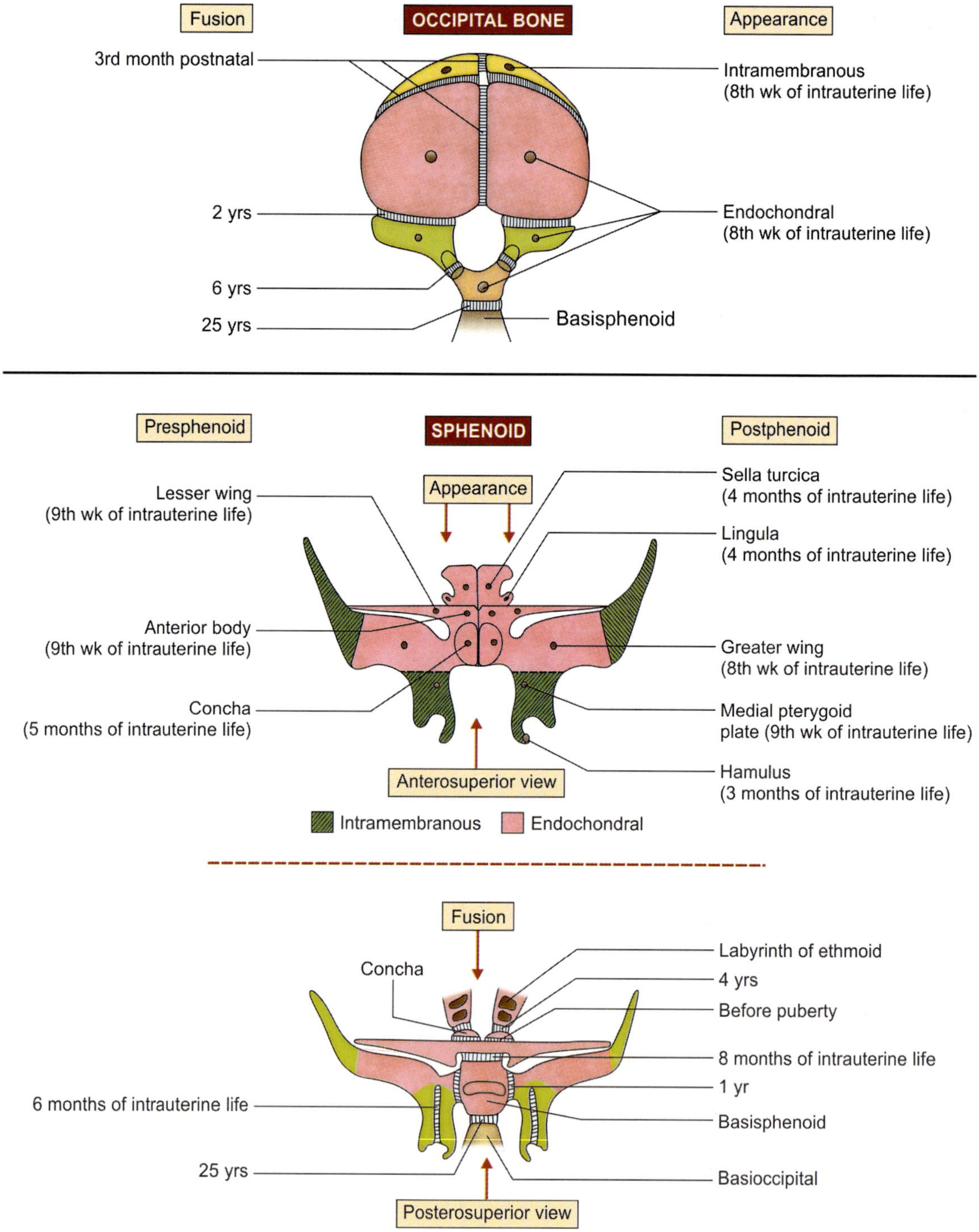

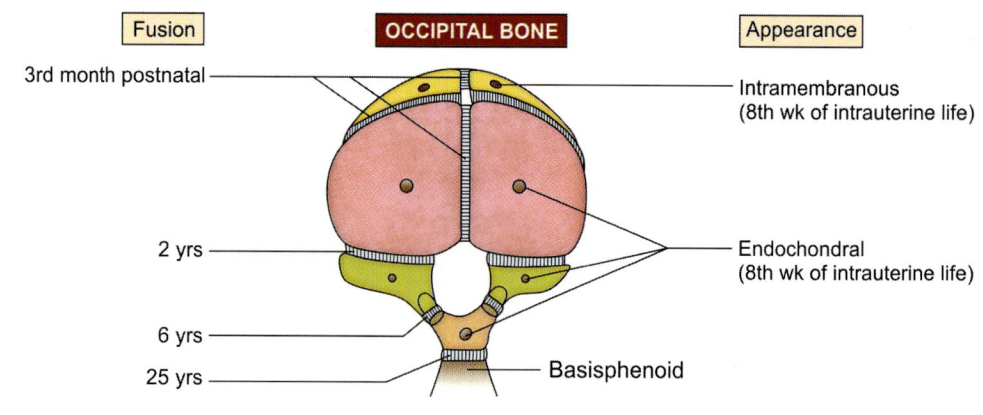

Fig. 44.7: Ossification of occipital bone and sphenoid

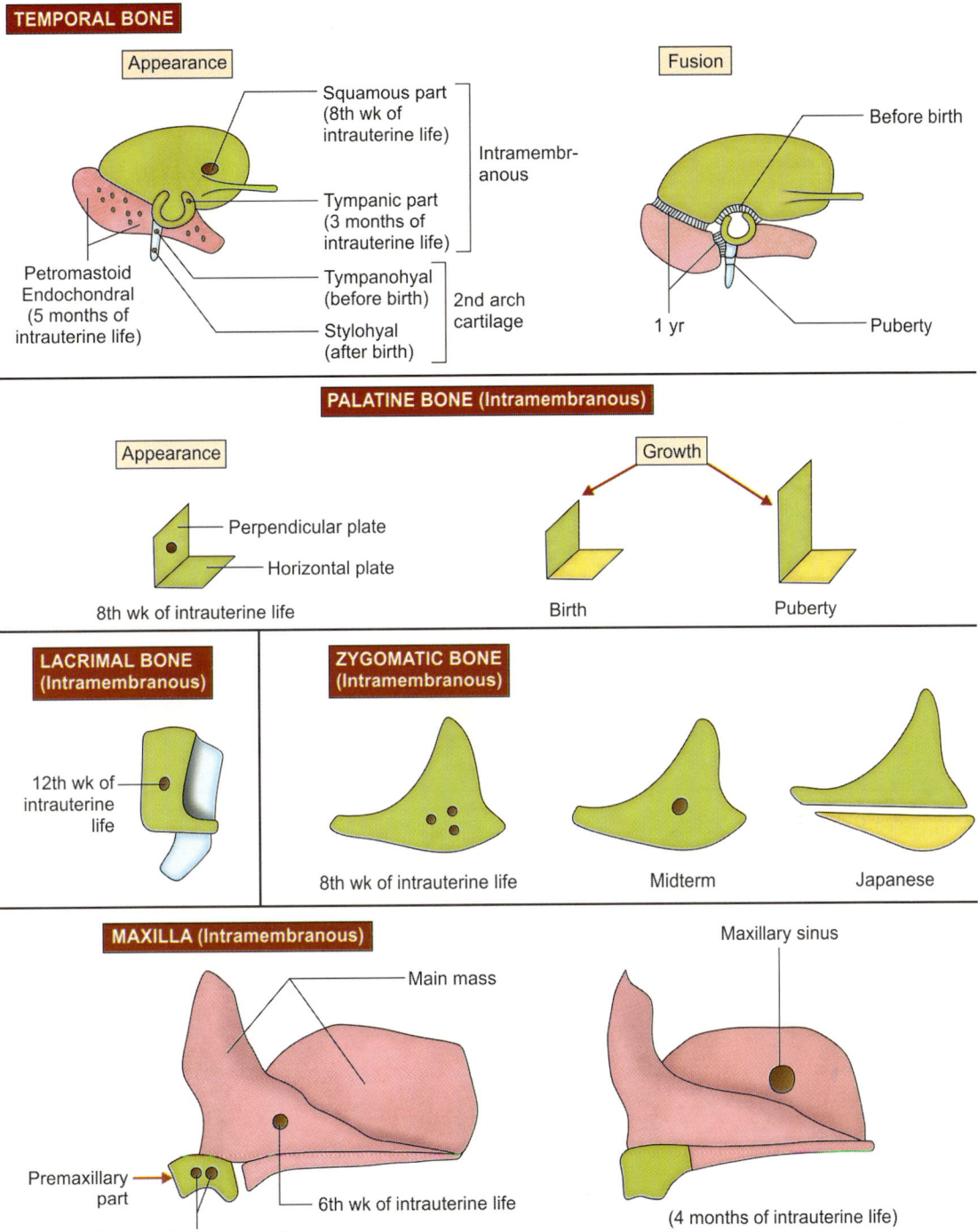

Fig. 44.8: Ossification of temporal bone, palatine bone, lacrimal bone, zygomatic bone and maxilla

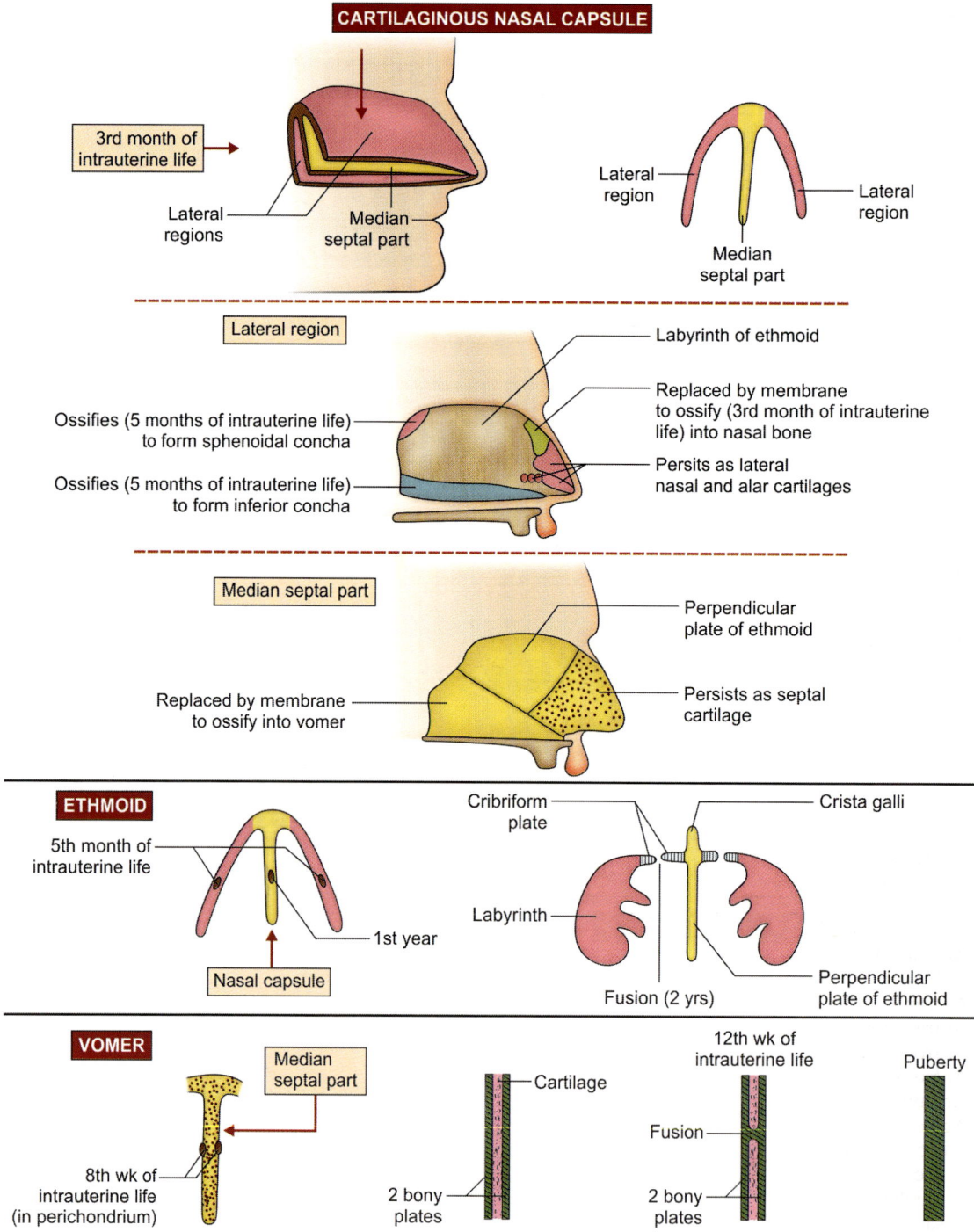

Fig. 44.9: Fate of cartilaginous nasal capsule

Index

A

Abduction injuries 115, 122
Abscess
  cold 169
  paravertebral 169
Acetabulum 73
Achondroplasia 276
Acromion 24
Acute synovitis 50
Adduction injuries 115, 122
Aerocele 225, 276, 293
Ainhum 141
Air cells
  ethmoidal 261
  mastoid 236
Ala of
  sacrum 158
  vomer 266
Ameloblastoma 210
Amenorrhea 331
Aneurysm, internal carotid artery 276
Angle of
  femoral torsion 88
  kyphosis 172
  lordosis 172
  rib 186
  scapula 22
  sternal 177, 178
Ankylosing spondylitis 84
Ankylosis of stapes 243
Anosmia 263, 317, 331
Antral puncture 318
Antrostomy 319
Antrum of Highmore 214
Antrum, mastoid 236
Apex of
  coccyx 163
  greater trochanter 90
  patella 103
  sacrum 158
Arch of atlas 147
    anterior 147
    posterior 148
  superciliary 291

  vertebral 144
  zygomatic 295
Arcuate line 75
Area
  intercondylar, of tibia 107
Artery
  epiphyseal 6
  metaphyseal 7
  nutrient 6
  periosteal 6
Articular surface 5
Atlas 147
Atlas, occipitalization 165
Auricular surface of hip bone 73
Avascular necrosis of
  head 12
    femur 96
    talus 128
  scaphoid 56
Axis 149

B

Base, of sacrum 158
Battle's sign 240
Bennett's fracture 60
Body of
  mandible 201
  maxilla 211
  sphenoid 269
  sternum 178
  talus 124
  vertebra 143
Bone
  accessory 4
  appendicular 4
  axial 4
  cancellous 1
  cartilaginous 3
  compact 2
  flat 3
  irregular 3
  long 3
  lymphatic drainage 7
  membranous 3

miniature long 3
nerve supply 3
ossification 7
pneumatic 7
sesamoid 3
short 3
spongy 1
sutural 4
Wormian 4
Bone marrow transplantation 12
Brain abscess 225, 293
Brain tumour 287
Bregma 286
Bulla ethmoidalis 262
Bump 17
Bumper fracture 114
Burr hole 297

C

Calcaneus 128
Calcaneal fracture 131
Calvaria 282
Canal 6
  carotid 232, 304
  condylar 305, 329
  craniopharyngeal 276
  greater palatine 212
  mandibular 205
  nasolacrimal 212
  palatovaginal 267, 275, 280
  sacral 161
Canaliculi 2
Capitate 51, 52, 54, 55
Caroticocavernous fistula 276, 330
Carpal bones 51
Cavity
  glenoid 22
  medullary 1
Central split of palate 281, 307, 318
Centres, of ossification 7
Cervical rib 164, 195
Chondromas 210, 307
Chondrosarcoma 197
Clavicle 13
Claw toe 141
Cleft sternum 180
Clivus 270, 327
Closed packed position 10
Coarctation of aorta 197
Coccydynia 85, 170
Coccyx 162
Codman's triangle 100
Cold abscess 169
Colles' fracture 40

Concha
  inferior 264, 316, 440
  middle 262, 316, 364, 440
  sphenoidal 271
  superior 262, 316, 364, 440
Condyle(s) of 5
  femur 93, 94
  tibia 106, 107
Congenital dislocation of the hip 84
Conjugate
  diagonal 78
  external 78
  obstetrical 78
  true 78
Conus medullaris 168
Cornu(a) 6
  coccygeal 162
  greater 198, 199
  hyoid 198
  lesser 198, 200
  sacral 160
Costotransverse bar 146
Craniostenosis 290
Cranium 282
Crest 6
  ethmoidal, of maxilla 213
  frontal 223
  infratemporal 272
  lacrimal
    anterior 213
    posterior 257
  nasal of
    maxilla 214
    nasal bone 255
    neck of rib 185
    palatine bone 278
  occipital
    external 246
    internal 247
  palatine of 277
    sphenoid 270
    supramastoid 227, 295
Crista galli 322
CSF otorrhea 240, 307, 331
CSF rhinorrhea 262, 317, 330
Cuboid bone 133
Cuneiform bones 135

D

Dacryocystorhinostomy 259, 318
Delayed union 17
Deficient acetabulum 84
Deafness, conductive 243
Deviation
  nasal bridge 293
  nasal septum 319

Diabetes insipidus 331
Diameter(s)
  conjugate 78
  Klein 77
  least diameter of pelvis 78
    cavity of pelvis 79
    inlet of pelvis 79
    outlet of pelvis 80
Diaphysis 5
Diastematomyelia 166
Diploic canals 297
Dislocation of
  cuboid 135
  cuneiform 136
  hip 97
  lunate 57
  patella 105
  shoulder 33
Dorsum sellae 325
Drooping of shoulder 17
Down's syndrome 195

E

Eminence
  canine 211, 292
  frontal 221, 292
  iliopubic 69
  parietal 218, 287
Endoskeleton 3
Eosinophilic granuloma 84
Epicondyle(s) of 5
  femur 94
  humerus 30
Epidural haematoma 220, 225, 249, 306, 330
Epiphyseal plate 5
Epiphysis 5
  aberrant 5
  atavistic 5
  pressure 5
  traction 5
Ethmoid bone 260
Ethmoidal malignancy 314
Ethmoidostomy 263
Ewing's tumour 197
Exoskeleton 3
Extradural haematoma 306

F

Facet 5
Facial paralysis 240, 428
Fascia, temporal 307
Femur 87
Fibula 117
Figure of 8 bandage 17

Fissure(s) 6
  orbital
    inferior 311
    superior 274, 312
  petrosquamous 228
  petrotympanic 228
  pterygomaxillary 296
  squamotympanic 228
Fistula, caroticocavernous 276, 330
Flail chest 196
Flat bones 3
Fontanelle, anterior 287
Foramen 6
  caecum 322
  greater palatine 300
  incisive 300
  jugular 305, 329, 457
  lacerum 303, 326
  lesser palatine 300
  magnum 244, 304, 328
  nutrient 6
  obturator 73
Fossa(e) 5
  cervical, of femur 89
  coronoid 30
  iliac 67
  infraspinous 19
  olecranon 30
  radial, of humerus 30
  subscapular 18
  supraspinous 19
  trochanteric 91
Fovea, of femoral head 88
Fracture(s) 10
  basal of 249, 306
    the base of 5th metacarpal bone 60
    the base of 5th metatarsal bone
  Colles' 40
  comminuted 208, 313
  coronoid process 50
  cribriform plate 263
  depressed 288, 298
  femoral neck 97, 98
  femur 96–99
  fibula 122, 123
  frontal bone 225
  green stick 11
  Guerin's 216, 280, 294
  lacrimal bone 258
  Le Fort I 216, 267, 276, 280, 294
  Le Fort II 216, 256, 263, 267, 276, 280, 294, 313
  Le Fort III 216, 253, 256, 258, 263, 267, 276, 280, 294, 313
  lunate 57
  mandible 208

maxillary   216
mid-facial skeleton   284
nasal bone   255
olecranon   50
orbital plate of ethmoid   262
parietal bone   219, 220
patella   105
pelvis   82, 83
phalanx   63, 141
pond   219
ribs   195
scaphoid   56
separation of the epiphysis   34
shaft of ulna   50
skull   293, 297, 298
Smith's   41
sphenoid bone   276
sternum   180
talus   127, 128
temporal bone   239, 240
the cuneiforms   136
tripod   252
triquetral   57
vault   288
zygoma   253
zygomatic arch   253
zygomatic bone   252, 253
zygomatic process   240
Funnel chest   181

G

Genu valgum   116
Genu varum   116
Giant cell tumours   307
Gout   139
Grafting   122
Granular foveolae   219
Graves' disease   313
Green stick fracture   11
Groove   6
  bicipital   27
  for popliteus   94

H

Haemorrhage into the orbit   313
Hallux valgus   139
Hamate   51, 52, 53, 54, 55
Hammer toe   141
Hamulus   6
Haversian systems   2
Hiatus   6
Hip bone   3, 164
Hip replacement   85, 86
Humerus   26

Hump   174
Hyoid bone   198
Hypertelorism   276
Hyperthyroidism   313

I

Idiopathic scoliosis   172
Ilium   65
Impotence   331
Incisure   6
Infracture, inferior concha   265, 318
Infrahyoid thyroid   200
Inion   289
Injuries, maxillofacial   298, 313
Ischium   70

J

Joints   7
Jugum sphenoidale   269, 323

K

Kienbock's disease   57
Klippel-Feil syndrome   165
Knee jerk   105
Kyphosis   169, 172

L

Labyrinth, ethmoid   261
Lacrimal bone   257
Lacunae   2
Lambda   287
Lamellae
  circumferential   2
  concentric   2
  interstitial   2
Lamina   6
Lateral mass of
  atlas   149
  sacrum   160
Leprosy   33
Levator glandulae thyroideae   200
Lingula, of mandible   205
Line(s)   75
  arcuate, of pelvis   75
  intertrochanteric   91
  nuchal
    highest   246, 289, 344, 402
    inferior   246, 344
    intercondylar, of femur   94
    superior   246, 289, 344, 400
  oblique
    anterior, of radius   37

of mandible 202
  posterior, of radius 37
  ulna 48
pectineal, of pubis 69
Reid's base 283
soleal 110
spiral, of femur 92
temporal 218, 294
Linea aspera 91
Lips of iliac crest 65, 66
Lordosis 167, 172
Lumbar ribs 165
Lumbarization of sacrum 165
Lunate bone 51, 52, 53, 54, 55, 57

M

Macrocephaly 288
Malar flush 252
Malleolus
  lateral 121
  medial 113
Mallet finger 62
Mandible 201
Mandibular fractures 208
Manubrium 176
March fracture 139
Mastoid
  acellular 237
  cellular 237
  diploic 237
Marrow
  red 2
  yellow 2
Maxilla 211
Maxillary
  sinusitis 215
  tumours 215
Maxillectomy 313
Meatus, acoustic
  external 233, 295
  internal 230, 239
Membranous bones 3
Meningitis 225, 293, 317
Metacarpal bones 58
Metaphysis 5
Metatarsalgia 139
Microcephaly 288
Midsternotomy 181
Myeloma 84
Myelomatosis 84

N

Nasal bone 254
Nasal ethmoidostomy 318

Navicular secundarium 133
Neck of
  femur 89
  fibula 122
  humerus 26, 27, 30
  mandible 205
  radius 37
  rib 185, 188
  talus 127
Nonunion 34
Norma
  basalis 298
  frontalis 290
  lateralis 294
  occipitalis 288
  verticalis 286
Notch 6
  acetabular 73
  fibular, of tibia 112
  radial, of ulna 46
  sciatic
    greater 67, 71
    lesser 71
  spinoglenoid 23
  suprascapular 21
  trochlear, of ulna 46
  ulnar, of radius 39
Nystagmus 240, 307, 331

O

Obelion 287
Occipital bone 244
Odontogenic tumours 210
Odontoma 210
Optic nerve decompression 258, 259, 263, 314
Orbit 308
Orbital tumour 314
Os
  odontoideum 166
  terminale 166
  trigonum 127, 128
Ossification 3
Osteochondritis 57, 131
Osteochondritis dissecans 99
Osteoarthritis of hip 84
Osteogenic tumours 210
Osteomalacia 11
Osteomas 307
Osteomyelitis 113, 196
Osteoporosis 11
Osteosarcoma 100
Otosclerosis 243

P

Paget's disease 115
Palate, hard 300

Palatine bone   277
Parietal bone   217
Patella   102
Pecten pubis   69
Pedicle, of vertebra   144
Pelvic
  axes   77
  cavity   76
  diameters   79
  girdle   74
  inclination   78
  inlet   75, 79
  outlet   76, 80
  segments   77
Pelvis
  false   74
  greater   74
  lesser   74
  major   74
  minor   74
  obstetric   74
  true   74
  type   78
Perforated septum   319
Periosteum   2
Pernicious anaemia   11
Perthes' disease   84
Phalanges of the
  foot   140
  hand   61
Pigeon chest   181
Pisiform   51, 52, 53, 54, 55
Pituitary tumour   276
Plaster immobilization   12
Plate(s)   6
  orbital, of frontal bone   223
  perpendicular of
    ethmoid   261
    palatine   278
  pterygoid
    lateral   274
    medial   274
Polyarthritis   84
Pond fracture   219
Postmenopausal osteoporosis   97
Pott's
  fracture   115, 116, 122, 128, 147, 158, 165
  spine   168, 169
Process(es)   6
  acromial   24
  alveolar, of maxilla   213
  articular, of vertebra   144, 146, 156
  clinoid
    anterior   274, 322
    posterior   270, 235

condylar   205
coracoid   24
coronoid of
  mandible   205
  ulna   45
ethmoidal, of inferior concha   265
frontal, of maxilla   213
jugular   245
lacrimal, of inferior concha   265
mamillary   157
mastoid   229
maxillary   265
odontoid   150
orbital, of palatine bone   279
pterygoid   274
spinous   22
styloid of
  fibula   118
  radius   36, 39
  temporal bone   233
  third metacarpal   58
  ulna   49
transverse   144, 146, 153, 156
uncinate, of ethmoid   262
xiphoid   180
zygomatic   213
Promontory of sacrum   158
Protuberance
  mental   201
  occipital
    external   246, 289, 400
    internal   247, 328, 456
Pterion   295
Pubic crest   68
Pulsating exophthalmos   276, 330

R

Radius   36
Ramus (rami)
  ischiopubic of   72
    ischium   72
    mandible   271
    pubis
      inferior   70
      superior   69
Recess, sphenoethmoidal   317
Reduction   12
Rhinion   291
Retrobulbar neuritis   313
Rib(s)   182
  atypical   183, 188
  bifid   195
  cervical   195

false 183
floating 183
lumbar 195
nonfloating 183
true 183
typical 183
vertebral 183
vertebrochondral 183
vertebrosternal 183
Rickets 11, 14
Rostrum, of sphenoid 270
Runner's knee 105
RVAD 172

S

Sacral promontory 75, 158
Sacralization of 5th lumbar vertebra 165
Sacroiliac joints 75
Sacroiliitis 85
Sacrum 157
Scaphoid bone 51, 52, 53, 54, 55, 56
Scaphoid scapula 25
Scapula 18
Scoliosis 165, 167, 172, 173, 174
Sella turcica 270, 325
Sesamoid bones 4
Sever's disease 131
Sharpey's fibres 2
Shin 108
Short bone 3
Sinuses 2
   ethmoidal 261
   frontal 224
   maxillary 212
   sphenoidal 272
Skull 282
Skull cap 2, 282
Smith's fracture 41
Sphenoid bone 269
Spina bifida 165
Spine(s) of 6
  Henle 228
  iliac
    anterior inferior 66
    anterior superior 65
    posterior inferior 67
    posterior superior 65
  ischial 71
  nasal
    anterior 291
    posterior 277
  of scapula 22
  vertebral 144
Spiral fracture 114
Spondylolisthesis 169

Squama 6
Sternal
  foramen 180
  puncture 11, 180
Sternebrae 178
Sternum 176
Still's disease 84
Stove-in-chest 196
Stress fracture 116, 133
Styloid process
  elongated of 239
    fibula 118
    radius 36, 39
    temporal bone 233
    third metacarpal 58
    ulna 49
Submucosal resection (S.M.R.) 268
Subpubic angle 76
Sudek's osteodystrophy 40
Sulcus 6
  calcanei 129
  tali 127
Supracondylar fracture 34, 97
Sustentaculum tali 130
Suprahyoid thyroid 200
Suture
  coronal 286
  frontal 221
  intermaxillary 290, 300
  lambdoid 286, 289
  metopic 221
  occipitomastoid 289
  parietomastoid 289
  sagittal 286
Symphysis menti 201
Syndrome
  cervical rib 195
  1st rib 195
  Naffziger's 195
  shoulder arm 195
  scalenus anticus 195
  thoracic outlet 195
  Treacher Collins' 243

T

'T' fracture 99
Table
  inner 2
  outer 2
Talus 124
Tarsus 124
Tegmen tympani 230
Temporal bone 226
Tantalum 288, 290

Tibia 106
Tietze's syndrome 196
Titanium 288, 290
Thyroglossal cyst 200
Torsion of
    femur 88
    humerus 31
Transitional cell carcinoma 307
Trapezium 51, 52, 53, 54, 55
Trapezoid 51, 52, 54, 55
Trephining 297
Triangle, suprameatal 227, 296
Trigeminal impression 229
Triquetral bone 51, 52, 54, 55, 57
Trochanter of 6
    femur
      greater 90
      lesser 91
      third 92
Trochlea of 6
  humerus 30
Tubercle(s) of 6
  adductor 94
  calcaneus 129
  greater 27
  humerus
  iliac crest 65
  infraglenoid 21
  intercondylar, of tibia 107
  lesser 27
  Lister 36, 39
  peroneal 129
  pubic 69
  scaphoid bone 52, 53
  supraglenoid 22
  talus 127

Trendelenburg's sign 83
Tuberculum sellae 270, 325
Tuberculosis 196
Tuberosity of 6
  deltoid 29
  gluteal 92
  iliac 68
  ischial 70
  navicular bone 132
  radial 37
  ulnar 45
Tumours of femur 100

U

Ulna 44
Ultrasonography 288

V

Vertebrae 142
Vertebral column 142, 143
Vertical compression fracture 115
Vertex of skull 286
Vertigo 240, 307, 331
Volkmann's canal 2
Volkmann's ischaemic contracture 34
Vomer 266

W

Wing of 6
  sphenoid 272
Winging of scapula 25

Z

Zygomatic bone 250